AF902800

Illustrated Anatomical Segmentectomy for Lung Cancer

Hiroaki Nomori • Morihito Okada

Illustrated Anatomical Segmentectomy for Lung Cancer

Springer

Hiroaki Nomori
Department of Surgery
Kameda Medical Center
Chiba, Japan

Morihito Okada
Department of Surgical Oncology
Hiroshima University
Hiroshima, Japan

ISBN 978-4-431-54143-1 ISBN 978-4-431-54144-8 (eBook)
DOI 10.1007/978-4-431-54144-8
Springer Tokyo Heidelberg New York Dordrecht London

Library of Congress Control Number: 2012948951

This English translation is based on the Japanese original
Kusetsu Atlas
© Hiroaki Nomori, Morihito Okada, 2011
Originally published in Japan in 2011 by BUNKODO CO., LTD.

© Springer Japan 2012
This work is subject to copyright. All rights are reserved by the Publisher, whether the whole or part of the material is concerned, specifically the rights of translation, reprinting, reuse of illustrations, recitation, broadcasting, reproduction on microfilms or in any other physical way, and transmission or information storage and retrieval, electronic adaptation, computer software, or by similar or dissimilar methodology now known or hereafter developed. Exempted from this legal reservation are brief excerpts in connection with reviews or scholarly analysis or material supplied specifically for the purpose of being entered and executed on a computer system, for exclusive use by the purchaser of the work. Duplication of this publication or parts thereof is permitted only under the provisions of the Copyright Law of the Publisher's location, in its current version, and permission for use must always be obtained from Springer. Permissions for use may be obtained through RightsLink at the Copyright Clearance Center. Violations are liable to prosecution under the respective Copyright Law.
The use of general descriptive names, registered names, trademarks, service marks, etc. in this publication does not imply, even in the absence of a specific statement, that such names are exempt from the relevant protective laws and regulations and therefore free for general use.
While the advice and information in this book are believed to be true and accurate at the date of publication, neither the authors nor the editors nor the publisher can accept any legal responsibility for any errors or omissions that may be made. The publisher makes no warranty, express or implied, with respect to the material contained herein.

Printed on acid-free paper

Springer is part of Springer Science+Business Media (www.springer.com)

Foreword

As stated in the Preface for the original "2011 Japanese Edition" of this book: "I am pleased and enthusiastic to have this opportunity to write an introductory preface to this book." I have yet greater enthusiasm for the opportunity of providing the Introductory Preface to the current English translation, which is provided and published by Springer. The English translation will reach a very much larger audience beyond Japan. Importantly, I believe these original contributions from Japanese thoracic surgeons are not widely known and appreciated throughout many of the pulmonary and thoracic programs throughout the world—including Europe and the Americas. This illustrated textbook contains significant, new, and original information which has worldwide importance and application in the management of primary non-small cell lung cancer (NSCLC). It is the product of a very long experience, carefully organized and planned, critically and impartially assessed, and meticulously documented.

Background and History

The anatomy and technique of segmental resection were first published by Churchill and Belsey in 1939 [1]. Shortly thereafter, the technique was popularized by the extensive experience of Overholt [2], another contemporary Boston surgeon. In 1959/60, I became a Senior House Officer with Ronald Belsey, then Head of the Regional Thoracic Unit at Frenchay & Bristol in the West of England. There, I was introduced to segmental resection, using the classical "finger tip stripping dissection of the intersegmental plane." This operation was relatively rough and difficult to teach.

In 1972, Noriaki Tsubota, recommended by Professor Nakamura in Kobe, Japan, became a Fellow for one year in our Division of Thoracic Surgery in Toronto, Canada. He learned the "Chamberlain/Belsey" technique of segmentectomy during that time. Following his return to Hyogo, a cancer center near Kobe, in Japan, he continued his experience with this method of anatomic segmental resection. He created important and practical technical modifications and shared this experience with his student, Morihito Okada. Tsubota (now retired) and his student, Okada, ultimately introduced further original modifications, which currently include: video-assisted segmentectomy, radical anatomic segmentectomy, sleeve segmentectomy, and a detailed documentation of local segmental and subsegmental anatomy. This detailed, well-illustrated anatomy is little, if at all known to a majority of thoracic surgeons elsewhere in the world. Their experience, however, has widely educated and influenced many of the leading thoracic surgeons throughout Japan. As a guest at the 51st meeting of the Japanese Association for Lung Cancer in November 2010, I was shown a draft of the Japanese edition of this illustrated text by two authors: Professor Hiroaki Nomori at Keio University in Tokyo and Morihito Okada of Hyogo, who was an appointed Professor in Hiroshima in 2010.

Current Japanese Clinical Experience

The Japanese Community of Thoracic Surgeons are now broadly experienced with a reproducible, relatively inexpensive technique of precise, video-assisted, anatomical radical segmentectomy. Morbidity and mortality rates are similar, or less, than those reported for lobectomy, wedge, or any other form of "lesser resection." Innovations include sleeve segmentectomy and subsegmental resection [3–11].

Okada, Tsubota et al. have published their clinical experience with segmentectomy for small (2 cm), NSCLC, and compared results with their experience with lobectomy for the same small, early NSCLC lesion [6–11]. Segmentectomy resulted in improved disease-free survival, improved preservation of pulmonary function, less morbidity, and lower procedural costs. The segmental plane is anatomically preserved—not folded and distorted by the "traditional" stapling used almost universally elsewhere. The segmental surface allows intraoperative smear cytology and is amenable to much improved management by the pathologist (e.g., tumor free margin assessment).

Although they have yet to complete a randomized trial of this comparison, such a trial is underway in multiple Japanese centers (P.I. Asamura and Okada) [12] and is more rapidly accruing patients than a similar American randomized trial (P.I. Altorki).

Other benefits worthy of comment are the absence of staplers for other than the larger vascular structures: using a 4 cm open "access incision," traditional open instruments may be used for "open" scissor dissection, segmental vessel clamping, and the use of old-fashioned ligatures for tying off the vessels. Staplers for small segmental arteries are often awkward and oversized.

Conclusion

It is probably evident from this appraisal that, in my opinion, thoracic surgeons who are not aware of this information and giving serious consideration for learning these techniques are "missing the boat."

F. Griffith Pearson
Toronto General Hospital
Toronto, Canada

References

1. Churchill ED, Belsey R. Segmental pneumonectomy in bronchiectasis: the lingula segment of the left upper lobe. Ann Surg. 1939;109(4):481–99.
2. Overholt RH, Woods FM, Ramsay BH. Segmental pulmonary resection: details of technique and results. J Thorac Surg. 1950;19(2):207–25.
3. Nomori H, Ikeda K, Mori T, et al. Sentinel node navigation segmentectomy for c-T1N0M0 non-small cell lung cancer. J Thorac Cardiovasc Surg. 2007;133:780–85.
4. Nomori H, Mori T, Izumi Y, et al. Is completion lobectomy merited for unanticipated nodal metastases after radical segmentectomy for cT1N0M0/pN1-2 non-small cell lung cancer? J Thorac Cardiovasc Surg. 2012;143:820–24.

5. Nomori H, Mori T, Ikeda K, et al. Segmentectomy for cT1N0M0 non-small cell lung cancer: a prospective study at a single institute. J Thorac Cardiovasc Surg. 2012;144:87–93.
6. Okada M, Tsutani Y, Ikeda T, et al. Radical hybrid video-assisted thoracic segmentectomy: long-term results of minimally invasive anatomical sublobar resection for treating lung cancer. Interact Cardiovasc Thorac Surg. 2012;14(1):5–11.
7. Okada M, Nakayama H, Okumura S, et al. Multicenter analysis of high-resolution computed tomography and positron emission tomography/computed tomography findings to choose therapeutic strategies for clinical stage IA lung adenocarcinoma. J Thorac Cardiovasc Surg. 2011;141(6):1384–91.
8. Okada M, Mimura T, Ikegaki J, et al. A novel video-assisted anatomic segmentectomy technique: selective segmental inflation via bronchofiberoptic jet followed by cautery cutting. J Thorac Cardiovasc Surg. 2007;133(3):753–8.
9. Okada M, Koike T, Higashiyama M, et al. Radical sublobar resection for small-sized non-small cell lung cancer: a multicenter study. J Thorac Cardiovasc Surg. 2006;132(4):769–75.
10. Okada M, Nishio W, Sakamoto T, et al. Effect of tumor size on prognosis in patients with non-small cell lung cancer: the role of segmentectomy as a type of lesser resection. J Thorac Cardiovasc Surg. 2005;129(1):87–93.
11. Okada M, Nishio W, Sakamoto T, et al. Sleeve segmentectomy for non-small cell lung carcinoma. J Thorac Cardiovasc Surg. 2004;128(3):420–4.
12. Nakamura K, Okada M, Asamura H, et al. A phase III randomized trial of lobectomy versus limited resection for small-sized peripheral non-small cell lung cancer (JCOG0802/WJOG4607L). Jpn J Clin Oncol. 2010;40(3):271–4.

Foreword

A new era of less invasive surgery for lung cancer has opened. There are two approaches: one of them is, needless to say, video-assisted thoracic surgery; the other is lesser resection for small, primary lung cancer. The former has already become a standard operation, but the latter is still controversial and has not yet achieved worldwide acceptance.

I started a pilot study on segmentectomy in 1992 and published the results and an improved method to find the intersegmental plane in the *Annals of Thoracic Surgery* (1998;66:1787, 2002;73:1055). During the past 20 years, many papers have been published from Japan on active indication of segmentectomy for early-stage lung cancer. Although many of those studies were retrospective, their results supported segmentectomy, and now that the era of less invasive surgery has arrived, accompanied by a rapid increase in the detection of small tumors, prospective studies are going on in America and Japan. I am thoroughly convinced that it will not take long for segmentectomy to become a standard procedure in the treatment of early-stage lung cancer.

The authors of this book, Dr. Hiroaki Nomori and Dr. Morihito Okada, are quite enthusiastic about the novel technique of segmentectomy for small lung cancer, and they continue to report their results. For many years, they have made a superb effort to develop their approach, which has finally borne fruit in the form of this textbook.

Chest surgeons who read this book will be surprised by its contents—the descriptions are so detailed, and the anatomical naming is so precise. The large, colorful figures will make it easy for them to understand how to accurately perform a segmentectomy and will help lessen their hesitation to tackle such a procedure.

In closing, I would like to point out that the concept of lung-saving surgery and the technique that makes this delicate procedure possible originated with Dr. F.G. Pearson, my mentor, during my fellowship days in Toronto back in 1973.

Enjoy the book. The connective tissue, blood vessels, and airways of the segment await.

Noriaki Tsubota
Kobe, Japan

Preface

When I was a trainee at the National Cancer Center in Tokyo, my mentors, thoracic surgeons, Drs. Shichiro Ishikawa and Tsuguo Naruke always cautioned me not to think that "I can do everything by myself". With this in mind, I accepted the kind offer of Professor Morihito Okada at the Department of Surgical Oncology, Hiroshima University to share with me his considerable expertise in segmental lung resection to help me produce this textbook. Thanks to his suggestions based on the philosophy of Dr. Noriaki Tsubota and the lessons learned from my mentors, I felt that I could present a balanced view of the current techniques of radical segmentectomy for treating lung cancer. I am grateful to Professor Okada for countless valuable discussions during more than 3 years required to complete this textbook.

My journey towards mastering the techniques of oncologically sound pulmonary segmentectomy started around the year 2000 when the incidence of small peripheral lung cancers started to increase in Japan based on the development of CT screening throughout the country. Despite understanding the radiographic anatomy of pulmonary segments obtained during my residency at the National Cancer Center in Tokyo under the guidance of Dr. Shigeto Ikeda, I discovered that the correct identification of the segmental anatomy of pulmonary arteries, veins, and bronchi during surgery was not as easy as I expected. In fact, I generally needed almost 5 hours to complete an anatomical segmentectomy during the beginning stages of acquiring the surgical techniques!

This textbook contains numerous color figures which are from among the 4,000 or so illustrations of the pulmonary anatomy that I sketched during more than 450 segmental lung resections over the past 7 years at Kumamoto and Keio Universities. I believe that this textbook addresses the technical details of all types of pulmonary segmentectomy. Although the techniques described herein will be modified and improved as surgical techniques evolve, I believe that this book will continue to help thoracic surgeons to understand the specific details of lung segmental anatomy that will always remain unchanged.

Hiroaki Nomori
Chiba, Japan

Preface

I find surgery fascinating, so a fateful encounter with surgery is a notable event in my life. The goal of surgery is to achieve maximal treatment effects with minimal invasiveness and to preserve more function for patients. In that sense, radical hybrid VATS segmentectomy is considered an ideal approach for treating small lung cancers, the rate of which has recently increased worldwide.

The art of surgery is absolutely sharp dissection. Dr. Ronald H.R. Belsey (Frenchay Hospital, Bristol, England), Dr. F. Griffith Pearson (University of Toronto, Toronto, Canada), and Dr. Noriaki Tsubota (Emeritus President of Hyogo Cancer Center, Japan) developed specialized techniques for sharp dissection in the depths of the thorax using long, heavy Allison scissors in the "upside down" position, with the thumb and index or middle finger through the loops. Their greatest impact on surgery for lung disease has been the increased competence of a legion of trainees from all over the globe. Dr. Pearson told me in 2005 that he had just attended the 22nd meeting of the Japanese Association for Chest Surgery in Kyoto, where he had witnessed a detailed presentation of the indications, clinical experience, and results of radical anatomical segmentectomy. He explained that the presentations had included a summary of an already large body of clinical experience, including indications and detailed results, that the illustrations and videos of my procedures were crystal clear and that he would try to persuade his North American colleagues to review and try this approach and technology. That remark stimulated my enthusiasm for the development of segmentectomy for lung cancer.

I am eternally grateful to Drs. Belsey, Pearson, Tsubota, and my co-editor, Dr. Hiroaki Nomori for encouraging me to write this book. I look forward to continuing to serve present and future generations of thoracic surgeons as a renewable resource.

Morihito Okada
Hiroshima, Japan

Contents

Part I

General Statement

1 Nomenclature of Segments

1.1 Nomenclature of Segmental and Subsegmental Lung

1.1.1 Right Upper Lobe

1. S^1 [Segmentum.apicale]
   (a) S^1a [Subsegmentum.apicale proprius]
   (b) S^1b [Subseg.ventrale]
2. S^2 [S.dorsale]
   (a) S^2a [Subseg.dorsale]
   (b) S^2b [Subseg.horizontale]
3. S^3 [S.ventrale]
   (a) S^3a [Subseg.laterale]
   (b) S^3b [Subseg.mediale]

1.1.2 Right Middle Lobe

1. S^4 [S.medium laterale]
   (a) S^4a [Subseg.laterale]
   (b) S^4b [Subseg.mediale]
2. S^5 [S.medium mediale]
   (a) S^5a [Subseg.laterale]
   (b) S^5b [Subseg.mediale]

1.1.3 Left Upper Lobe

1.1.3.1 Upper Division ($S^{1+2}+S^3$)

1. S^{1+2} [S.apicodorsale]
   (a) $S^{1+2}a$ [Subseg.apicale]
   (b) $S^{1+2}b$ [Subseg.dorsale]
   (c) $S^{1+2}c$ [Subseg.horizontale]
2. S^3 [S.ventrale]
   (a) S^3a [Subseg.laterale]
   (b) S^3b [Subseg.mediale]
   (c) S^3c [Subseg.superius]

1.1.3.2 Lingular Division (S^4+S^5)

1. S^4 [S.lingulare superius]
   (a) S^4a [Subseg.laterale]
   (b) S^4b [Subseg.mediale]
2. S^5 [S.lingulare inferius]
   (a) S^5a [Subseg.superius]
   (b) S^5b [Subseg.inferius]

1.1.4 Lower Lobe

1. S^6 [S.superius]
   (a) S^6a [Subseg.superius]
   (b) S^6b [Subseg.laterale]
   (c) S^6c [Subseg.mediale]
2. S^* [S.subsuperius]
3. S^7 [S.mediobasale] (only right side)
   (a) S^7a [Subseg.dorsale]
   (b) S^7b [Subseg.ventrale]
4. S^8 [S.ventrobasale]
   (a) S^8a [Subseg.laterale]
   (b) S^8b [Subseg.basale]
5. S^9 [S.laterobasale]
   (a) S^8a [Subseg.laterale]
   (b) S^8b [Subseg.basale]
6. S^{10} [S.dorsobasale]
   (a) $S^{10}a$ [Subseg.dorsale]
   (b) $S^{10}b$ [Subseg.laterale]
   (c) $S^{10}c$ [Subseg.mediale]

H. Nomori and M. Okada, *Illustrated Anatomical Segmentectomy for Lung Cancer*,
DOI 10.1007/978-4-431-54144-8_1, © Springer Japan 2012

1.2 Nomenclature of Segmental and Subsegmental Bronchus

1.2.1 Right Upper Lobe

1. B^1 [R.apicalis]
   (a) B^1a [Rm.apicalis proprius]
   (b) B^1b [Rm.ventralis]
2. B^2 [R.dorsalis]
   (a) B^2a [Rm.dorsalis]
   (b) B^2b [Rm.horizontalis]
3. B^3 [R.ventralis]
   (a) B^3a [Rm.latelasis]
   (b) B^3b [Rm.medialis]

1.2.2 Right Middle Lobe

1. B^4 [R.medius lateralis]
   (a) B^4a [Rm.lateralis]
   (b) B^4b [Rm.medialis]
2. B^5 [R.medius medialis]
   (a) B^5a [Rm.lateralis]
   (b) B^5b [Rm.medialis]

1.2.3 Left Upper Lobe

1.2.3.1 Upper Division Bronchus

1. B^{1+2} [R.apicodorsalis]
   (a) $B^{1+2}a$ [Rm.apicalis]
   (b) $B^{1+2}b$ [Rm.dorsalis]
   (c) $B^{1+2}c$ [Rm.horizontalis]
2. B^3 [R.ventralis]
   (a) B^3a [Rm.lateralis]
   (b) B^3b [Rm.medialis]
   (c) B^3c [Rm.superior]

1.2.3.2 Lingular Division Bronchus

1. B^4 [R.lingualis superior]
   (a) B^4a [Rm.lateralis]
   (b) B^4b [Rm.medialis]
2. B^5 [R.lingualis inferior]
   (a) B^5a [Rm.superior]
   (b) B^5b [Rm.inferior]

1.2.4 Lower Lobes

1. B^6 [R.superior]
   (a) B^6a [Rm.superior]
   (b) B^6b [Rm.lateralis]
   (c) B^6c [Rm.medialis]
2. B^* [R.subsuperior]
3. B^7 [R.mediobasalis] (only right side)
   (a) B^7a [Rm.dorsalis]
   (b) B^7b [Rm.ventralis]
4. B^8 [R.ventrobasalis]
   (a) B^8a [Rm.lateralis]
   (b) B^8b [Rm.basalis]
5. B^9 [R.laterobasalis]
   (a) B^9a [Rm.lateralis]
   (b) B^9b [Rm.basalis]
6. B^{10} [R.dorsobasalis]
   (a) $B^{10}a$ [Rm.dorsalis]
   (b) $B^{10}b$ [Rm.lateralis]
   (c) $B^{10}c$ [Rm.medialis]

1.3 Nomenclature of Segmental and Subsegmental Artery

1.3.1 Right Upper Lobe

1. A^1 [R.apicalis]
   (a) A^1a [Rm.apicalis proprius]
   (b) A^1b [Rm.ventralis]
2. A^2 [R.dorsalis]
   (a) A^2a [Rm.dorsalis]
   (b) A^2b [Rm.horizontalis]
3. A^3 [R.ventralis]
   (a) A^3a [Rm.latelasis]
   (b) A^3b [Rm.medialis]

1.3.2 Right Middle Lobe

1. A^4 [R.medius lateralis]
   (a) A^4a [Rm.lateralis]
   (b) A^4b [Rm.medialis]
2. A^5 [R.medius medialis]
   (a) A^5a [Rm.lateralis]
   (b) A^5b [Rm.medialis]

1.3.3 Left Upper Lobe

1.3.3.1 Upper Division Artery

1. A^{1+2} [R.apicodorsalis]
   (a) $A^{1+2}a$ [Rm.apicalis]
   (b) $A^{1+2}b$ [Rm.dorsalis]
   (c) $A^{1+2}c$ [Rm.horizontalis]
2. A^3 [R.ventralis]
   (a) A^3a [Rm.lateralis]
   (b) A^3b [Rm.medialis]
   (c) A^3c [Rm.superior]

1.3.3.2 Lingular Division Artery

1. A^4 [R.lingualis superior]
   (a) A^4a [Rm.lateralis]
   (b) A^4b [Rm.medialis]
2. A^5 [R.lingualis inferior]
   (a) A^5a [Rm.superior]
   (b) A^5b [Rm.inferior]

1.3.4 Lower Lobes

1. A^6 [R.superior]
   (a) A^6a [Rm.superior]
   (b) A^6b [Rm.lateralis]
   (c) A^6c [Rm.medialis]
2. A^* [R.subsuperior]
3. A^7 [R.mediobasalis] (only right side)
   (a) A^7a [Rm.dorsalis]
   (b) A^7b [Rm.ventralis]
4. A^8 [R.ventrobasalis]
   (a) A^8a [Rm.lateralis]
   (b) A^8b [Rm.basalis]
5. A^9 [R.laterobasalis]
   (a) A^9a [Rm.lateralis]
   (b) A^9b [Rm.basalis]
6. A^{10} [R.dorsobasalis]
   (a) $A^{10}a$ [Rm.dorsalis]
   (b) $A^{10}b$ [Rm.lateralis]
   (c) $A^{10}c$ [Rm.medialis]

1.4 Nomenclature of Segmental and Subsegmental Vein

1.4.1 Right Upper Lobe

1. V^1 (V.apicalis)
   (a) V^1a: between S^1a and S^1b
   (b) V^1b: between S^1b and S^3b
2. V^2 (V.dorsalis)
   (a) V^2a: between S^1a and S^2a
   (b) V^2b: between S^2a and S^2b
   (c) V^2c: between S^2b and S^3a
   (d) V^2t: below S^2a
3. V^3 (V.ventralis)
   (a) V^3a: between S^3a and S^3b
   (b) V^3b: below S^3b
   (c) V^3c between S^3bi and S^3bii
4. Central vein: $V^2a+V^2b+V^2c(+V^3a)$

1.4.2 Right Middle Lobe

1. V^4 (V.media.lateralis)
   (a) V^4a: between S^4a and S^4b
   (b) V^4b: between S^4b and S^5b
2. V^5 (V.media.medialis)
   (a) V^5a: between S^5a and S^5b
   (b) V^5b: below S^5b

1.4.3 Left Upper Lobe

1. V^{1+2} (V.apicodorsalis)
   (a) $V^{1+2}a$: between $S^{1+2}a$ and S^3c
   (b) $V^{1+2}b$: between $S^{1+2}a$ and $S^{1+2}b$
   (c) $V^{1+2}c$: between $S^{1+2}b$ and $S^{1+2}c$
   (d) $V^{1+2}d$: between $S^{1+2}c$ and S^3a
2. V^3 (V.ventralis)
   (a) V^3a: between S^3a and S^3b
   (b) V^3b: between S^3b and S^4b
   (c) V^3c: between S^3b and S^3c
3. V^4 (V.lingualis superior)
   (a) V^4a: between S^4a and S^4b
   (b) V^4b: between S^4b and S^5a
4. V^5 (V.lingualis inferior)
   (a) V^5a: between S^5a and S^5b
   (b) V^5b: below S^5b

1.4.4 Lower Lobes

1. V^6 (V.superior)
   (a) V^6a: between S^6a and S^6b+c
   (b) V^6b: between S^6b and S^6c, and between S^6 and S^{8+9}
   (c) V^6c: between S^6c and $S^{10}a$ (or S^7a only in the right side)
2. V^7 (V.mediobasalis) (only right side)
   (a) V^7a: between S^7a and S^7b
   (b) V^7b: between S^7b and S^8b

3. V^8 (V.ventrobasalis)
   (a) V^8a: between S^8a and S^8b
   (b) V^8b: between S^8b and S^9b
4. V^9 (V.laterobasalis)
   (a) V^9a: between S^9a and S^9b
   (b) V^9b: between S^9b and $S^{10}b$
5. V^{10} (V.dorsobasalis)
   (a) $V^{10}a$: between $S^{10}a$ and $S^{10}c$
   (b) $V^{10}b$: between $S^{10}b$ and $S^{10}c$
   (c) $V^{10}c$: among $S^{10}c$

Front view

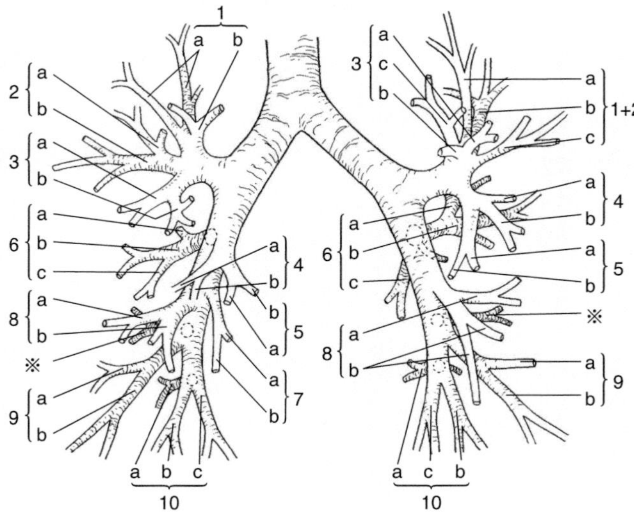

Lateral view

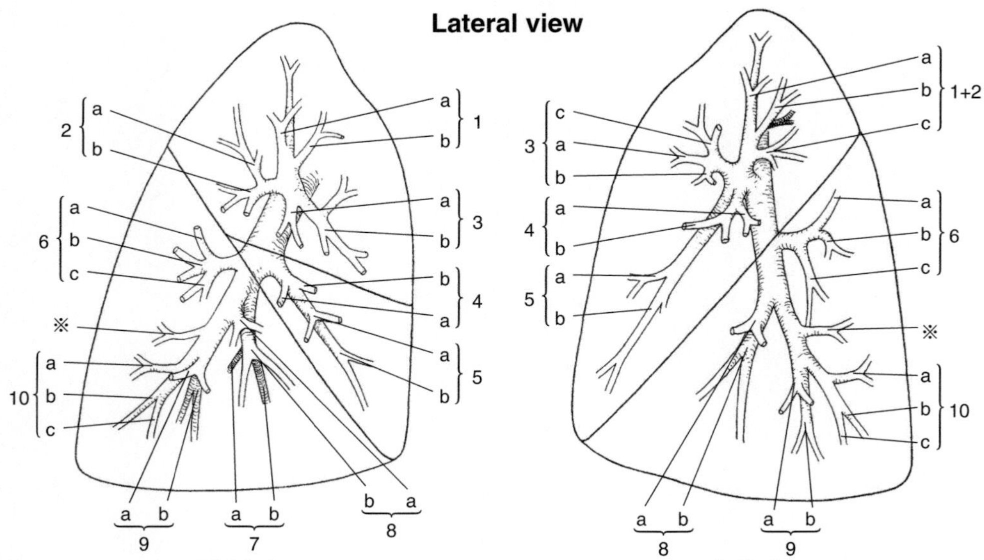

Right view **Left view**

Location of numbered segments

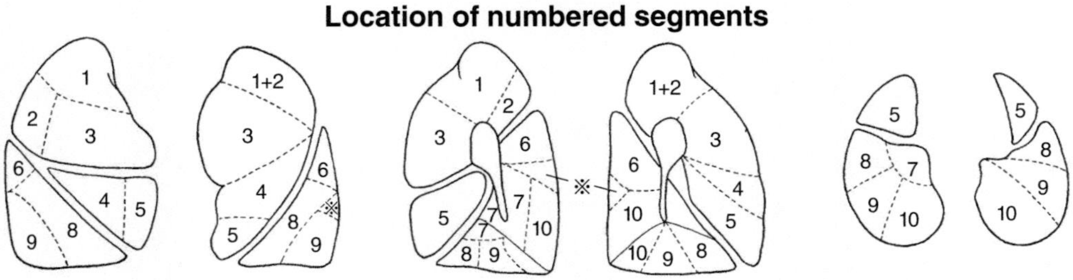

External view **Internal view** **Caudal view**

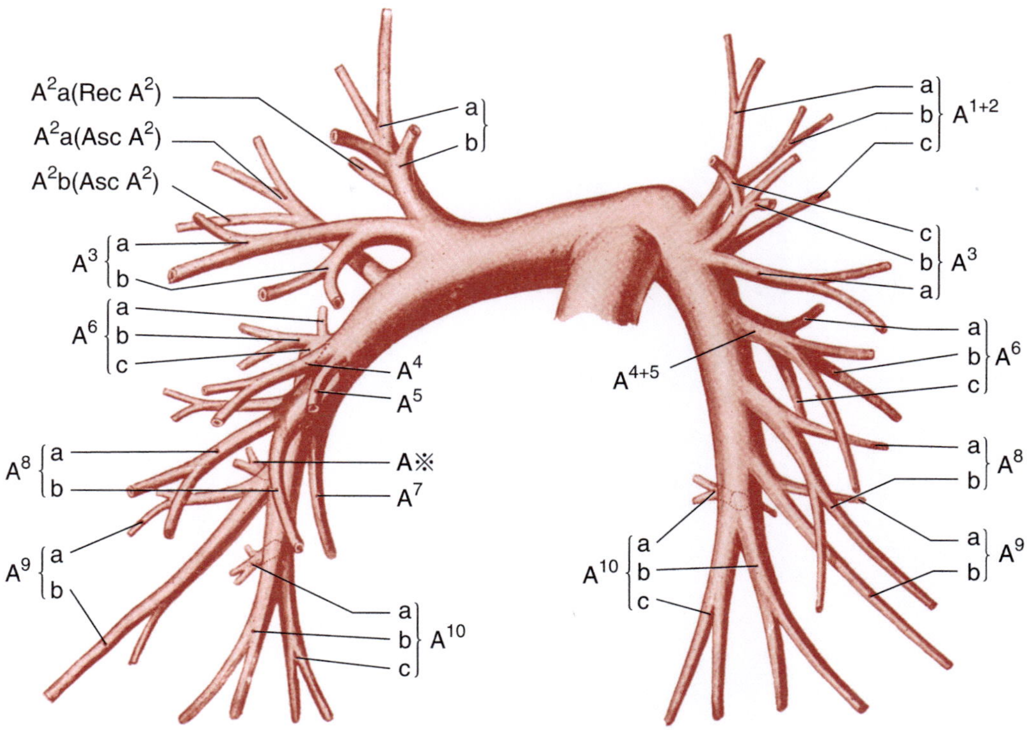

A^2a(Rec A^2)
A^2a(Asc A^2)
A^2b(Asc A^2)
a
b
A^3 a b
A^6 a b c
A^4
A^5
A^8 a b
A※
A^7
A^9 a b
a b c A^{10}
a b c A^{1+2}
c b a A^3
A^{4+5}
a b c A^6
a b A^8
a b A^9
A^{10} a b c

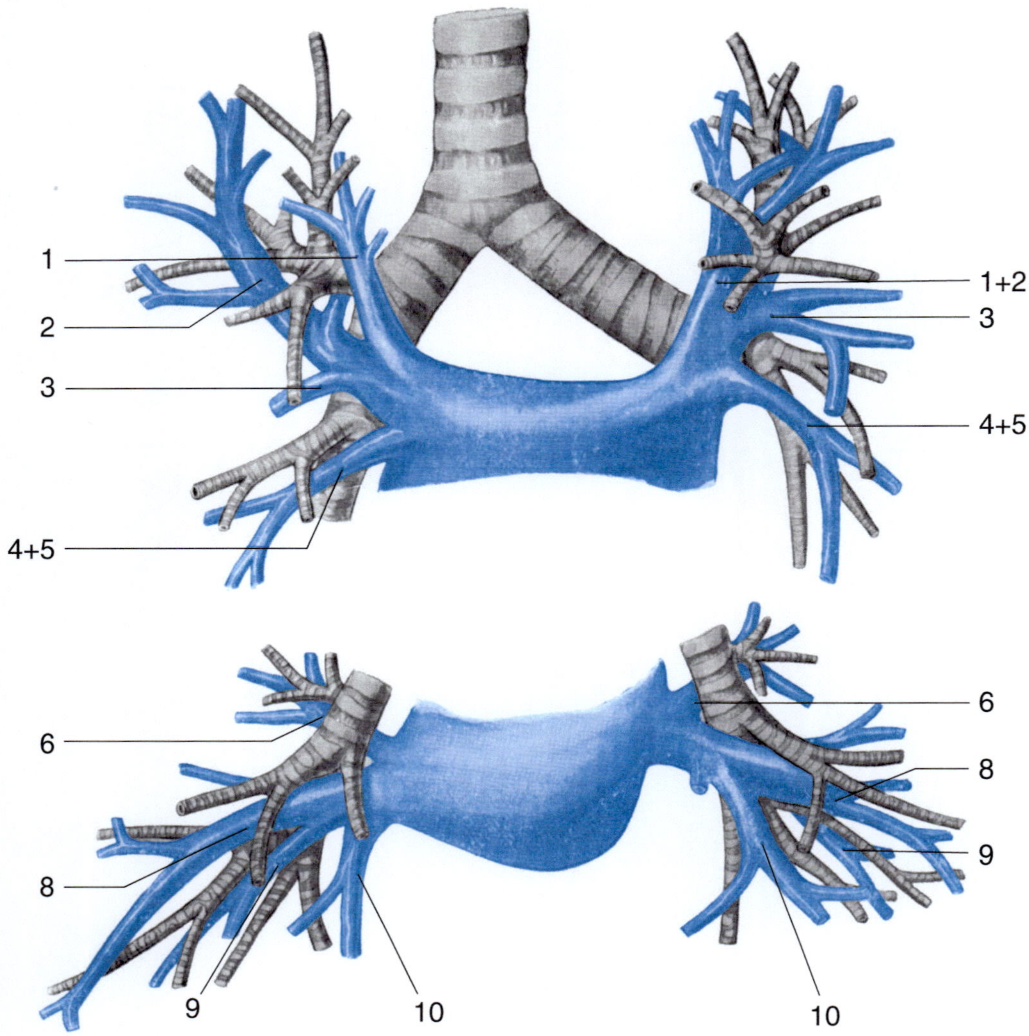
1
2
3
4+5
1+2
3
4+5
6
8
9
10
6
8
9
10

2 General Knack of Segmentectomy

2.1 Preoperative Interpretation of MDCT

The tumor location and the anatomy of branches of the bronchus, arteries, and veins are defined using axial, coronal, and sagittal views of MDCT. Because the lung should be resected at least 2 cm away from the tumor during segmentectomy, vessels or the bronchus within 2 cm of the tumor should be identified on MDCT. If the lung tissue within 2 cm from the tumor is not limited within one segment, the additional resection of subsegment or segment would be necessary. The branching pattern and size of the bronchus, arteries, and veins on MDCT should be identified before segmentectomy.

2.2 Exposing the Segmental Bronchus (Figs. 2.1 and 2.2)

The segmental bronchus is exposed and then the bronchus is grasped with tweezers. The lateral side and back of the segmental bronchus are peeled from the segmental vein, lymph nodes, and other tissues using scissors or a cotton bar, and then encircled with thread.

2.3 Obtaining a Sufficient Surgical Margin (Fig. 2.3)

A sufficient surgical margin is critical to successful segmentectomy. While the malignant aggressiveness of small tumors can be evaluated from high-resolution CT and PET/CT images [1–8], a surgical margin should be taken sufficiently regardless of the tumor aggressiveness. The study based on HRCT reported that approximately 30% of c-T1aN0M0 NSCLCs extend beyond one segment [9]. Therefore, cutting lung tissue during segmentectomy only along the segmental vein and inflated–deflated line would not take a sufficient surgical margin. To take a sufficient surgical margin, when a tumor is relatively close to the cutting line of the lung tissue, the tumor is grasped within a ring-shaped forceps 3~5 cm in diameter, and then lung tissue is cut away from the forceps [10]. When the cutting line is beyond the intersegmental plane, a stapler is required to resect a part of neighboring segment together.

2.4 Lifting the Distal Stump of Bronchus (Figs. 2.4–2.6)

The distal stump of the cut segmental bronchus is lifted. The back of distal stump of the bronchus is denuded in the peripheral direction using a cotton bar, which moves the stump away from the hilum and then enables the resection of hilar part of the segment (Fig. 2.4). Lifting the distal stump also exposes vein branches running into the segment, which is cut. Cutting the vein branches further elevates the distal stump of the bronchus together with lung tissues at both sides of the stump, which is cut towards the inflation–deflation line using electrocautery (Fig. 2.5). Thereafter, the lung is cut along the inflation–deflation line from the periphery, which is cut from various directions to facilitate simple and accurate cutting along the segmental border (Fig. 2.6).

H. Nomori and M. Okada, *Illustrated Anatomical Segmentectomy for Lung Cancer*,
DOI 10.1007/978-4-431-54144-8_2, © Springer Japan 2012

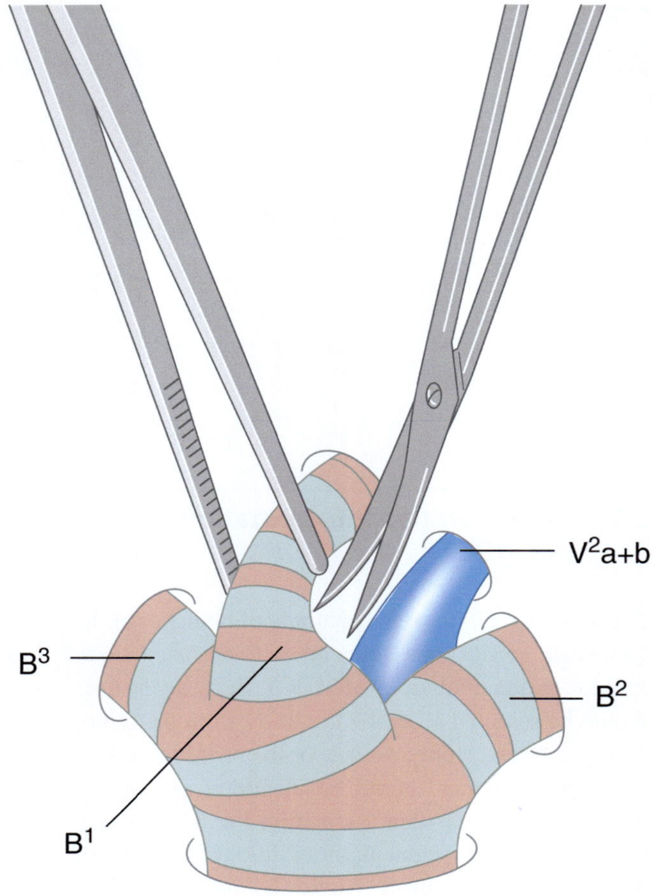

Fig. 2.1 Exposing the bronchus using scissors.

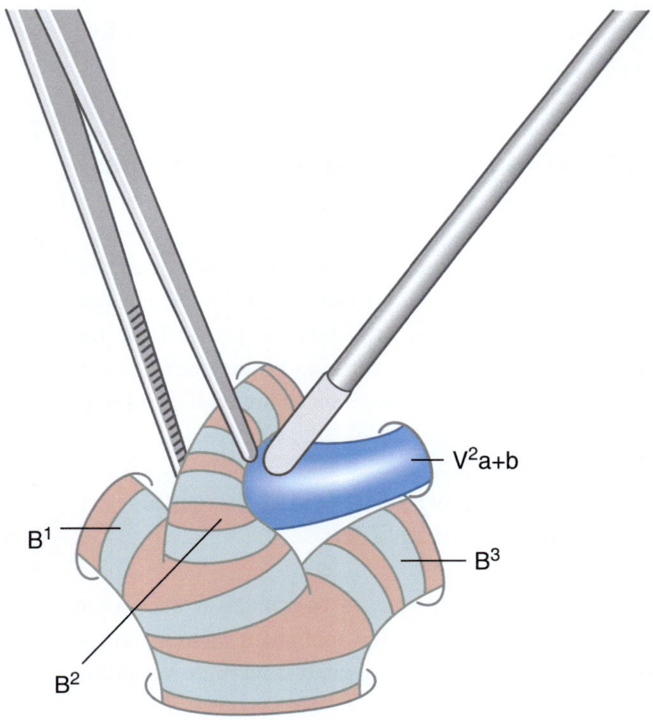

Fig. 2.2 Exposing the bronchus using cotton bar.

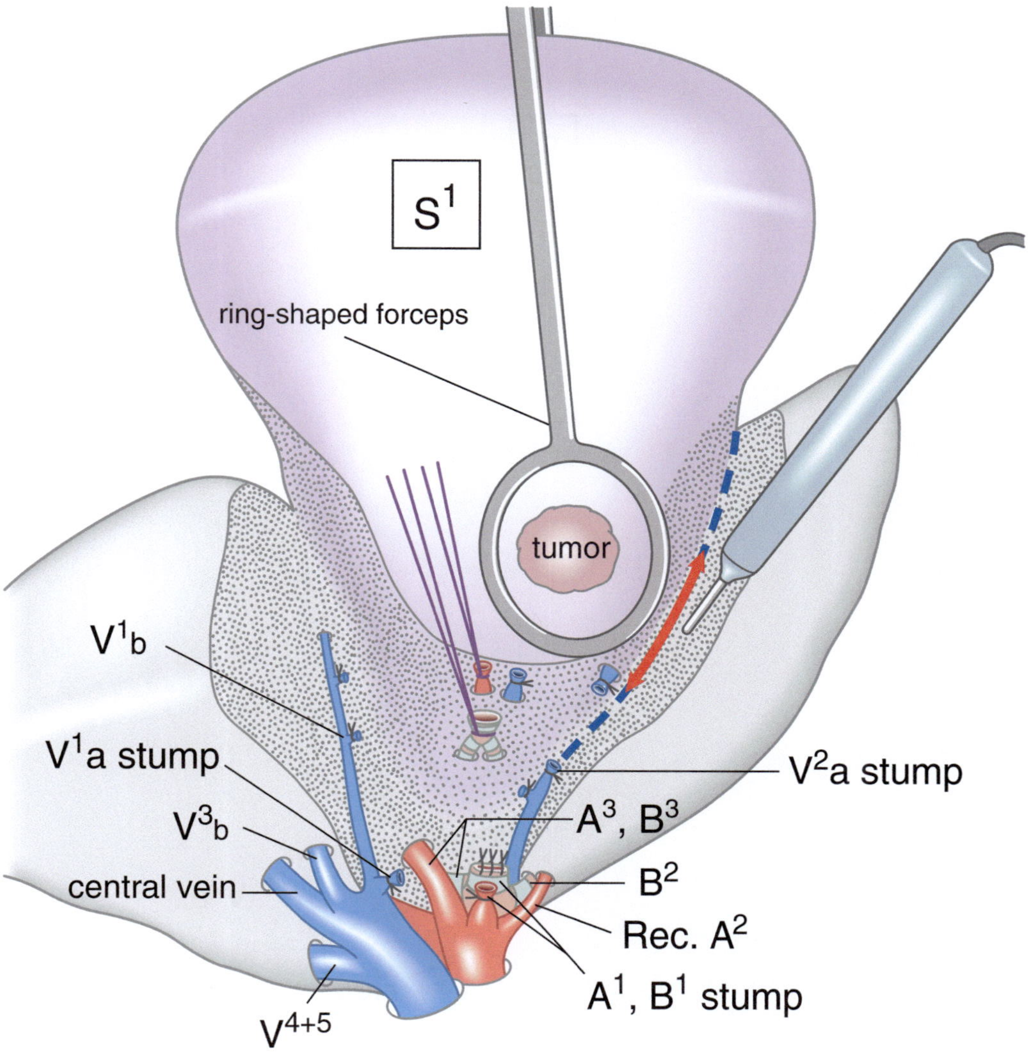

Fig. 2.3 Obtaining a sufficient surgical margin.

2.5 Cutting Along the Intersegmental Plane (Figs. 2.7 and 2.8)

We detect the intersegmental plane during segmentectomy using selective jet ventilation under bronchoscopy (Fig. 2.7). The segment scheduled for removal can be inflated, whereas the segments to be preserved are maintained to be deflated. This technique is diametrically opposite to the conventional method and allows clear visualization of the intersegmental line between the two segments. The actual surgical margin can be visualized by the inflated-deflated line and a good surgical field can be achieved even through video-assisted thoracic surgery (VATS) without the need to suppress the other segments and lobes with an instrument. In addition, dissection of the anatomic intersegmental plane by electrocautery (but not by stapling) reduces unfavorable recurrent local failure at the margin and allows full expansion of the preserved adjacent segments to result in maximal pulmonary function.

Recognition of the intersegmental plane (Fig. 2.8) is accomplished by differential inflation with jet ventilation [11]. After the segmental bronchi are isolated, an anesthesiologist inserts a 3.5-mm bronchoscope through a double-lumen tube into the orifice of the targeted segmental bronchus. The light at the tip of the

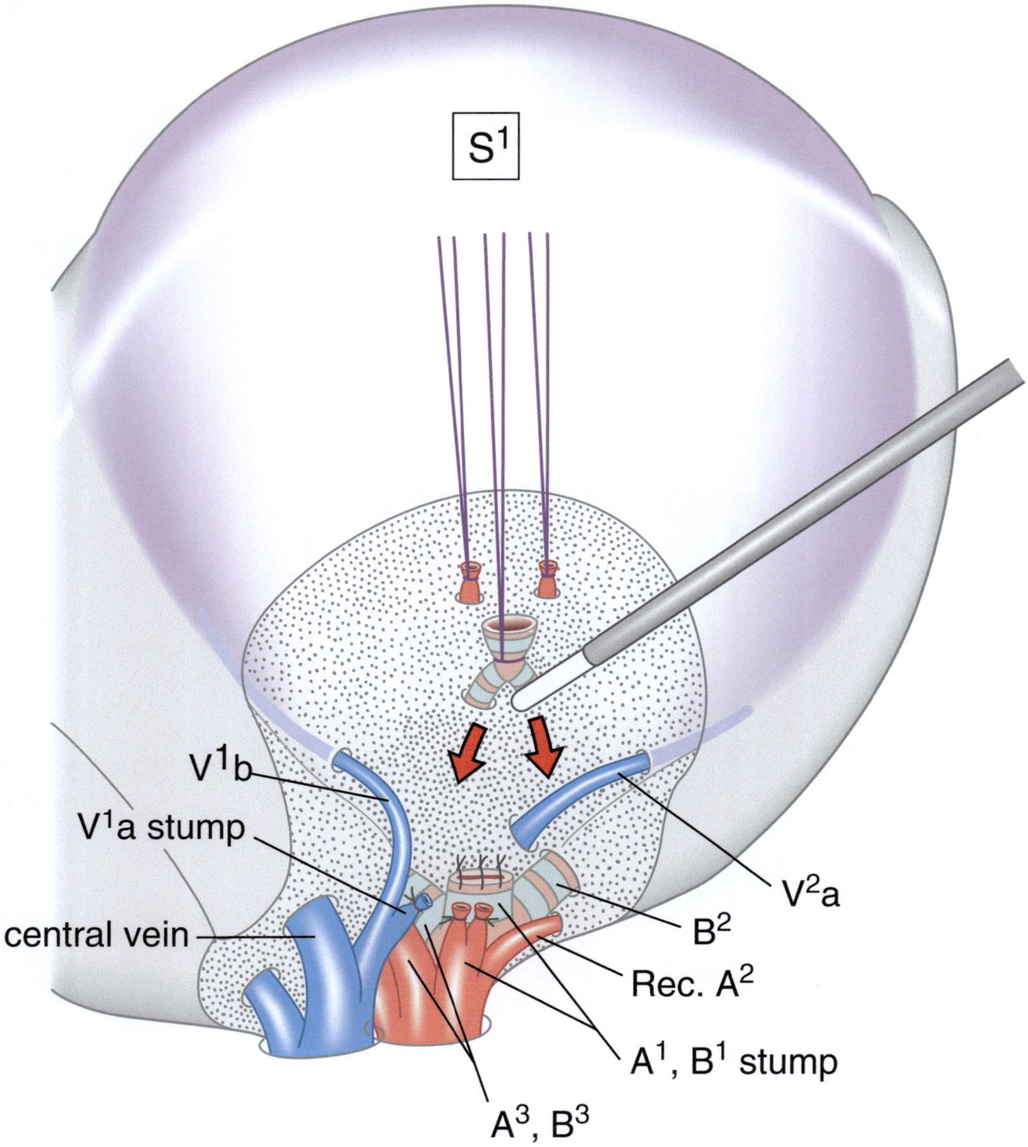

Fig. 2.4 Denuding along the intersegmental plane.

bronchoscope is visible in the surgical field and the surgeon can guide it to a desirable location at the targeted bronchus, where high-frequency oscillation is started (40 Hz, working pressure 2 kg/cm^2, HFO Jet Ventilator). The diseased segment is inflated while the preserved segments appear collapsed, and the line that forms between the inflated and deflated lung parenchyma indicates the anatomical intersegmental plane. This technique allows the development of a defined plane without the need for air transmission via collateral ventilation, unlike the conventional method. After jet ventilation fills the targeted segment, the distal site of the bronchus is tied to keep the segment inflated, and the site proximal to the tied point is transected to leave a stump of sufficient length so that closure will not occlude other segmental orifices. When more than one segment is to be removed, the surgeon can selectively insert the tip of the bronchoscope into each segmental bronchus and sequentially inflate each segment. At the central portion around the hilum, the intersegmental plane is approached along the intersegmental vein,

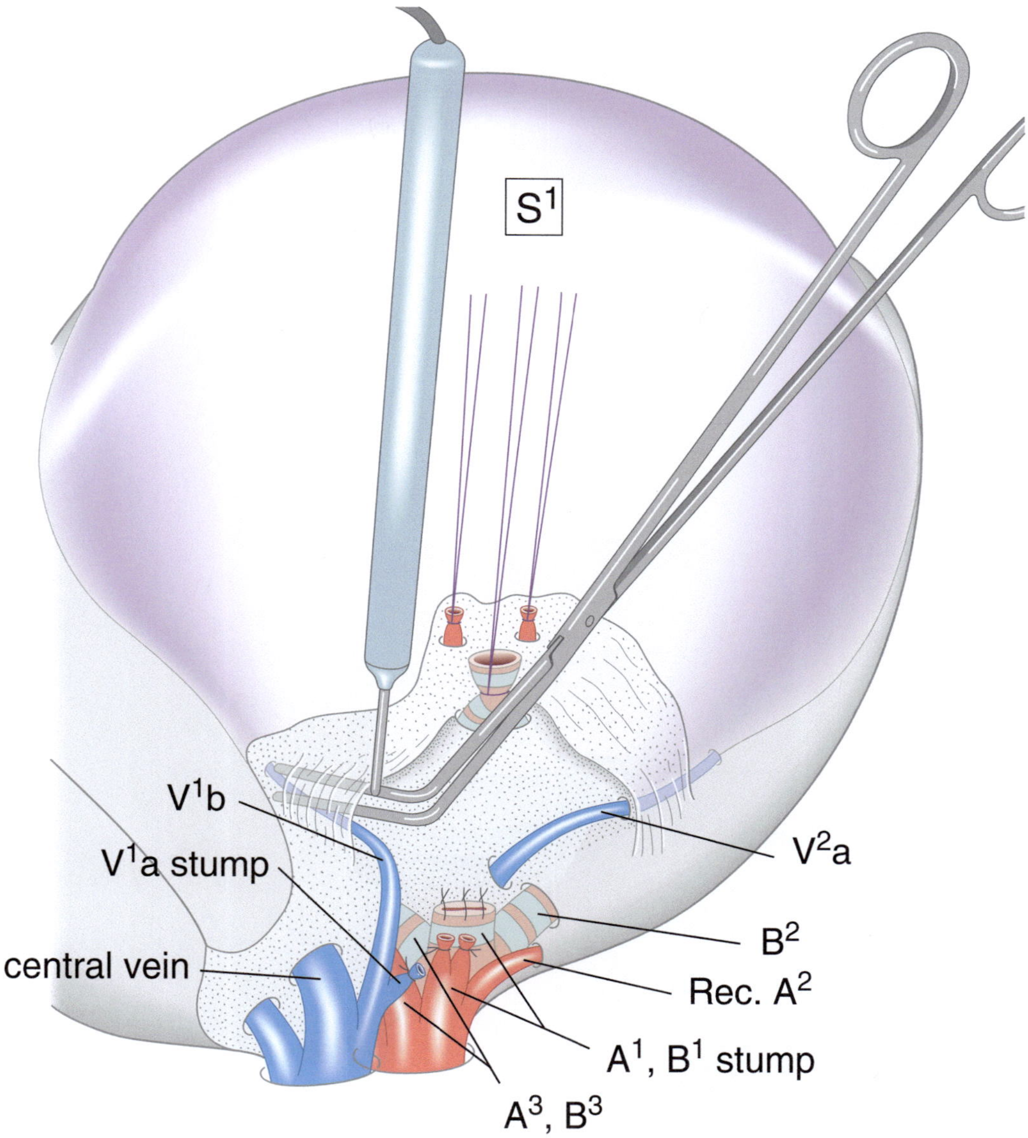

Fig. 2.5 Cutting along the intersegmental plane.

and electrocautery is applied at the peripheral site along the inflation–deflation line. The raw surface of the remaining lung is covered with a fibrin sealant composed of fibrinogen and thrombin and an absorbable polyglycolic acid (PGA) felt prevents air leakage after cutting by electrocautery. Air leakage can be minimized using staplers to divide the intersegmental plane when the lung is emphysematous. Since the margin is not greater than the tumor diameter, that is, at least 2 cm of healthy lung tissue is present, the resection line can be placed on the segment adjacent to the affected segment, or portions of a few adjacent segments or subsegments can be extirpated (Fig. 2.8). The applicability of segmentectomy must be determined by sampling or dissection of segmental, lobar, hilar, and mediastinal lymph nodes followed by frozen-section analysis. When patients are actually indicated for radical segmentectomy, lobectomy should be performed instead when the surgical margin is judged imperfect or a diseased lymph node is found. The chest is routinely drained with a single chest tube under a water seal that is inserted through the incision initially established for thoracoscopy.

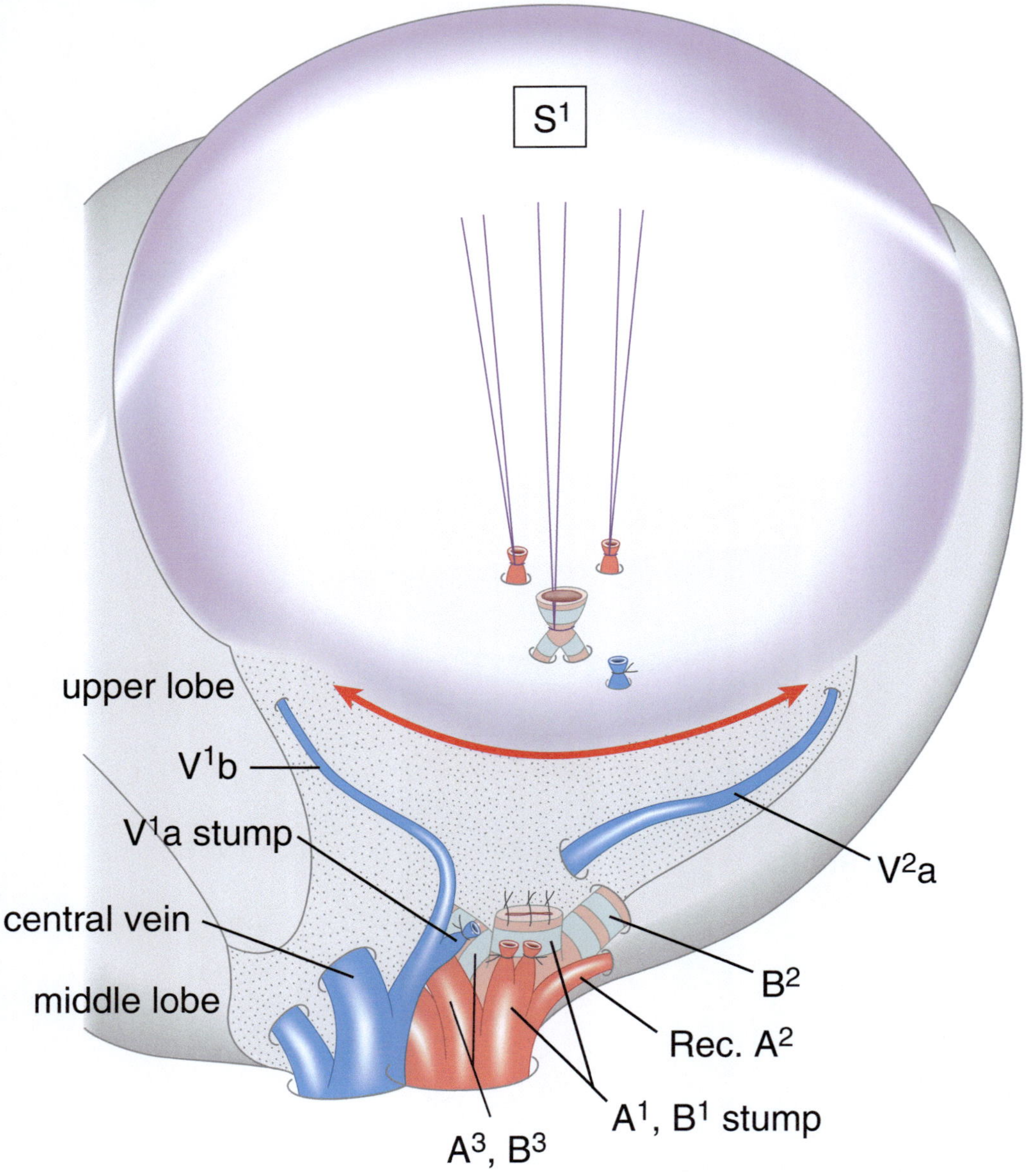

Fig. 2.6 Direction of cutting along the intersegmental plane.

2.6 Lymph Node Dissection

Lymph node dissection plays an important role in radical segmentectomy. The frequency of lymph node metastasis in patients with cT1aN0M0 non-small-cell lung cancer according to the 2004 Japanese registry of surgical lung cancers is about 10% [12]. Even if the PET/CT showed N0 stage, final pathological N-stage should be confirmed by pathological examination, because PET cannot detect metastasis lesion less than 4 mm within lymph node [13].

2.6.1 Lymph Node Dissection at the Hilum

After segmental resection, the #10–12 lymph nodes should be dissected, which is simple and safe when

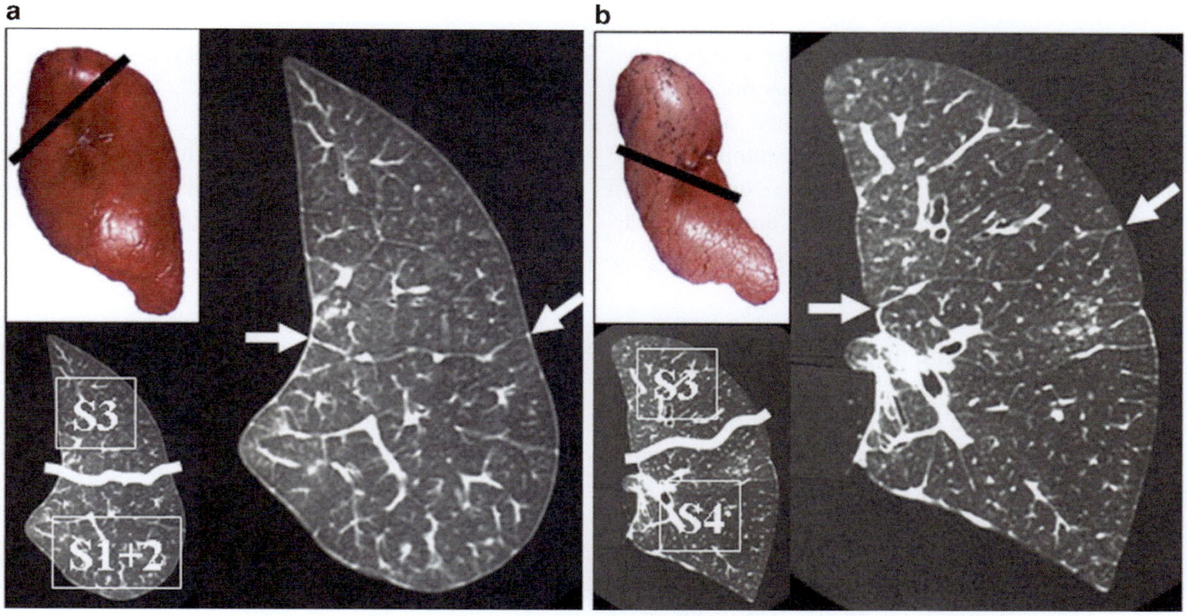

Fig. 2.7 Transaxial (**a**) and coronal (**b**) CT views of left upper lobe tissue specimen. Anatomical intersegmental lines between S^{1+2} (apical and posterior segments) and S3 (anterior segment) (**a**), and between S^3 and S^4 (superior segment) (**b**) are considered as inflation–deflation lines [11].

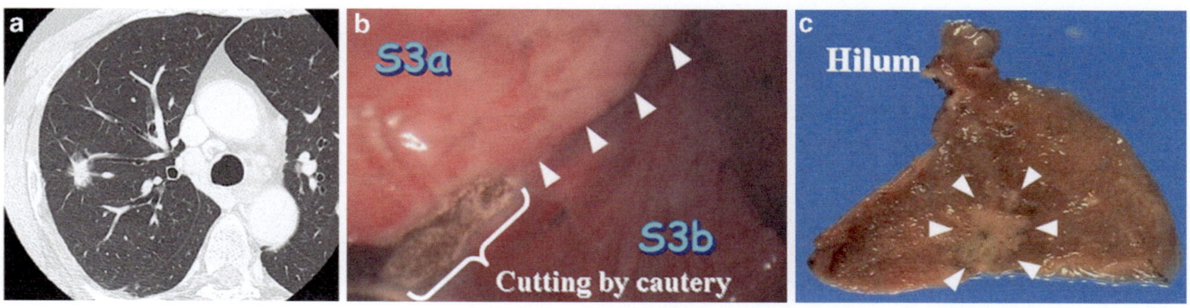

Fig. 2.8 Representative atypical segmentectomy: S^2b (anterior subsegment of posterior segment) + S^3a (posterior subsegment of anterior segment) resection of the right upper lobe. (**a**) High-resolution CT image shows tumor located at S^2b and S^3a border. (**b**) Intraoperative findings show inflation–deflation line (*arrowheads*) between inflated (resected) S^3a and deflated (preserved) S^3b segments. (**c**) Resected surgical specimen shows tumor (*arrowheads*) with sufficient margin [11].

the segmental bronchus and vessels are encircled with tape.

However, it is controversial whether the #13 nodes in the preserved segment should be dissected or not. To clarify this question, Nomori et al. mapped sentinel nodes (SN) in the segmental lymph nodes of patients who underwent segmentectomy by using radioisotope [14]. When the segments were classified as anterior and posterior ones, segmental (#13) SNs were more prevalent in the posterior segment. For example, SN of the tumor located in S^8 (anterior segment) often presents not only in the #13 node around B^8 but also in the #13 around B^6, which locates in the posterior site of chest cavity. This finding suggests that lymphatic flow often passes not only to their own segmental nodes but also to the segmental nodes of posteriorly located segments, probably because the lobar bronchi are located in the posterior part of the chest cavity. Therefore, the #13 nodes of the posterior segments should be dissected, especially when a tumor is located in the anterior segment. For example, the #13 node around the B^6 should be dissected in S^8-segmentectomy, whereas the #13 around B^8 does not always require dissection in S^6-segmentectomy.

2.6.2 Mediastinal Lymph Node Dissection

Skip metastasis to the mediastinal lymph node occurs in 20–40% of patients with N2-NSCLC, possibly because some lymphatic flow from the lung goes directly to the mediastinum but not to the hilar lymph node stations. Therefore, mediastinal lymph nodes should be dissected even if metastasis is not evident in frozen sections of hilar nodes. Metastasis in mediastinal nodes is usually lobe specific, that is, lower paratracheal node (#4R) in the right upper lobe, subaortic one (#5) in the left upper lobe, and subcarinal nodes (#7) in both sides of lower lobes [15–23]. Therefore, at least, these lobe-specific mediastinal lymph nodes should be dissected during segmentectomy.

2.6.3 Selection of Lymph Nodes for Intraoperative Frozen Section

It is hard to submit all dissected lymph nodes for frozen sections. Based on sentinel node mapping, we recommend that lymph nodes for frozen section should be selected as follows. The frequency of SN is higher in the #12 (39%) and #13 (57%) nodes in the hilar region than in the #10 (10%) and #11 (16%) nodes and thus the former two might be more appropriate for frozen section. Regarding mediastinal nodes, at least lobe-specific mediastinal nodes described in the previous session (2.6.2) are submitted for frozen section during segmentectomy [15–23]. Among each mediastinal stations, the largest lymph node is preferable to be submitted for frozen section, because the frequency of metastasis has been reported to be the highest (94%) in this node whereas that in the next largest node is 6% in N2-disease [24]. The report also describes that there is no metastasis in the 3rd largest nodes or smaller nodes. Therefore, frozen sections of the largest or second-largest nodes obtained intraoperatively at each mediastinal station are sufficient to find N2-disease.

2.7 Hybrid VATS and Sharp Dissection (Figs. 2.9 and 2.10)

In principle, complete VATS performed indirectly using a monitor is limited to relatively simple lung resections and cannot be applied to all lung cancer operations including segmentectomy and bronchoplasty. From the viewpoint of treating various malignancies using minimally invasive techniques, we have widely applied hybrid VATS, which is an integrated surgical combination of a muscle-sparing minithoracotomy without rib spreading, a thoracoscopic hole prepared under television monitoring and direct visualization [25–28]. The primary target of ideal minimally invasive surgery is to preserve the pulmonary parenchyma, and the secondary aim is to reduce trauma through selecting the most suitable surgical approach. The three-dimensional view provided by direct visualization via hybrid VATS enables surgeons to understand appropriate margins, thus minimizing the likelihood of missing diseased lung tissue or removing an excessive amount of healthy tissue. The advantages of using VATS to treat lung cancer using only a monitor for visualization are arguable, although surgeons can appreciate a sense of achievement. Whether or not direct vision is used in VATS is essentially a peripheral matter. Thoracic surgeons need to balance the strengths and weaknesses of complete VATS, for example, to avoid a lobectomy to treat a tiny undiagnosed tumor. The most important aspects of cancer surgery are total removal of a malignancy and preserved functionality for patients.

The hybrid VATS approach generally requires two skin incisions without cutting through muscles or ribs. One incision should be 4–5 cm long to allow access and manipulation and the other should be 1 cm long to allow the insertion of a thoracoscope (Fig. 2.9). The surgeon directly observes the hilum of the diseased lobe through the main access port using a silicon rubber wound retractor without rib spreading, and individually isolates and severs all bronchi and vessels of the segment in question. Television monitor guidance is applied during the procedure when dissecting an area outside the direct view. The skin incision must be extended if difficulties are encountered with the surgical view. We prefer a backhand grip to hold 30-cm scissors (Model 101-8098-30; Mayo-Harrington; Stille, Sweden) for sharp dissection, long needle holders and upside-down forceps.

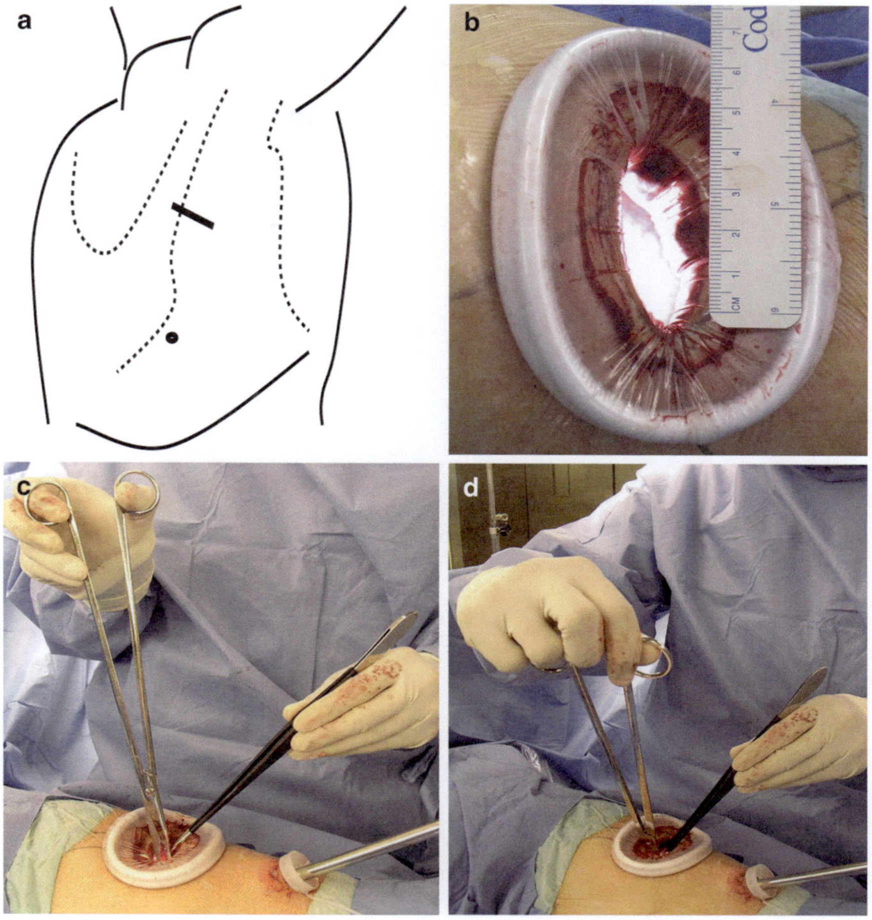

Fig. 2.9 Hybrid VATS approach. (**a**) Skin incisions for thoracoscopic (*circle*) access and for thoracotomy (*solid line*) are positioned over the mid-axillary line in fourth interspace for upper or middle lobe tumors. Lower lobe tumors are approached through the auscultatory triangle in the fifth interspace. (**b**) Operative field widened about 2-cm using wound retractor. Rib spreading is not required. (**c** and **d**) Sharp dissection in depths of directly visualized open thorax using upside-down grip on 30-cm scissors manipulated with the thumb and index finger through the loops and turning the wrist. The ulnar side of the hands rests comfortably alongside the margins of the incision to avoid awkward elevation of the forearms or elbows [27].

Although the easiest to the most difficult segments to remove are in the order of the upper division (S^{1-3}) and lingular segment (S^{4+5}) of the left upper lobe, and the superior (S^6) and basal (right S^{7-10} or left S^{8-10}) segments of either lower lobe, we have performed aggressive and complicated resections such as the left S^3 segment + S^{1+2} sub-segment (Fig. 2.10).

The key to achieving excellence using the hybrid VATS approach is the upside-down backhand grip on long scissors for incisive dissection, and the long needle holder for bronchoplasty or angioplasty developed by Belsey (Frenchay Hospital; Bristol, UK), Pearson (Toronto General Hospital; Toronto, ON, Canada), and Tsubota (Hyogo Cancer Center; Akashi, Hyogo, Japan) to facilitate deep maneuvering. This skill was advanced before the introduction of VATS, and we still find it suitable for maneuvering through a small access thoracotomy during the VATS era. In general, segmentectomy is technically more demanding than lobectomy because a thorough three-dimensional understanding of all relevant bronchoarterial relationships is required along with possible anomalies of the arterial branches. Sharp dissection with scissors that can accurately and rapidly expose the segmental hilar structures is important for radical hybrid VATS segmentectomy.

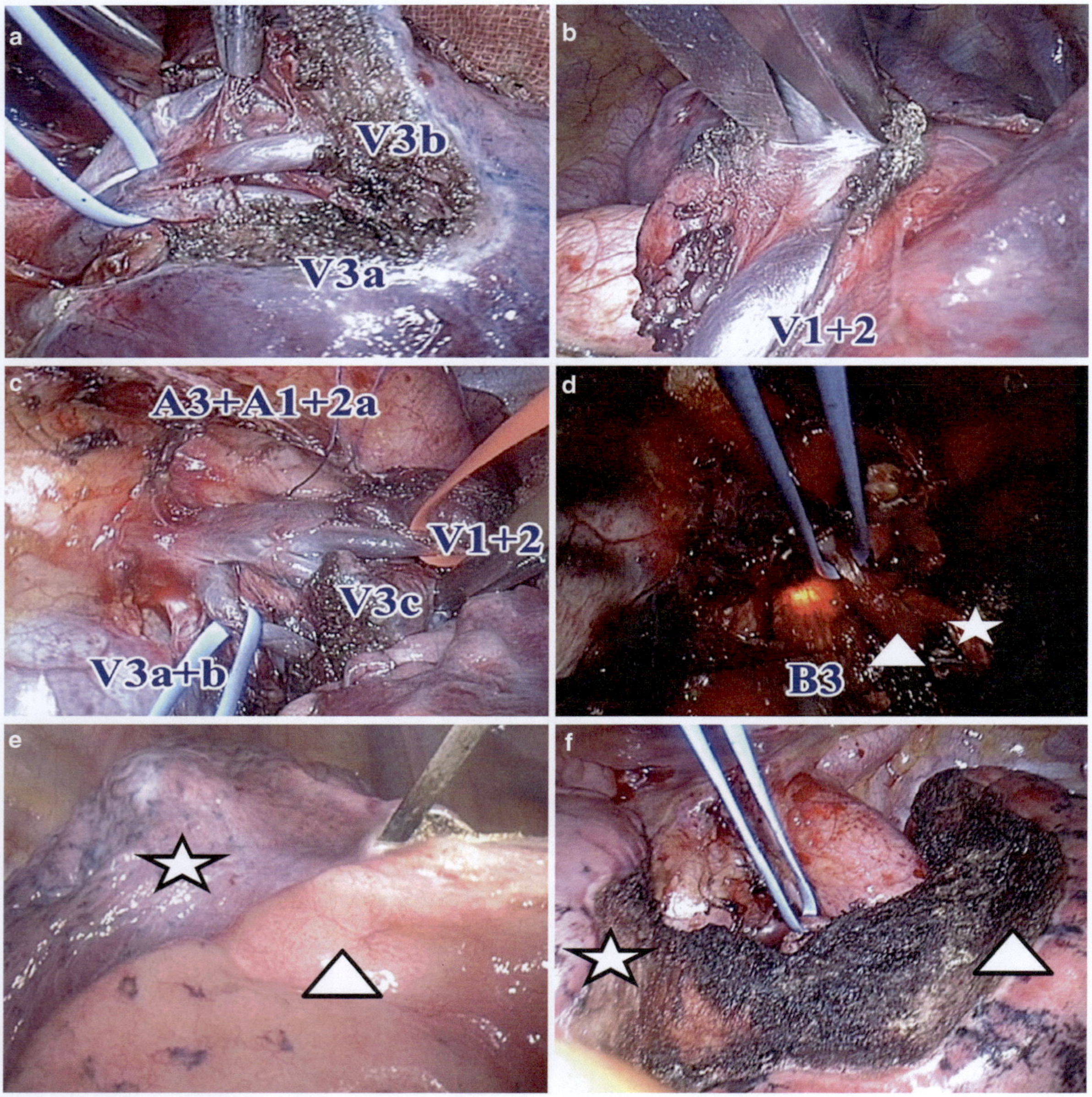

Fig. 2.10 Left $S^3+S^{1+2}a$ segmentectomy. (**a**) V^3a and V^3b branches of vein running between upper division and lingular segment are identified and exposed distally. (**b**) V^{1+2} vein branch is also exposed distally and $V^{1+2}a$, $V^{1+2}b+c$ and V^{1+2}superior branches are identified. $V^{1+2}a$ runs between S^3c and $S^{1+2}a$ and $V^{1+2}b+c$ runs between $S^{1+2}a$ and $S^{1+2}b+c$. (**c**) The first two branches of the artery (A^3 and $A^{1+2}a$) and vein ($V^{1+2}a$, $V^{1+2}b+c$, V^3a, V^3b and V^3c) are uncovered. $V^{1+2}b+c$, V^3b intersegmental branches of the vein are saved for venous return from preserved adjacent segments. (**d**) Bronchofiberscope inserted through a double-lumen tube into the orifice of a targeted segmental bronchus (B^3) and $B^{1+2}a$ (*asterisks*), where high-frequency oscillation is applied. $V^{1+2}b+c$ (*triangle*) is preserved. (**e**) Inflation–deflation line between inflated (resected) $S^{1+2}a$ and deflated (preserved) $S^{1+2}b+c$ subsegments, along which the anatomical intersubsegmental plane is dissected with cautery. (**f**) Saved parenchyma of $S^{1+2}b+c$ (*triangle*) and S^4 (*asterisks*) is fully inflated after $S^3+S^{1+2}a$ is removed [27].

2.8 Covering the Intersegmental Plane (Fig. 2.11)

After segment resection, lung inflation without immersing the lung in water can reveal peripheral bronchial fistulas, which should be closed by suture. Air leakage is then investigated by immersing the cut plane in water–under approximately 10 cm H_2O. Leaks comprising only small bubbles of 2–3 mm can be stopped as follows: the cut surface of the intersegmental plane is

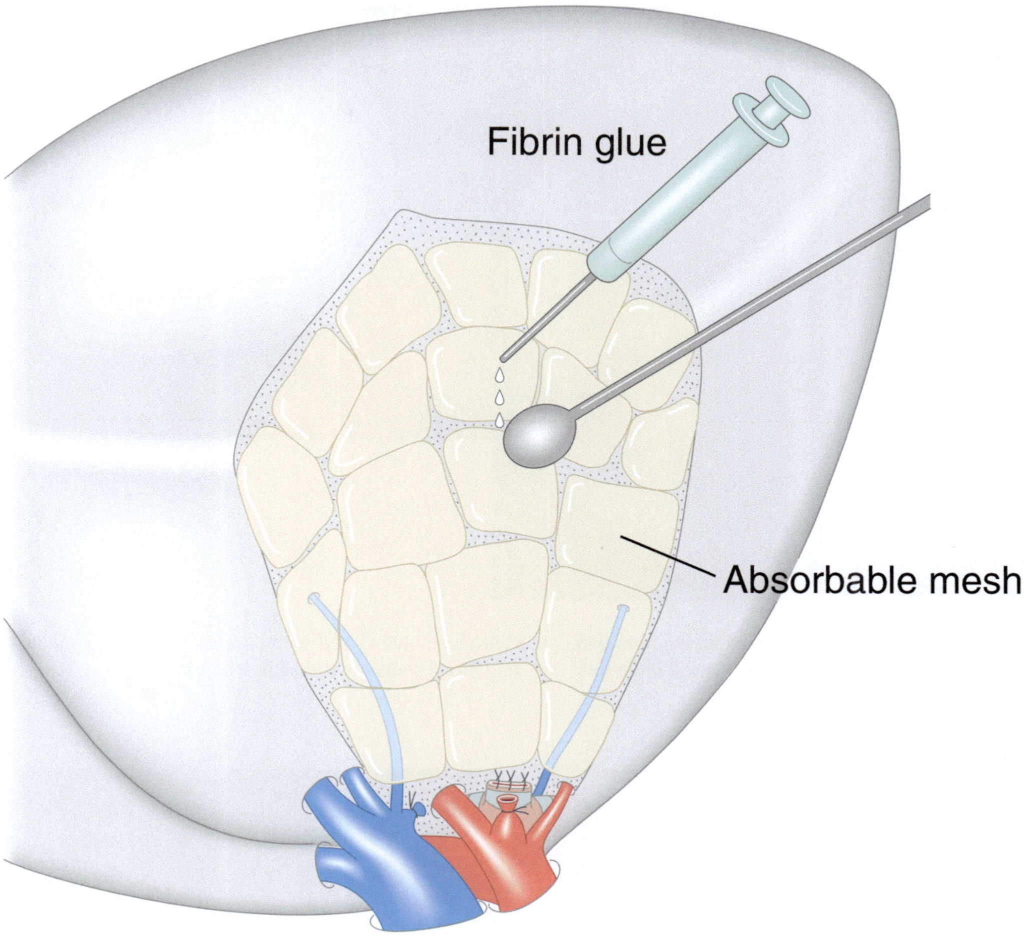

Fig. 2.11 Covering the dissected intersegmental plane.

covered under slight inflation with a 1~2-cm^2 absorbable mesh such as PGA sheet and fibrin glue (Fig. 2.11) [29].

2.9 Marking Segments with Dye (Fig. 2.12)

Although not always necessary, staining can help to identify the segmental artery especially during complicated procedures such as subsegmentectomy. To mark the segments, a conventional tracheal tube (not a double-lumen tube) is inserted in the operation room. A needle biopsy catheter is inserted into the subsegmental bronchus through a bronchoscope and then about 1 mL of indigo carmine dye mixed with contrast medium (using for angiography) is injected into the lung tissue under fluoroscopy. If the catheter is inserted too deeply, the dye might be injected into the thoracic wall. If the needle of the forceps is too shallow, the dye might leak into the central bronchus. When injected into the appropriate position, the contrast medium mixture with dye can be visualized on fluoroscopy that moves with breathing. However, because the dye usually disappears within 1 h, the surface of the stained lung tissue is marked by suture immediately after thoracotomy (Fig. 2.12).

2.10 Marking a Nodule Using Contrast Medium (Fig. 2.13)

Bronchioloalveolar carcinoma or small tumors located deeply within the lung tissue sometimes cannot be localized by visual inspection or palpation during surgery, which could also cause local recurrence at the surgical margin after segmentectomy. Preoperative

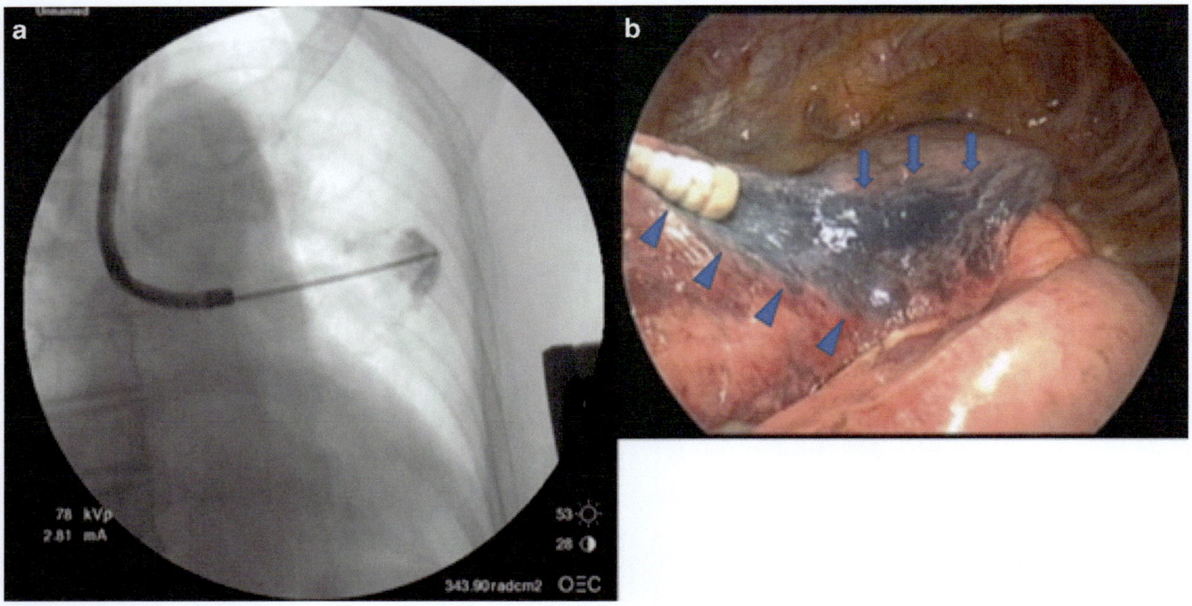

Fig. 2.12 Staining lung tissue with contrast medium and dye. Methylene blue mixed with contrast medium is injected into lung tissue under fluoroscopic guidance after tracheal intubation (**a**) Lung tissue stained with methylene blue (**b**).

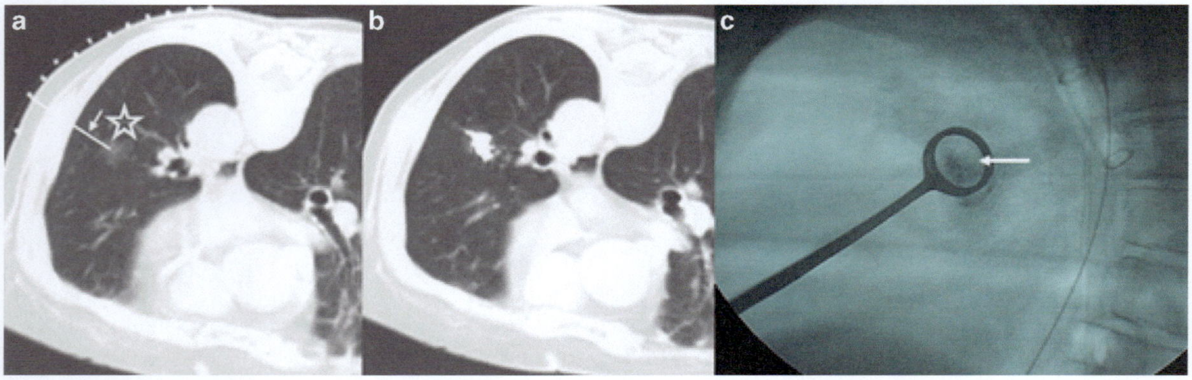

Fig. 2.13 Marking a nodule with ground grass opacity (GGO) finding. A needle is inserted into a GGO lesion under CT fluoroscopy (**a**) Lesion stained with lipiodol (**b**) is intraoperatively grasped with a ring-shaped forceps under fluoroscopic guidance (**c**).

marking using a needle marker or contrast medium under CT is sometimes necessary for such tumors. Lipiodol (Lipiodol Ultrafluid, Laboratoire Guerbet, Aulnay-Sous-Bois, France), which is generally used as a contrast medium for lymphatic vessels, can be used for this procedure [30, 31]. Under CT guide, the needle is inserted into the lesion by percutaneous way and lipiodol about 0.5 mL in volume is injected. Before injection, the syringe is pulled to confirm that no blood flows backward. During surgery, the lesion marked with lipiodol can be visualized under fluoroscopy. The lesion marked with lipiodol is grasped within a ring-shaped forceps under fluoroscopy (Fig. 2.13). Lipiodol persists at the injection site for over 1 month because of its lipid solubility. Because it is not generally accepted for use in surgery involving lung tissue, an institutional ethics committee must approve its use before application for this purpose.

References

1. Okada M, Tauchi S, Iwanaga K, et al. Associations among bronchioloalveolar carcinoma component, positron emission tomographic, computed tomographic findings and malignant behavior in small lung adenocarcinomas. J Thorac Cardiovasc Surg. 2007;133:1448–54.
2. Nakayama H, Okumura S, Okada M, et al. Value of integrated positron emission tomography revised using a phantom to evaluate malignancy grade of lung adenocarcinoma: a multicenter study. Cancer. 2010;111:3170–7.
3. Okada M, Nakayama H, Okumura S, et al. Multicenter analysis of high-resolution computed tomography and positron emission tomography/computed tomography findings to choose therapeutic strategies for clinical stage IA lung adenocarcinoma. J Thorac Cardiovasc Surg. 2011;141:1384–91.
4. Nomori H, Ohtsuka T, Naruke T, et al. Histogram analysis of computed tomography numbers of clinical T1N0M0 lung adenocarcinoma, with special reference to lymph node metastasis and tumor invasiveness. J Thorac Cardiovasc Surg. 2003;126:1584–9.
5. Nomori H, Watanabe K, Ohtsuka T, et al. Evaluation of F-18 fluorodeoxyglucose (FDG) PET scanning for pulmonary nodules less than 3 cm in diameter, with special reference to the CT images. Lung Cancer. 2004;45:19–27.
6. Nomori H, Watanabe K, Ohtsuka T, et al. Fluorine 18-tagged fluorodeoxyglucose positron emission tomographic scanning to predict lymph node metastasis, invasiveness, or both, in clinical T1N0M0 lung adenocarcinoma. J Thorac Cardiovasc Surg. 2004;128(3):396–401.
7. Tsutani Y, Miyata Y, Okada M, et al. Difference in prognostic significance of maximum standardized uptake value on [18F]-fluoro-2-deoxyglucose positron emission tomography between adenocarcinoma and squamous cell carcinoma of the lung. Jpn J Clin Oncol. 2011;41:890–6.
8. Tsutani Y, Miyata Y, Okada M, et al. Prognostic significance of using solid versus whole tumor size on high-resolution computed tomography for predicting pathologic malignant grade of tumors in clinical stage IA lung adenocarcinoma: a multicenter study. J Thorac Cardiovasc Surg. 2012 (in press).
9. Horinouchi H, Nomori H, Nakayama T, et al. How many pathological T1N0M0 non-small cell lung cancers can be completely resected in one segment? Special reference to high-resolution computed tomography findings. Surg Today. 2011;41:1062–6.
10. Nomori H, Mori T, Izumi Y, et al. Is completion lobectomy merited for unanticipated nodal metastases after radical segmentectomy for cT1N0M0/pN1–2 non-small cell lung cancer? J Thorac Cardiovasc Surg. 2012;143:820–4.
11. Okada M, Mimura Y, Ikegaki J, et al. A novel video-assisted anatomical segmentectomy technique: selective segmental inflation via bronchofiberoptic jet followed by cautery cutting. J Thorac Cardiovasc Surg. 2007;133:753–8.
12. Sawabata N, Miyaoka E, Asamura H, et al. Japanese lung cancer registry study of 11,663 surgical cases in 2004: demographic and prognosis changes over decade. Japanese Joint Committee for Lung Cancer Registration. J Thorac Oncol. 2011;6:1229–35.
13. Nomori H, Watanabe K, Ohtsuka T, et al. The size of metastatic foci and lymph nodes yielding false-negative and false-positive lymph node staging with positron emission tomography in patients with lung cancer. J Thorac Cardiovasc Surg. 2004;127(4):1087–92.
14. Nomori H, Ohba Y, Shibata H, et al. Required area of lymph node sampling during segmentectomy for clinical stage IA non-small cell lung cancer. J Thorac Cardiovasc Surg. 2010;139:38–42.
15. Okada M, Tsubota N, Yoshimura M, et al. Proposal for reasonable mediastinal lymphadenectomy in bronchogenic carcinomas. J Thorac Cardiovasc Surg. 1998;116:949–53.
16. Naruke T, Tsuchiya R, Kondo H, et al. Lymph node sampling in lung cancer: how should it be done? Eur J Cardiovasc Surg. 1999;16:S17–24.
17. Asamura H, Nakayama H, Kondo H, et al. Lobe-specific extent of systematic lymph node dissection for non-small cell lung carcinomas according to a retrospective study of metastasis and prognosis. J Thorac Cardiovasc Surg. 1999;117:1102–11.
18. Okada M, Sakamoto T, Yuki T, et al. Selective mediastinal lymphadenectomy for clinico-surgical stage I non-small cell lung cancer. Ann Thorac Surg. 2006;81:1028–32.
19. Nomori H, Horio H, Naruke T, et al. Use of technetium-99m tin colloid for sentinel lymph node identification in non-small cell lung cancer. J Thorac Cardiovasc Surg. 2002;24:486–92.
20. Nomori H, Ikeda K, Mori T, et al. Sentinel node navigation segmentectomy for c-T1N0M0 non-small cell lung cancer. J Thorac Cardiovasc Surg. 2007;133:780–5.
21. Nomori H, Ikeda K, Mori T, et al. Sentinel node identification in clinical stage Ia non-small cell lung cancer by a combined single photon emission computed tomography/computed tomography system. J Thorac Cardiovasc Surg. 2007;134:182–7.
22. Nomori H, Ohba Y, Yoshimoto K, et al. Difference of sentinel lymph node identification between tin colloid and phytate in patients with non-small cell lung cancer. Ann Thorac Surg. 2009;87:906–10.
23. Nomori H. Sentinel node mapping in lung cancer. The Japanese experience. Semin Thorac Cardiovasc Surg. 2009;21:316–22.
24. Ikeda K, Nomori H, Mori T, et al. Size of metastatic and non-metastatic mediastinal lymph nodes in non-small cell lung cancer. J Thorac Oncol. 2006;1:949–52.
25. Okada M, Sakamoto T, Yuki T, et al. Hybrid surgical approach of video-assisted minithoracotomy for lung cancer. Chest. 2005;128:2696–701.
26. Patterson, Cooper, Deslauriers, Lerut, Luketich, Rice, editors. Pearson's Thoracic & Esophageal Surgery, Vol. 1, 3rd ed. Churchill Livingstone (Elsevier). 2008 p. 5.
27. Okada M, Tsutani Y, Ikeda T, et al. Radical hybrid video-assisted thoracic segmentectomy: long-term results of minimally invasive anatomical sublobar resection for treating lung cancer. Interact Cardiovasc Thorac Surg. 2012;14:5–11.
28. Miyata Y, Okada M. Hybrid video-assisted thoracic surgery basilar (S9-10) segmentectomy. Semin Thorac Cardiovasc Surg. 2011;23:73–7.
29. Asakura K, Izumi Y, Nomori H, et al. Effect of cutting technique at the intersegmental plane during segmentectomy on expansion of the preserved segment: comparison between staplers and scissors in ex vivo pig lung. Eur J Cardiothorac Surg. 2011;40:34–8.
30. Nomori H, Horio H, Naruke T, et al. Fluoroscopy-assisted thoracoscopic resection of lung nodules marked with lipiodol. Ann Thorac Surg. 2001;74:170–3.
31. Watanabe K, Nomori H, Ohtsuka T, et al. Usefulness and complications of computed tomography-guided lipiodol marking for fluoroscopy-assisted thoracoscopic resection of small pulmonary nodules: experience with 174 nodules. J Thorac Cardiovasc Surg. 2006;132:320–4.

Part II

Details of Technique

3 Segmentectomy of the Right Upper Lobe

The major branches of the right pulmonary artery are defined herein as follows:
Truncus superior: pulmonary artery of the first major branch to the right upper lobe.
Truncus intermedius: pulmonary artery between the truncus superior artery and A^6.
Basal artery: A^{7-10}.

			Frequency (%)
Bronchus	Three branches into B^1, B^2, and B^3		40
	Two branches into B^{1+3} and B^2		24
	B^{1+2} and B^3		14
	B^1+B^{2+3}		10
	Four branches into others		12
Artery	A^1	Both A^1a and A^1b from truncus superior artery	68
		A^1a branches independently, A^1b from truncus superior artery	32
	A^2	A^2a from recurrent artery; A^2b from ascending artery	72
		Both A^2a and A^2b from ascending artery	16
		Both A^2a and A^2b from recurrent artery	12
	A^3	Both A^3a and A^3b from truncus superior artery	48
		A^3a from truncus intermedius; A^3b from truncus superior artery	34
		A^3a from truncus superior; A^3b from truncus intermedius	18
Vein	Both apical (V^1) and central (V^2) veins		70
	Apical vein without central vein: V^1 and V^2 form common branch, running ventral to the hilum. V^2 branches along this route, running into the lung and between ascending and truncus superior arteries.		22
	Central vein without apical vein: common branch comprising V^1 and V^2 runs as central vein. V^1 branches along this route running cranially inside the lung.		8

H. Nomori and M. Okada, *Illustrated Anatomical Segmentectomy for Lung Cancer*,
DOI 10.1007/978-4-431-54144-8_3, © Springer Japan 2012

3.1 Right S^1 Segmentectomy

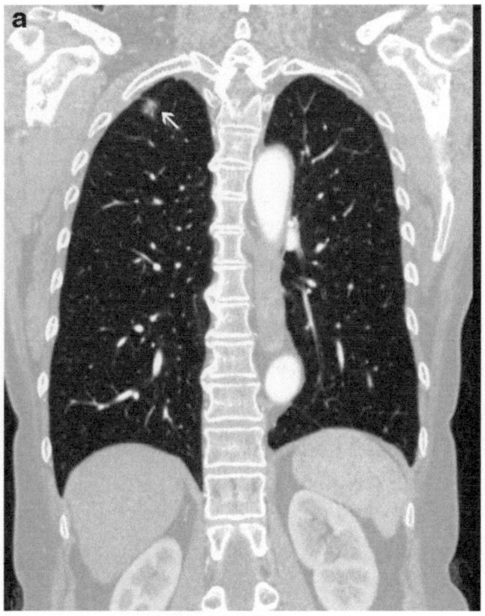

coronal view (CT scan)

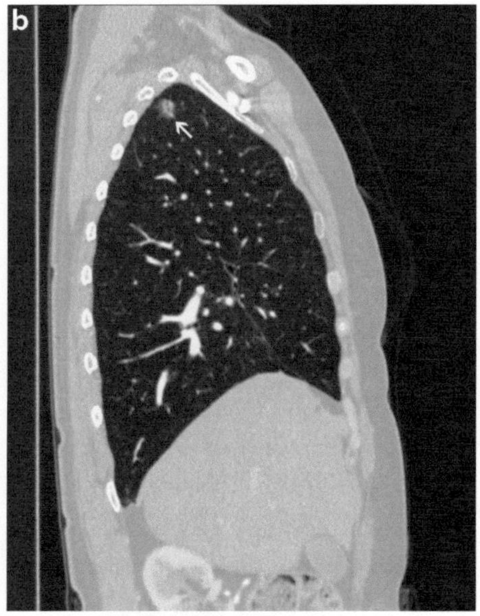

sagittal view (CT scan)

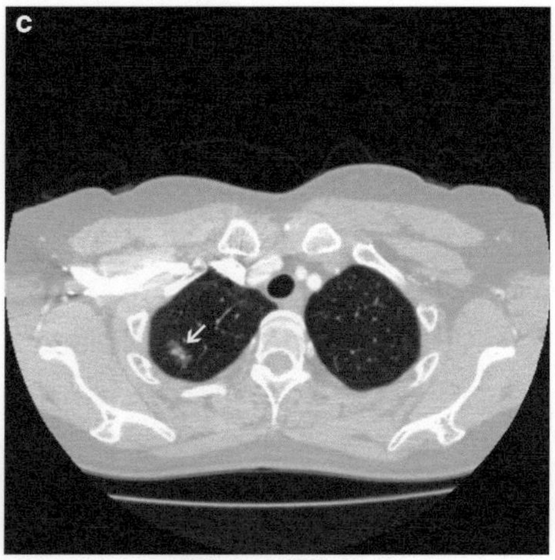

axial view (CT scan)

A follow-up CT scan after a left lower lobectomy to treat lung adenocarcinoma a few years before in a 60-year-old female revealed a 1.6-cm nodule with mixed GGO at the right S^1 that was diagnosed as lung adenocarcinoma from a CT-guided needle biopsy specimen. S^1-segmentectomy was undertaken. The final pathological diagnosis was pT1aN0M0 papillary adenocarcinoma.

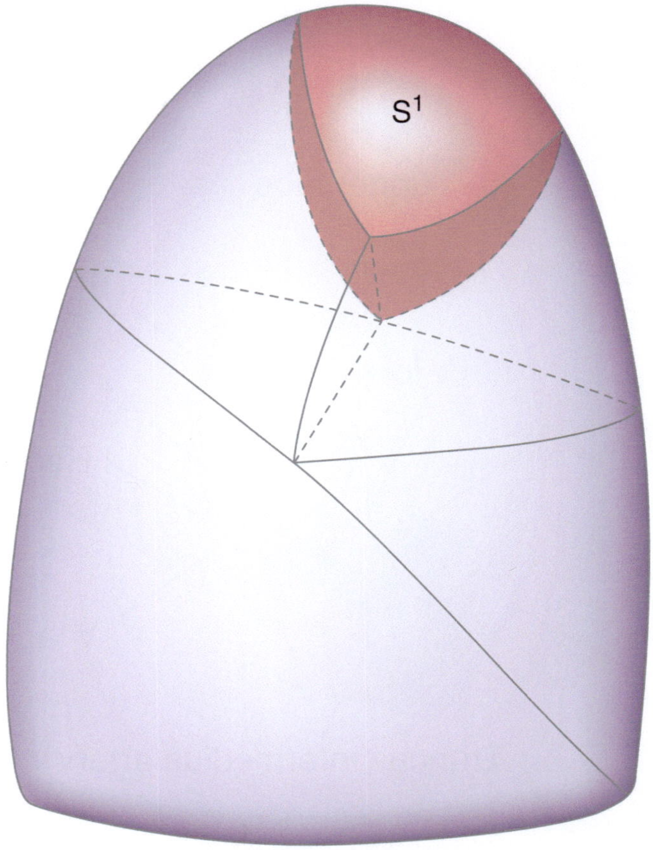

Fig. 3.1.1 The artery, vein, and bronchus branching profiles are confirmed from axial, coronal, and sagittal HRCT views. Branching pattern and size of B^1, B^2, and B^3 are further reconfirmed using bronchoscopy after tracheal intubation. The anatomical configuration of the segmental bronchus, artery, and vein in the figures of this session was the most frequent type as follows: the right upper bronchus branches into B^1, B^2, and B^3; A^1 and A^3 segmental arteries branch from the truncus superior artery; A^2a branches as a recurrent A^2 from the truncus superior artery and A^2b branches as an ascending A^2; and the segmental vein branches with the apical and central profile. The third intercostal space is recommended for thoracotomy in S^1-segmentectomy.

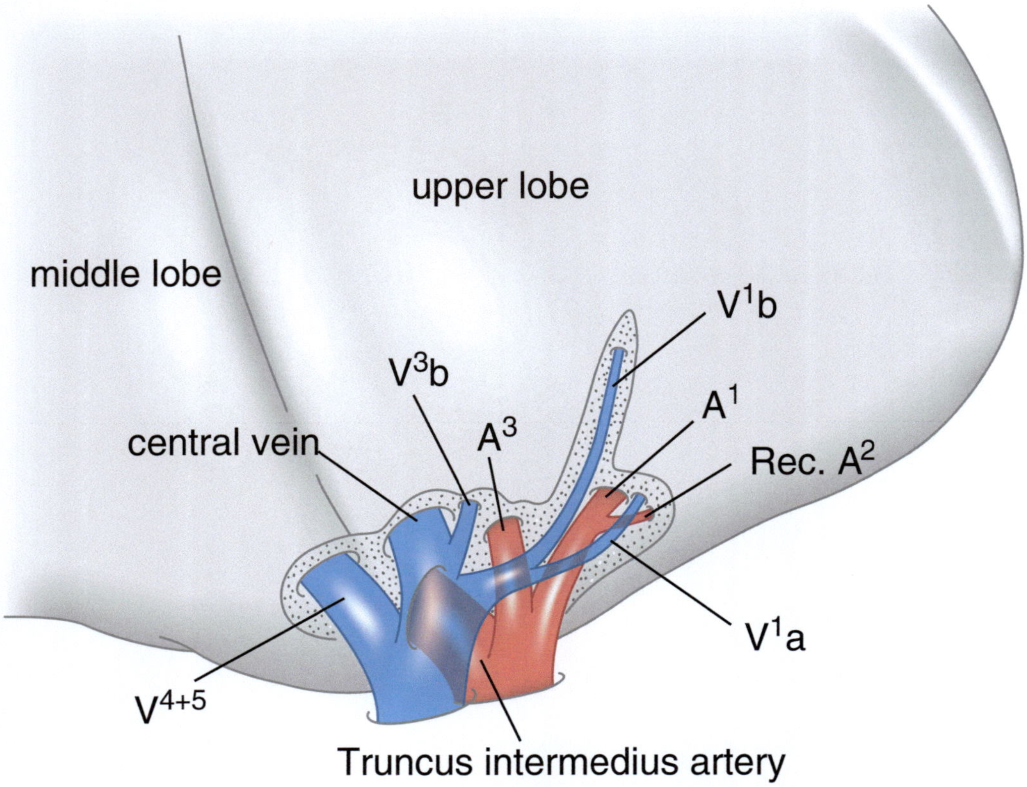

Fig. 3.1.2 The hilum of the right upper lobe is exposed from the ventral to the dorsal side to reveal the superior pulmonary vein, truncus superior artery, upper lobar bronchus, and the bifurcation between the upper lobar bronchus and truncus intermedius bronchus. If possible, the dorsal site of the upper lobar bronchus is exposed peripherally to the bifurcation of B^1 and B^2, which facilitates later identification of recurrent A^2. The V^1 is encircled with tape and exposed peripherally to identify V^1a and V^1b. The V^1b runs near the surface and towards the apex of the lung. When V^3c (vein between S^3bi and S^3bii) which branches at the central side of the V^1b is seen, it should be differentiated from V^1b. While V^1b runs towards the apex and near the lung surface, V^3c runs towards the ventral side and deeply into the lung. The V^1b is exposed peripherally. V^1a (vein between S^1a and S^1b) is cut. Exposing V^1b enables the identification of A^1 and A^3 that run dorsally and ventrally to V^1b, respectively.

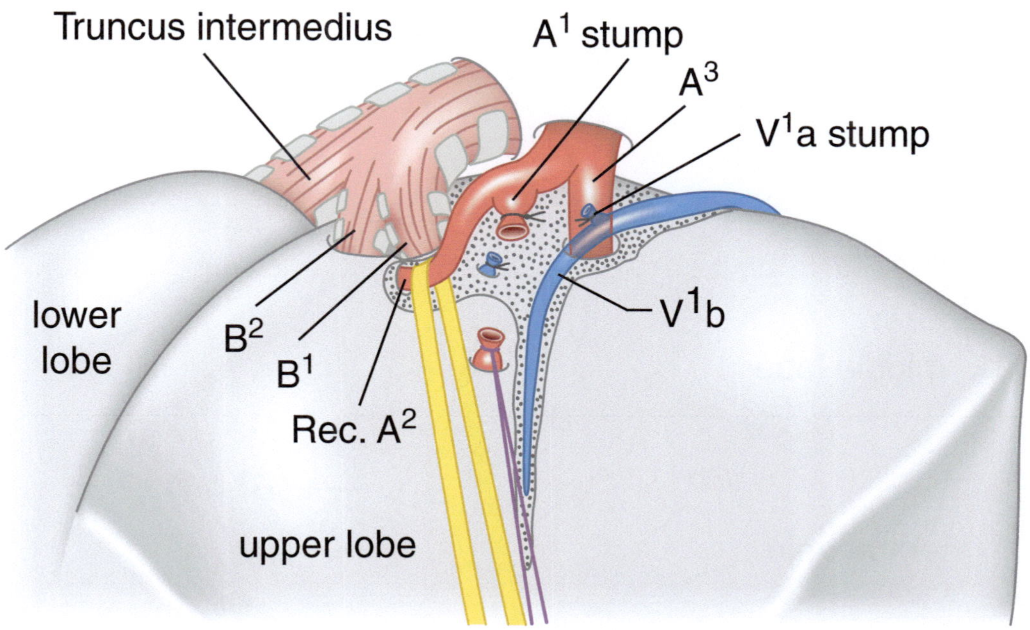

Fig. 3.1.3 A recurrent A^2 is verified after cutting V^1a. However, this is not usually easy to identify at this point. Reports indicate that 84 % of patients have a recurrent A^2. If there is a difficulty to differentiate between A^1-branch and recurrent A^2, the dorsal branch of A^1 is preserved because it might be a recurrent A^2. The ventral branches of A^1 are cut first, which must not be recurrent A^2. A recurrent A^2 is easy to be identified after cutting the B^1 or by creating an inflation–deflation line later. A recurrent A^2 runs away from distal stump of B^1, whereas A^1-branch runs towards it. This technique avoids misidentification of the segmental artery also in other types of segmentectomy.

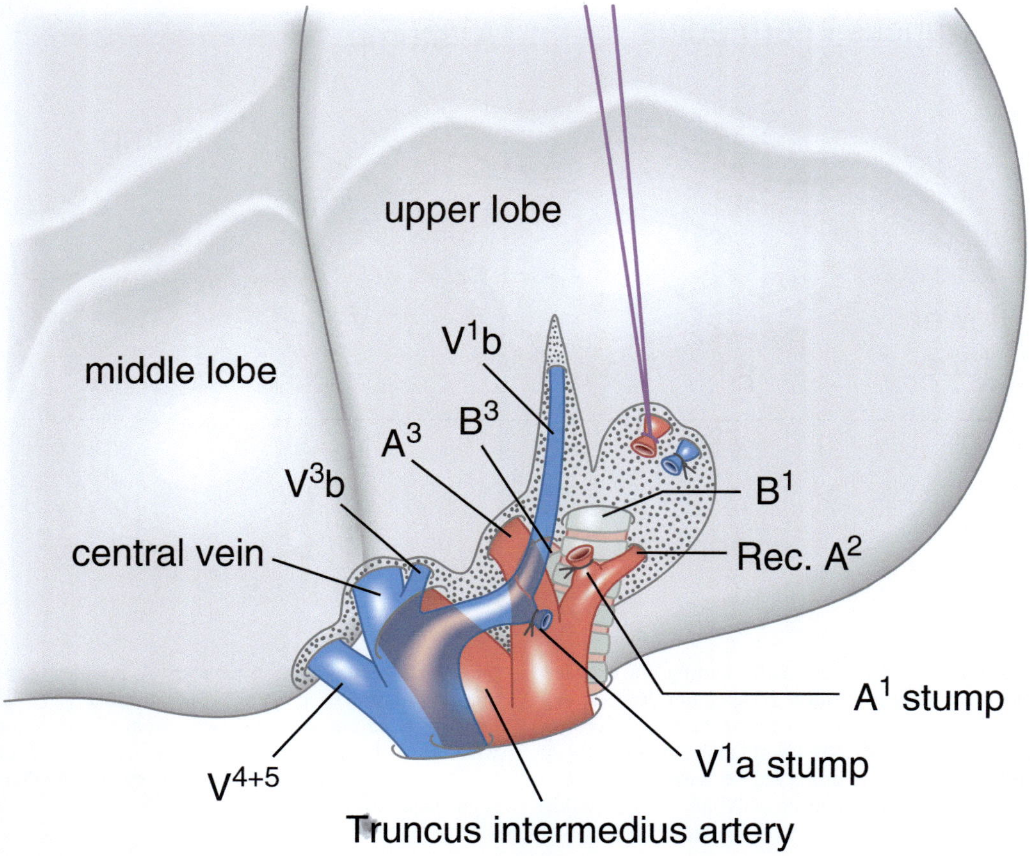

Fig. 3.1.4 After cutting A^1, a few lymph nodes in front of B^1 are dissected to expose B^1. Because V^2a runs behind B^1, B^1 is carefully encircled with thread to avoid damaging the V^2a. When B^1 cannot be identified definitely, illumination from a bronchoscope inserted into the B^1, B^2, and B^3 can help it.

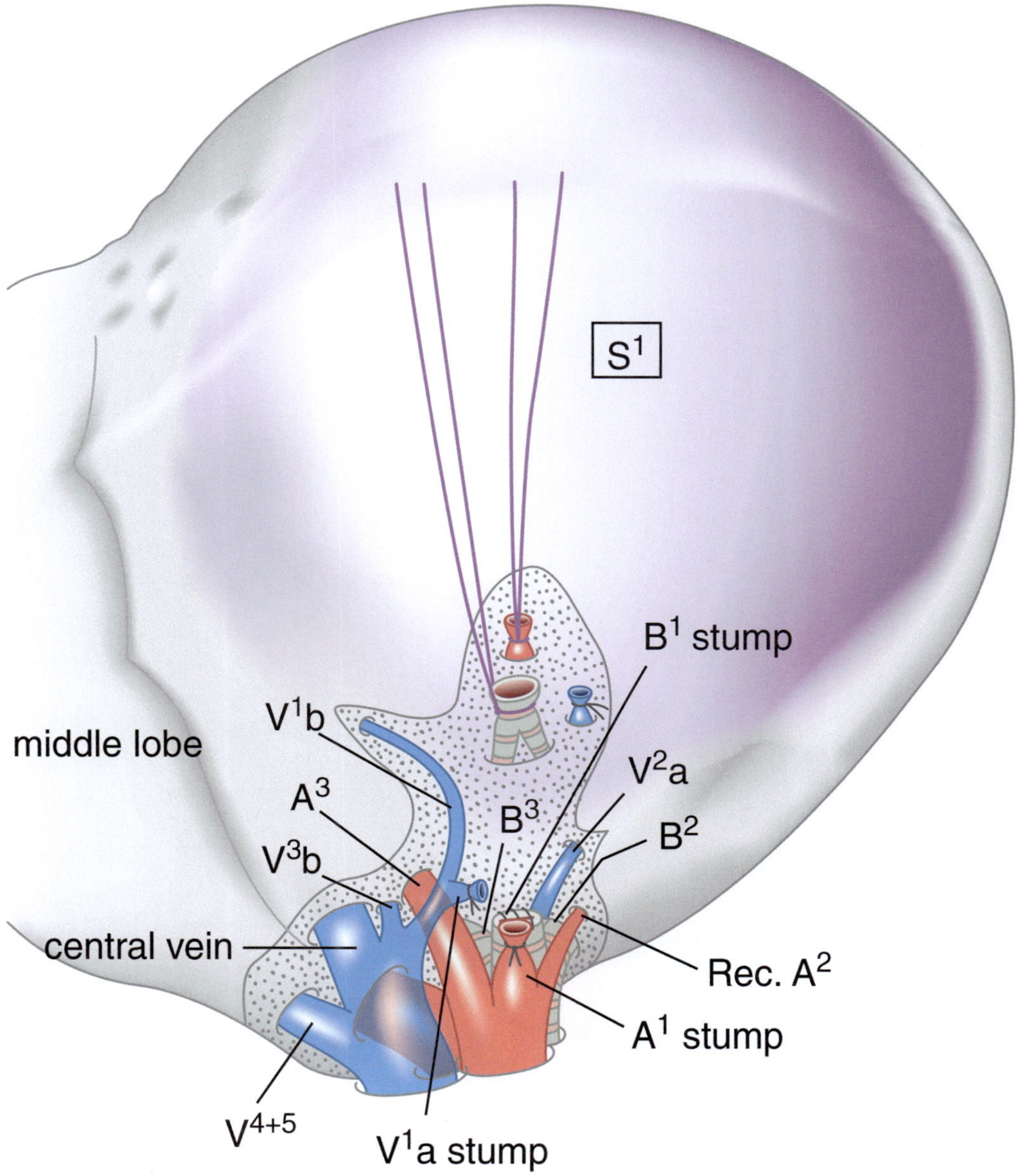

Fig. 3.1.5 S^1 can be selectively inflated by inserting a bronchoscope into the B^1 followed by jet ventilation, or by cutting the B^1 and inserting a catheter into the distal stump followed by air inflation. The distal stump is closed to trap air within S^1. The proximal stump of B^1 is closed with suture or ligation. B^1 can be cut using a stapler when S^1 is inflated by jet ventilation via bronchoscope. The distal stump of B^1 is lifted, and the back of it is peripherally denuded to move the stump away from the hilum. Lifting the distal B^1 stump also elevates lung tissue at both sides of it, which is cut towards the inflation–deflation line using electrocautery.

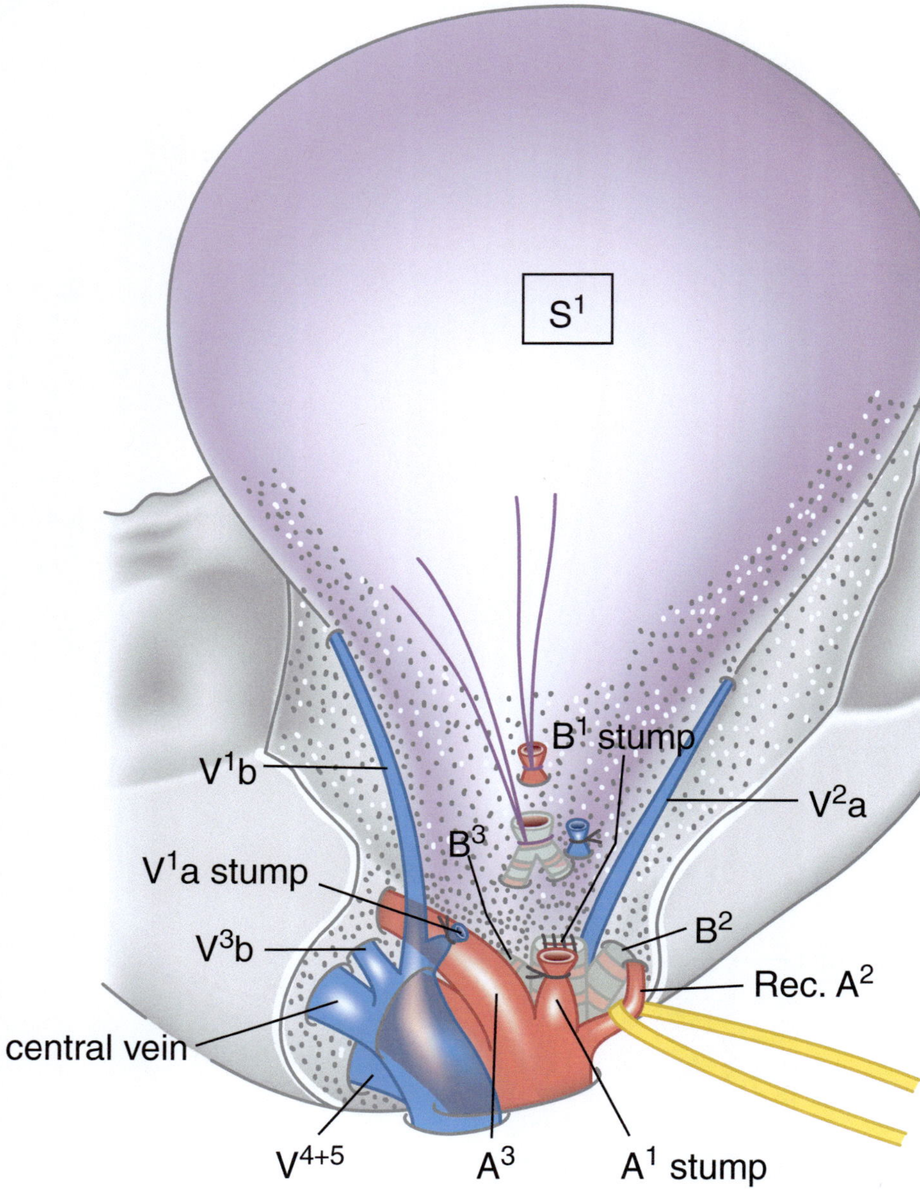

Fig. 3.1.6 At this point, V^2a is visible behind B^1, which runs between S^1 and S^2. Lung tissue is then cut along the V^1b and V^2a and also along the inflation–deflation line using electrocautery. In principle, V^1b and V^2a are preserved on the S^3 and S^2, respectively, to use for the guide of intersegmental plane and preserve venous flow, if the surgical margin is sufficient. The intersegmental plane is cut from various directions to facilitate simple and accurate intersegmental cutting.

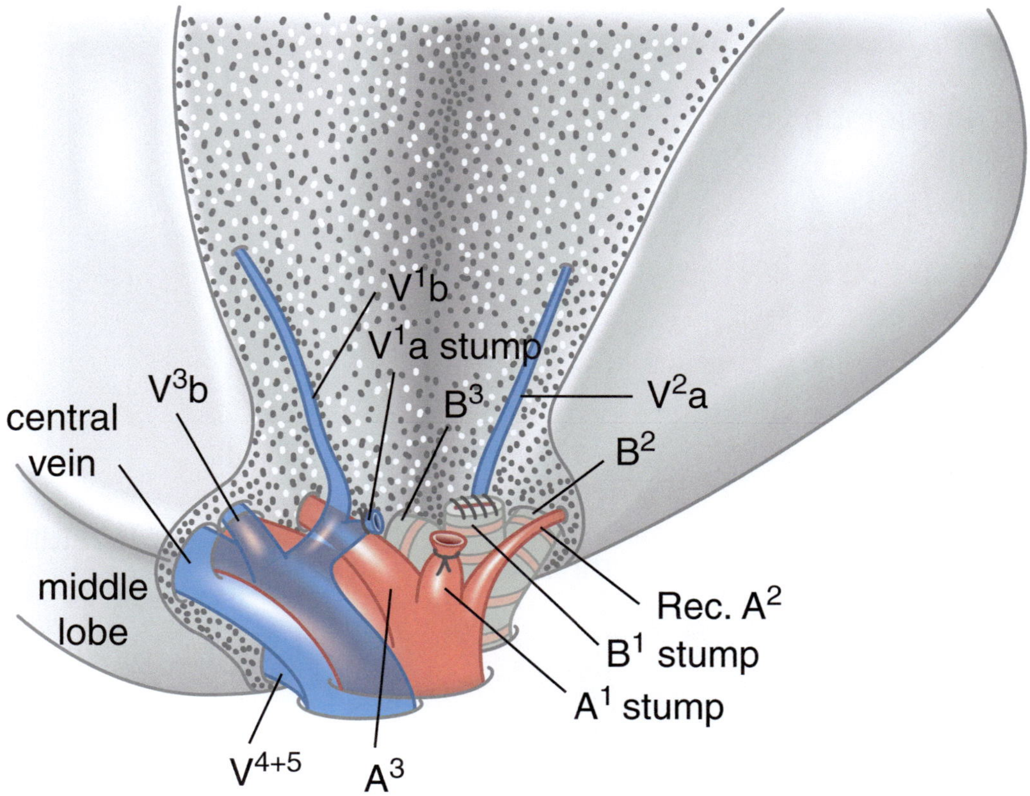

Fig. 3.1.7 V^1b and V^2a run on the segmental planes of S^3 and S^2, respectively.

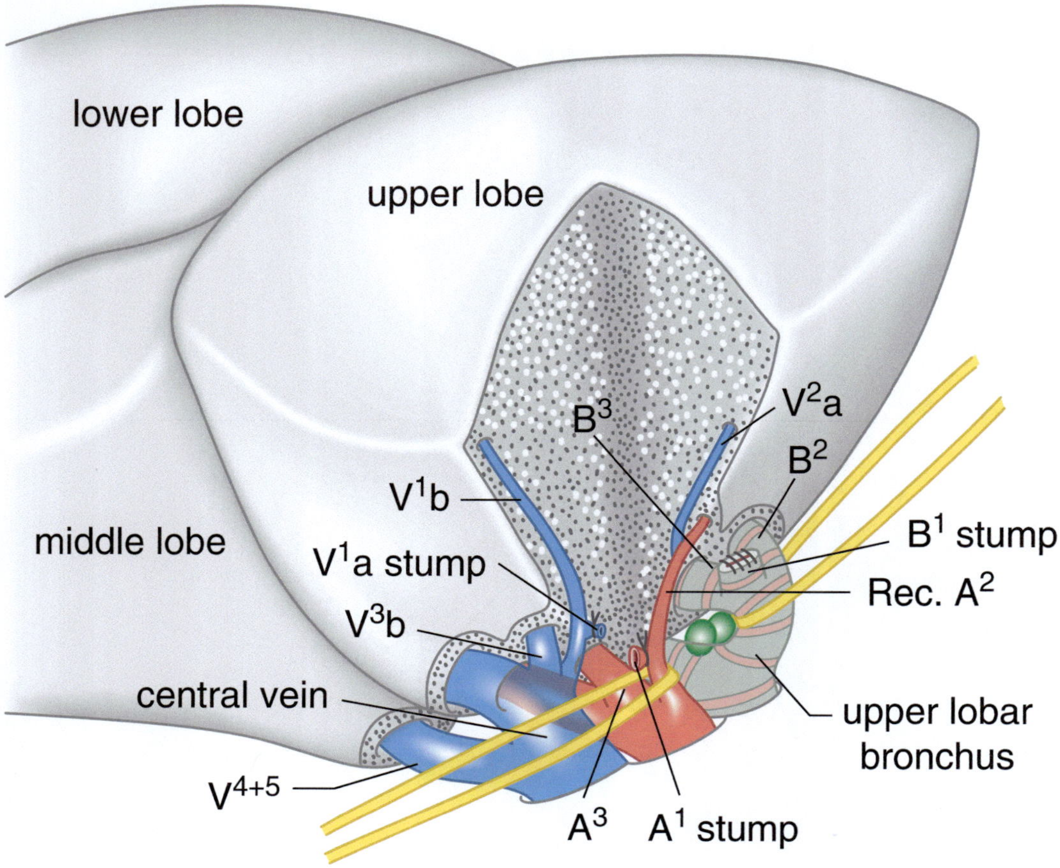

Fig. 3.1.8 The procedures of hilar lymph node dissection in S^1-segmentectomy differ from those in S^2- or S^3-segmentectomy. The #11s and #12u lymph nodes are hardly visible during S^1-segmentectomy, because the fissure between the right upper and lower lobes is not opened. The ascending A^2 is adjacent to the #11s lymph node. Therefore, damage to the ascending A^2 during dissection of the #11s lymph node should be carefully avoided. The following procedures would be useful for #11s and #12u dissection: the truncus superior artery and upper lobar bronchus are encircled with tape, the #11s lymph node is sufficiently peeled from the bronchus from the dorsal side. Finally #11s and #12u are taken away from the interspace between the truncus superior artery and upper lobar bronchus from the apical side.

3.2 Right S^2 Segmentectomy

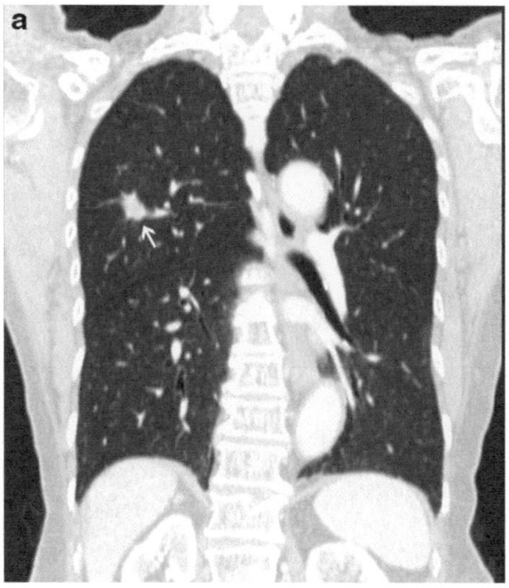

coronal view (CT scan)

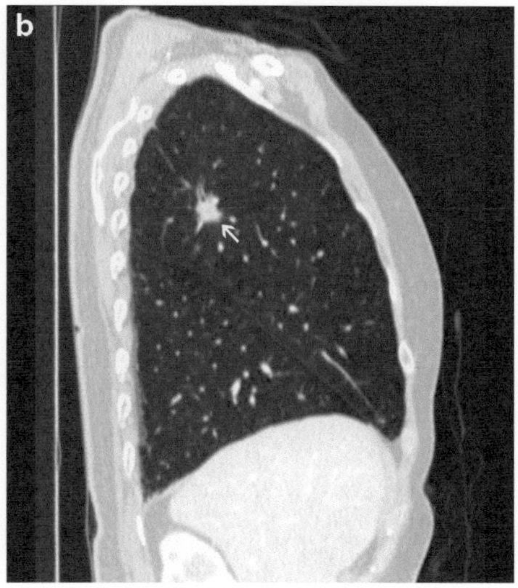

sagittal view (CT scan)

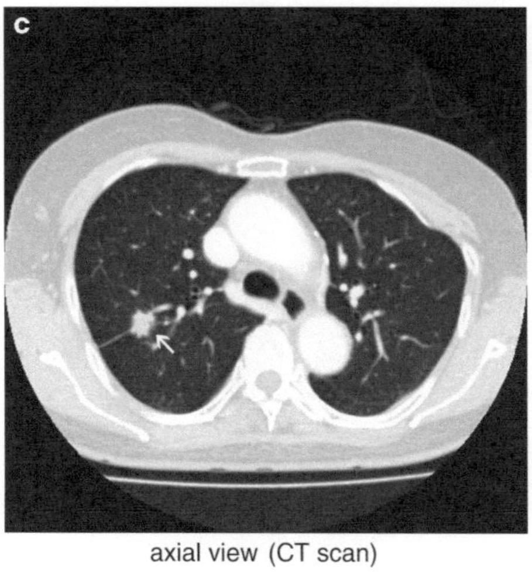

axial view (CT scan)

A GGO lesion at the right S^2 in an 81-year-old female that had been identified 3 years previously had increased and transformed to a solid type during follow-up. Computed tomography revealed a 1.5-cm solid nodule with spicular formation and pleural indentation at the right S^2b. Bronchoscopic biopsy diagnosed it as adenocarcinoma. Because the tumor was close to the V^2c (between S^2b and S^3a), S^2 segmentectomy was proceeded with cutting the V^2c and resecting a part of S^3a to obtain a sufficient surgical margin.

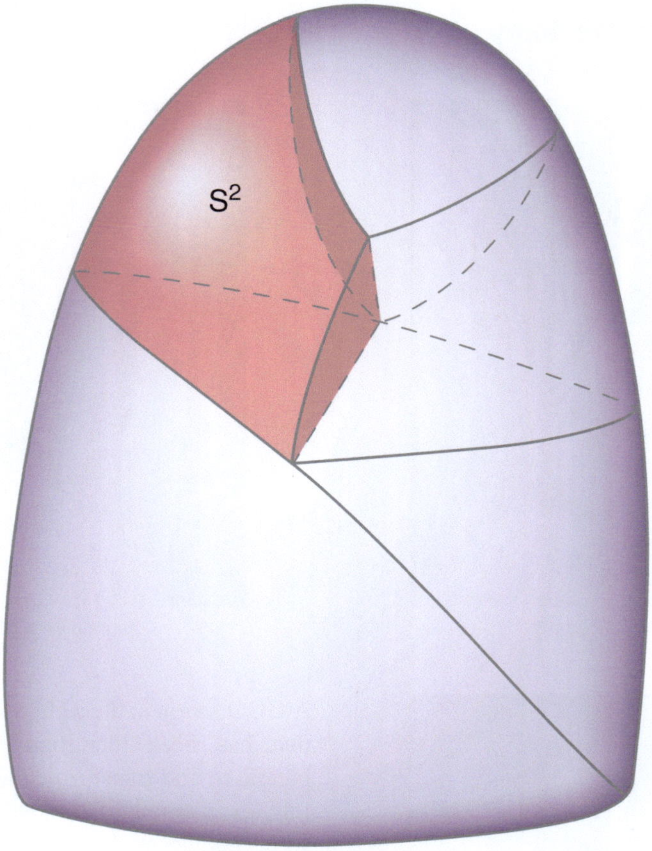

Fig. 3.2.1 The artery, vein, and bronchus branching profiles are confirmed from axial, coronal, and sagittal HRCT views. Branching pattern and size of B^1, B^2, and B^3 are further reconfirmed by bronchoscopy after tracheal intubation. The anatomical configuration of the segmental bronchus, artery in the figures of this session is the most frequent type as follows: the upper lobar bronchus branches into B^1, B^2, and B^3, the A^1 and A^3 branches from the truncus superior artery; the A^2a is a recurrent A^2 branching from the truncus superior artery; A^2b branches as an ascending A^2; and the segmental vein branches with apical and central profiles. The third intercostal space is generally an appropriate site for thoracotomy for S^2-segmentectomy.

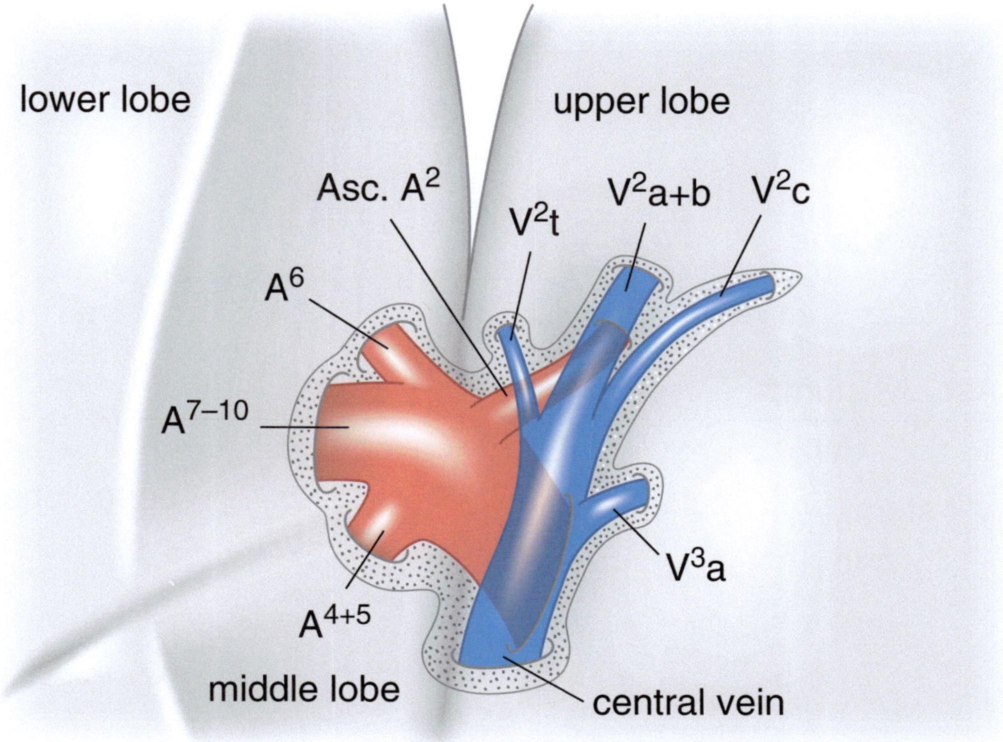

Fig. 3.2.2 The fissure between the right upper and lower lobes is divided using electrocautery but not a stapler, because a staple line would complicate identification of V^2 branches and of the intersegmental plane between the S^2 and S^3. The following procedure facilitates the fissure identification: a bronchoscope is inserted into B^2 followed by jet ventilation, which forms an inflation–deflation line between the inflated S^2 and the deflated lower lobe. The fissure can be divided along the inflation–deflation line using electrocautery. The central vein is exposed at the fissure.

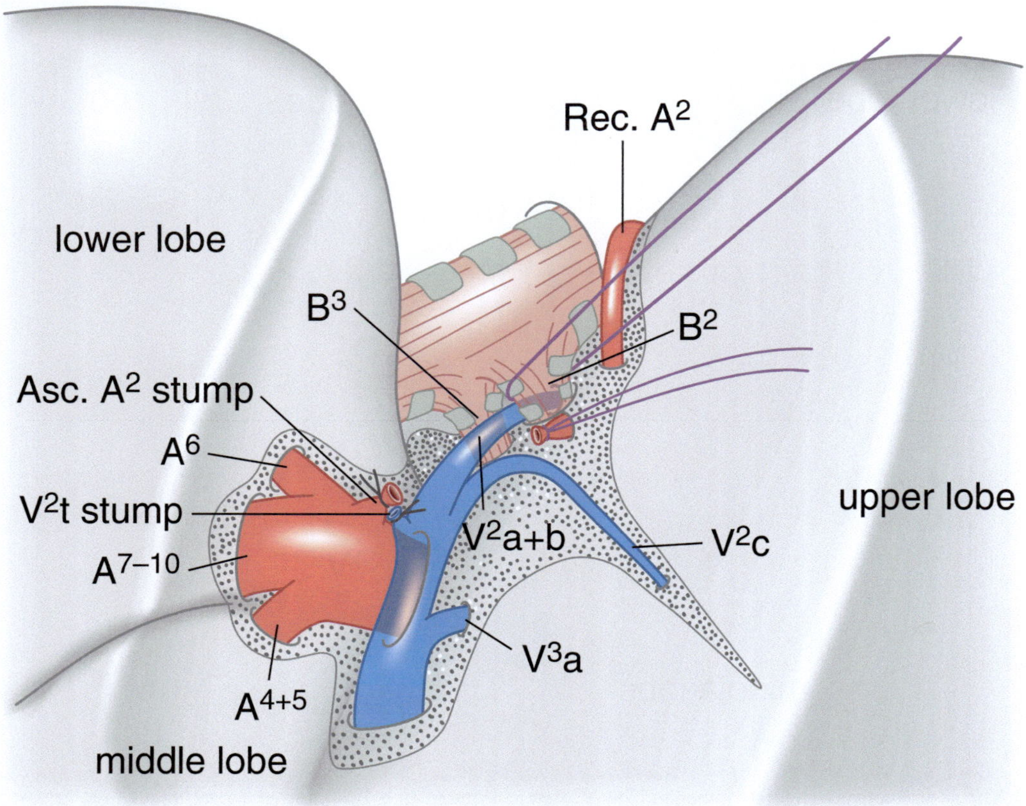

Fig. 3.2.3 V^2 is encircled with tape and exposed in the peripheral direction. V^2t running along the inferior border of the upper lobe is cut. V^2c, which runs between S^2 and S^3, is identified and exposed peripherally. V^2c generally runs alongside V^2a+b immediately after branching, where the former runs in the front and the latter runs behind in this operative field. Thereafter, V^2c runs towards the lateral side of the upper lobe near the lung surface. V^2c is exposed peripherally, which can clarify the border between S^2 and S^3. V^3a is occasionally mistaken for V^2c, which can be differentiated as follows: V^2c branches at the posterior side of the interlobar fissure and often runs alongside V^2a+b immediately after branching, whereas V^3a often branches vertically from the central vein at the center of the fissure. The ascending A^2 is exposed. Because an ascending A^2 and ascending A^3a sometimes form a common truncus, the ascending artery is exposed peripherally to confirm the presence or absence of the ascending A^3a which runs toward the ventral side of V^2c. The ascending A^3a is preserved.

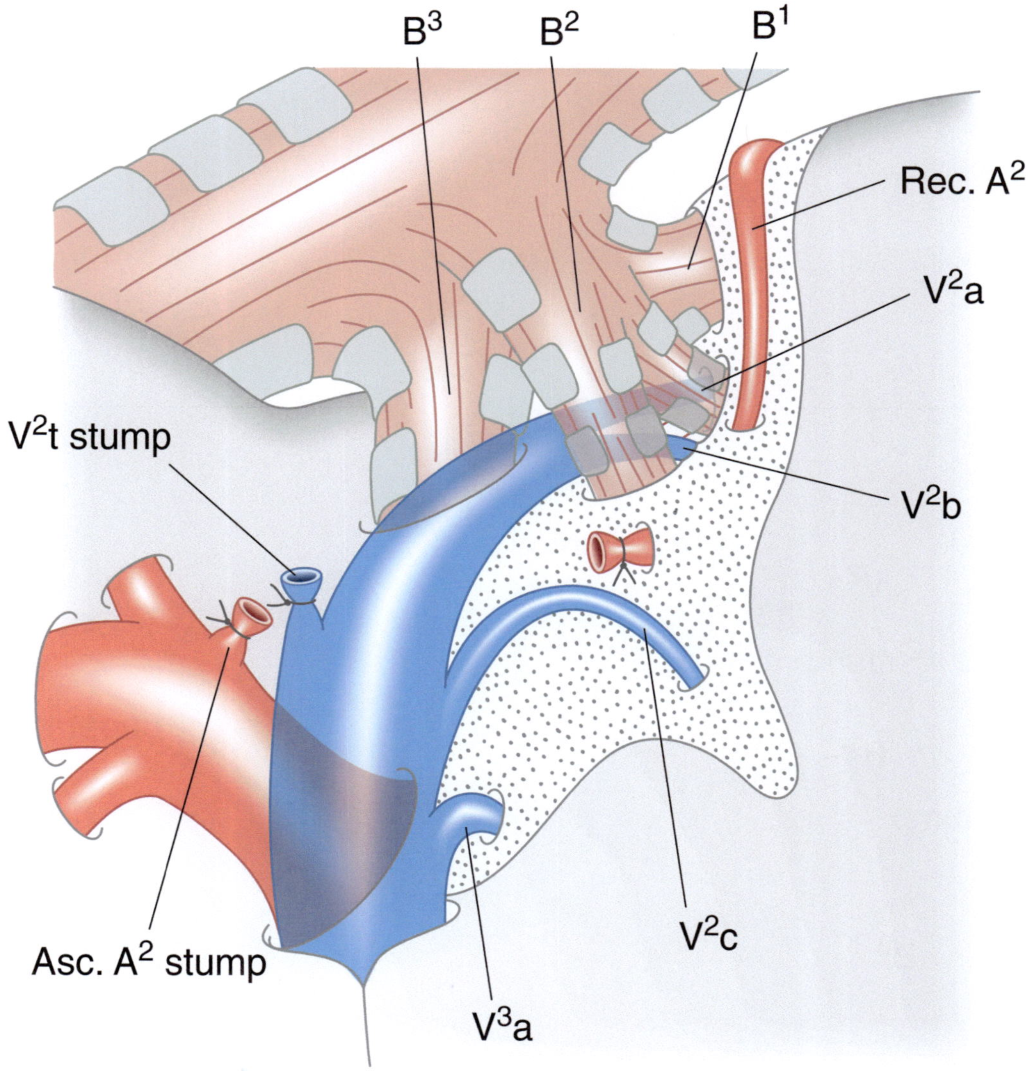

Fig. 3.2.4 B^2 is identified after cutting the ascending A^2. B^2 runs in front of V^2a+b in this surgical field, while B^3 runs behind V^2a+b, which enables the identification of B^2 and B^3. In addition, the right upper lobar bronchus is exposed peripherally from the apical side, which enables the identification of B^1 and B^2. The B^2 is encircled with thread. A recurrent A^2 and A^1a may be difficult to differentiate at this point, but this is unnecessary because it can be easily identified later after cutting B^2 or creating an inflation–deflation line. A recurrent A^2 runs towards the distal stump of B^2, whereas A^1-branch runs away from it. Illumination from a bronchoscope can help to reconfirm the identifying B^1, B^2, and B^3.

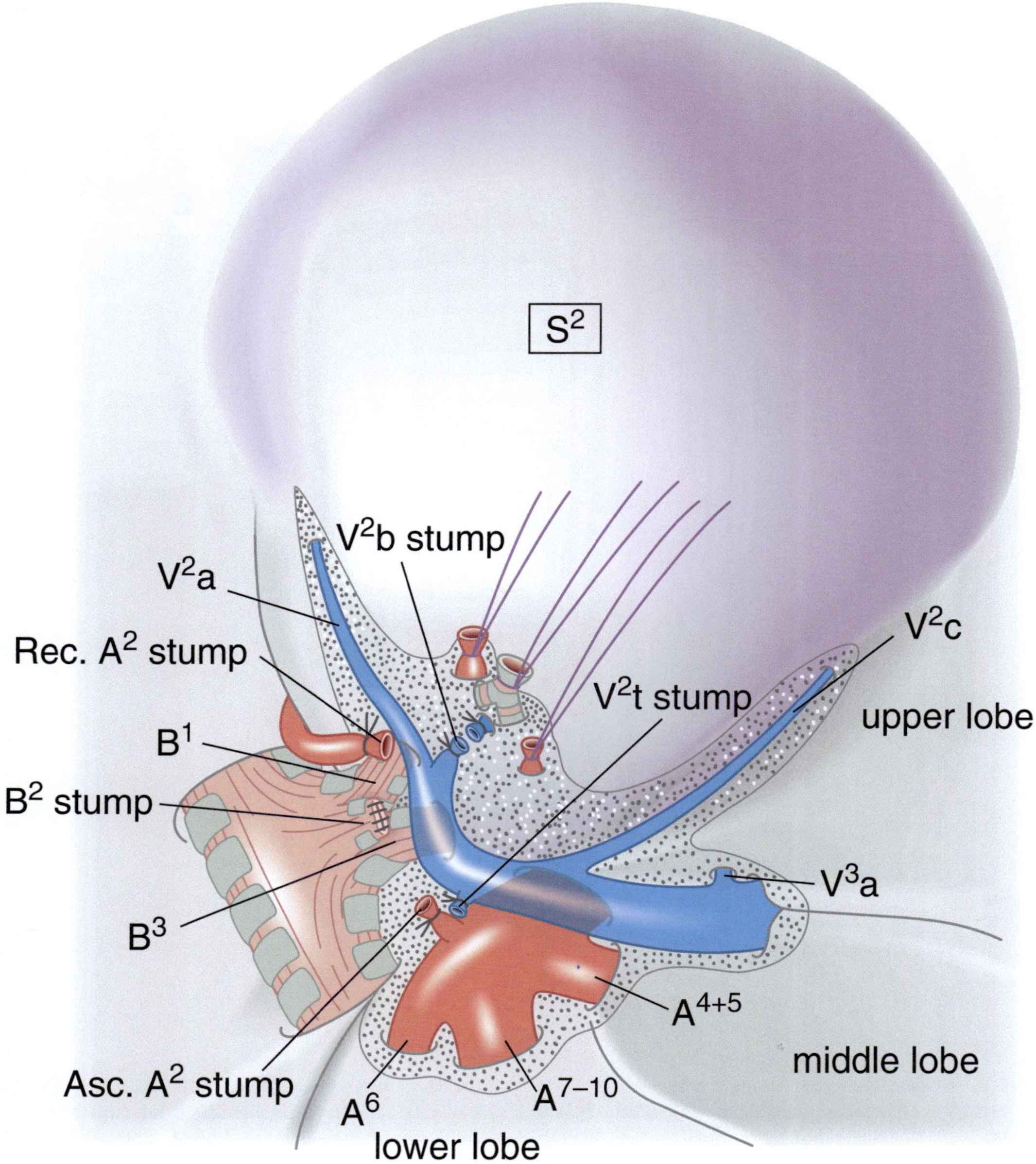

Fig. 3.2.5 The S^2 is selectively inflated by either inserting a bronchoscope into B^2 followed by jet ventilation, or by cutting the B^2 and inserting a catheter into the distal stump followed by air inflation. The distal stump is closed to trap air within S^2. The proximal stump of B^2 is closed with suture or ligation. B^2 can also be cut using a stapler when S^2 is inflated using jet ventilation via bronchoscope. The distal stump of B^2 is lifted, and the back is denuded peripherally to move the distal B^2 stump away from the hilum. A recurrent A^2 can be easily identified at this point, because it runs towards the distal B^2 stump, which is cut. V^2b running towards and behind the distal B^2 stump is cut, that further lifts the stump together with lung tissue on both sides. The lung tissue on both side of the distal stump of B^2 is then cut towards the inflation–deflation line using electrocautery. The V^2a (between S^1a and S^2a) and V^2c (between S^2b and S^3a) veins are important landmarks for accurately cutting the intersegmental plane. Lung tissue is cut along the inflated–deflated line using electrocautery and also along V^2a and V^2c, which are preserved on the S^1 and S^3 segments, if the surgical margin is sufficient. The intersegmental plane is cut from various directions to facilitate simple and accurate intersegmental cutting.

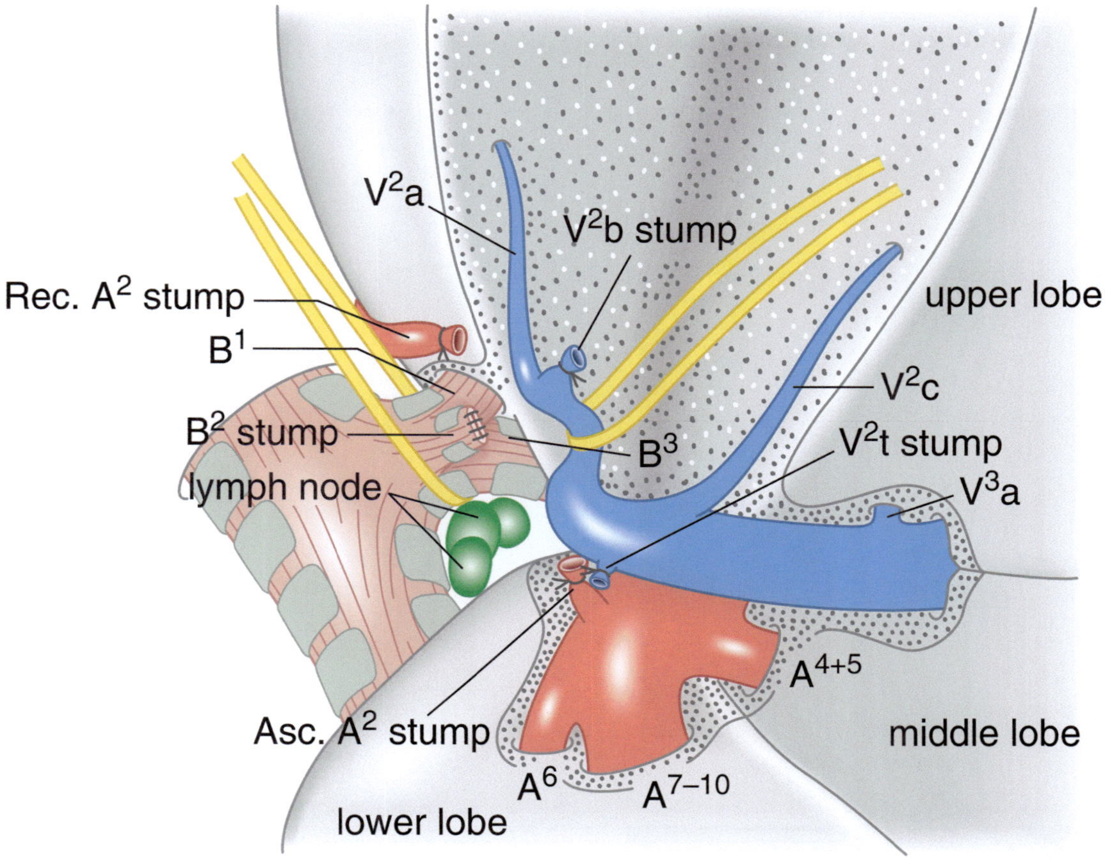

Fig. 3.2.6 V^2a and V^2c run on the segmental plane of S^1 and S^3, respectively. Hilar lymph node dissection during S^2-segmentectomy is relatively simple because the dorsal side of the hilum is already opened. The V^2, upper lobar bronchus, and truncus superior artery are encircled with tape, which exposes the #11s and #12 lymph nodes. These nodes are peeled from the upper lobar bronchus and intermediate bronchus at the dorsal site, but they had better not be taken out at this point. The #11s and #12 nodes are then passed through the interspace between upper lobar bronchus and truncus superior artery, and dissected from the apical side, which facilitates complete dissection of these nodes.

3.3 Right S^3 Segmentectomy

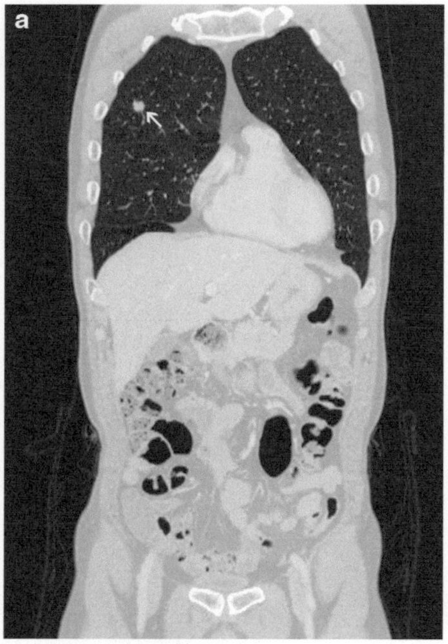

coronal view (CT scan)

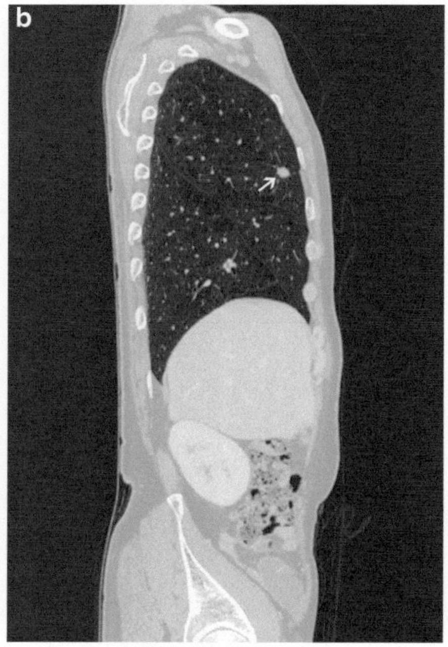

axial view (CT scan)

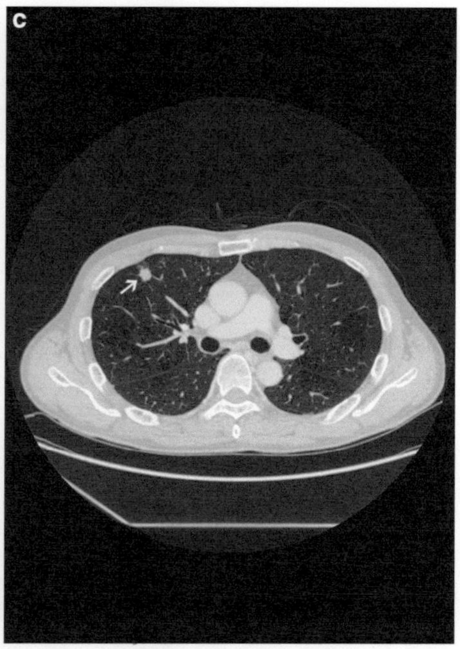

sagittal view (CT scan)

A routine chest X-ray of a 58-year-old male uncovered a nodule, which CT defined as a 1-cm nodule with spicular formation at S^3b. The nodule was diagnosed as adenocarcinoma from a CT-guided needle biopsy. S^3-segmentectomy was proceeded. The final pathological diagnosis was pT1aN0M0 papillary adenocarcinoma.

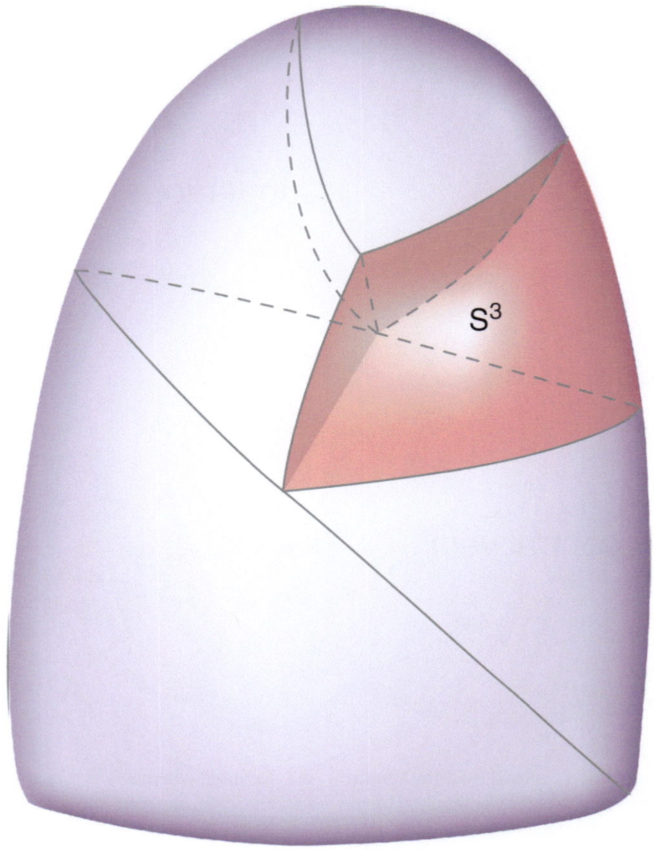

Fig. 3.3.1 The branching profile of segmental artery, vein, and bronchus is confirmed from axial, coronal, and sagittal HRCT views. Branching pattern and size of B^1, B^2, and B^3 are further reconfirmed using bronchoscope after tracheal intubation. The anatomical configuration of the segmental bronchus, vein, and artery in the figures of this session is the most frequent type as follows: the upper lobar bronchus branches into B^1, B^2, and B^3; the artery branches into A^1, A^3, and recurrent A^2a from the truncus superior artery; the A^2b branches as ascending A^2; and the segmental vein branches into apical and central veins. The optimal site of thoracotomy is generally the third intercostal space.

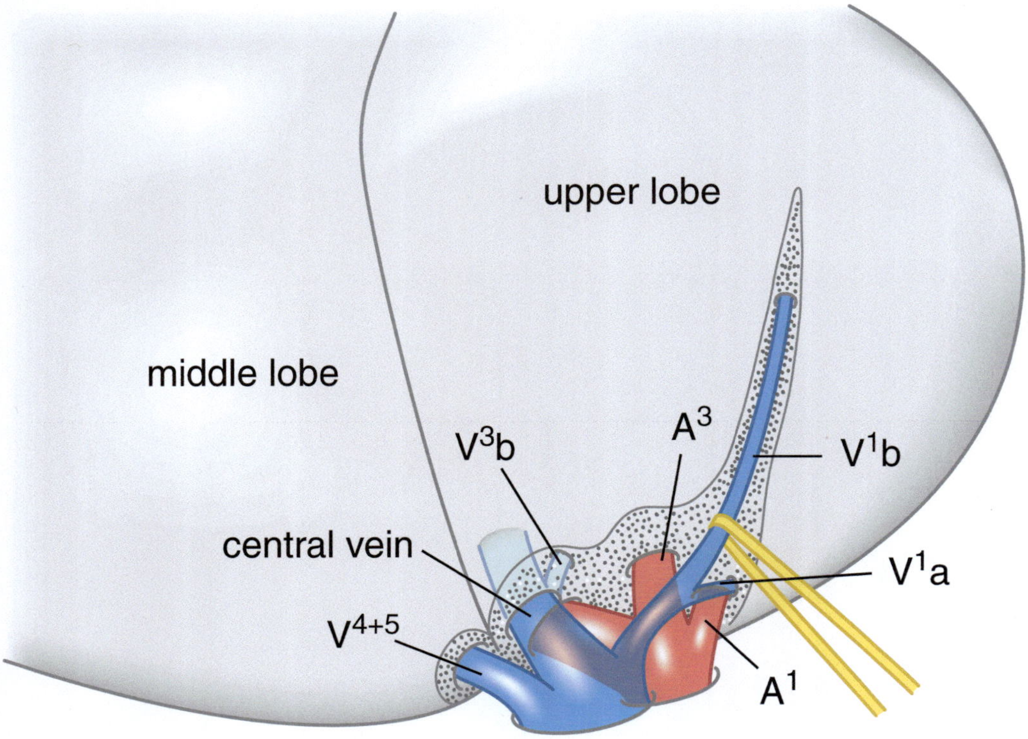

Fig. 3.3.2 The hilum of the upper lobe is exposed from the ventral to the dorsal side to reveal the superior pulmonary vein, the truncus superior artery, the upper lobar bronchus, the bifurcation between upper lobar bronchus and the truncus intermedius bronchus. The dorsal site of the upper lobar bronchus is exposed to the peripheral side, enabling simple identification of B^1, B^2, and B^3 later. The V^1 is encircled with tape and exposed peripherally to identify V^1a and V^1b. The V^1b is the intersegmental vein between S^1 and S^3, running near the surface of the lung and towards the lung apex. The V^1b is exposed peripherally. While V^3c (between S^3bi and S^3bii) sometimes branches at proximal site of V^1 and runs like V^1b, they can be differentiated because V^3c runs along the ventral side and deeply into the lung, whereas V^1b runs towards the apex and near the lung surface. Identifying the V^1b makes it possible to identify the A^1 and A^3, i.e. the former runs dorsal and the latter runs ventral to V^1b. However, this position relation is not usually correct depending on the direction of the lung traction, i.e. A^1 sometimes seems to run ventral to the V^1b and A^3 sometimes seems to run dorsal to it. Therefore, it should be taken care to identify the A^1 and A^3, even after identifying the V^1b. To identify them accurately, indistinguishable posterior arterial branch of A^3 is preserved, which might be A^1-branch. After cutting B^3, the A^1 - and A^3-branches can be easily discriminated, because A^3-branch runs towards the distal stump of B^3, whereas A^1-branch runs away from it.

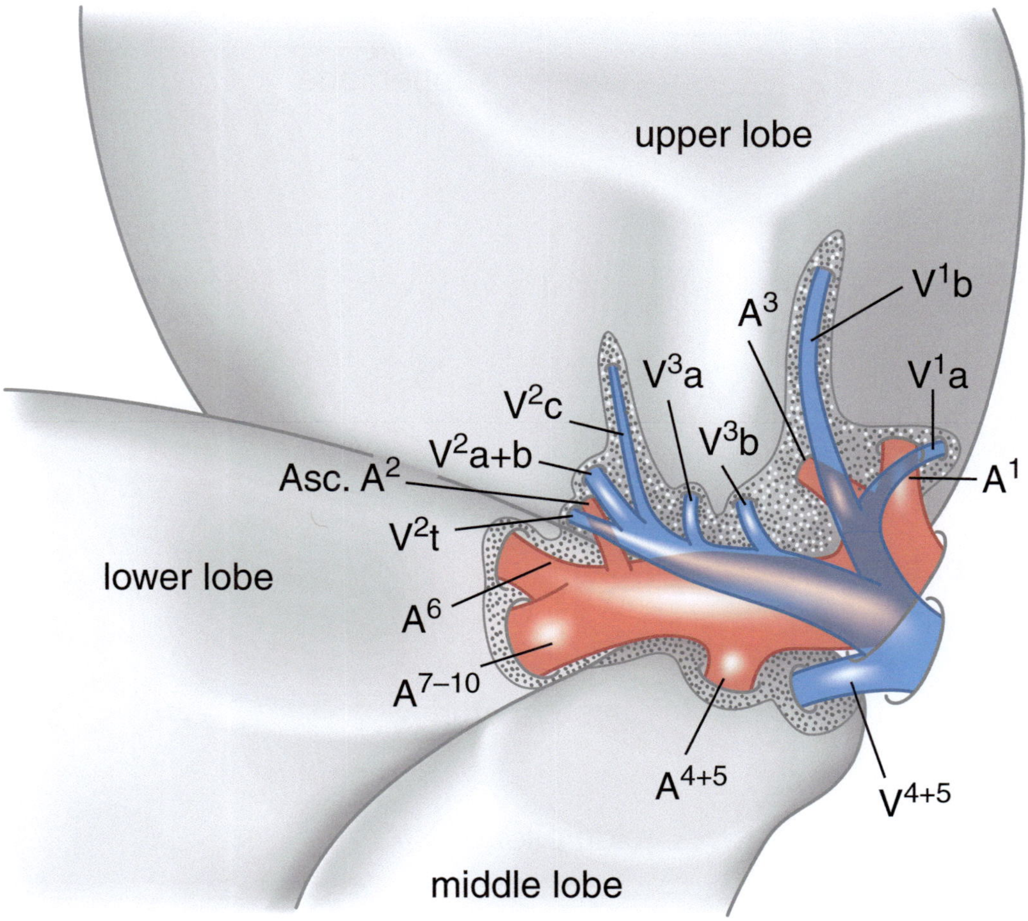

Fig. 3.3.3 The fissure between the right upper and middle lobes that is frequently fused is divided during S^3-segmentectomy by using electrocautery. A stapler should not be used for this because a staple line would complicate identifying the intersegmental plane between S^2 and S^3. One way to identify a largely fused fissure is to insert a bronchoscope into B^3 and then apply jet ventilation, which creates an inflation–deflation line between the inflated S^3 and deflated middle lobe. The fissure can be easily divided along the inflation–deflation line using electrocautery. The central vein is visualized after dividing the fissure and exposed to peripheral direction, which in turn reveals V^3b, V^3a, and V^2c. Sometimes, V^3a and V^2c are difficult to be distinguished each other, which can be differentiated by the followings: (1) while the V^2c often branches at the dorsal side of the interlobar fissure, V^3a branches at the central portion of it; and (2) V^2c runs side by side with V^2a+b immediately after its branching; and (3) V^3a often branches vertically from the central vein. V^2c is encircled with tape and exposed peripherally to define the intersegmental plane between S^2 and S^3. After these vessel branches are identified, A^3, V^3a, V^3b, and V^3c are cut.

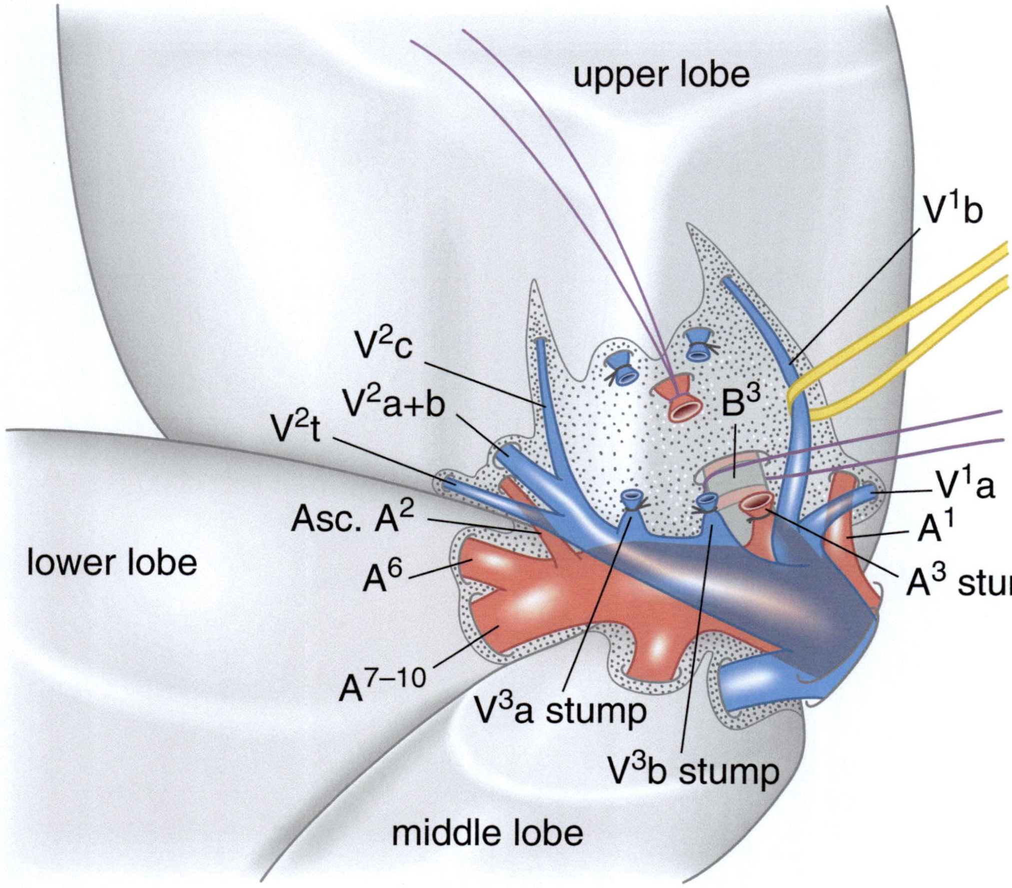

Fig. 3.3.4 After cutting A^3, a few lymph nodes in front of B^3 are dissected to disclose B^3, which is then encircled with thread. B^3a and B^3b sometimes branch near the root of B^3, which renders B^3a difficult to be exposed from the ventral side. In this situation, B^3a is exposed by pulling the thread on B^3b, followed by additionally encircling the root of B^3 by thread. The identification of B^3 can be confirmed by illumination from a bronchoscope inserted into the bronchus.

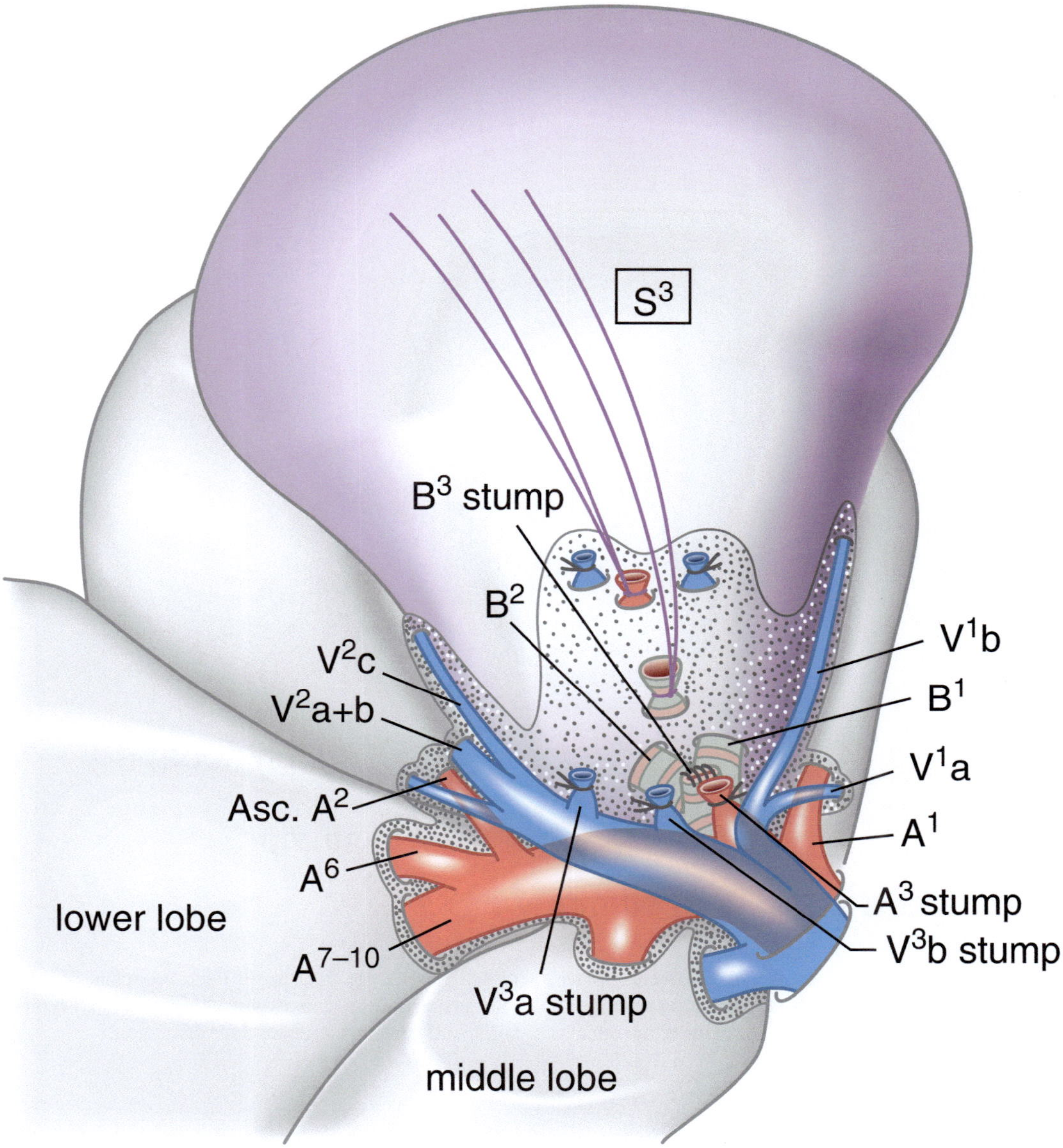

Fig. 3.3.5 The S^3 can then be selectively inflated by either inserting a bronchoscope into B^3 followed by jet ventilation into B^3, or by cutting the B^3 and inserting a catheter into the peripheral stump followed by air inflation. The distal stump is closed to trap air within S^3. The proximal stump of B^3 is then closed by suture or ligation. When S^3 is inflated by jet ventilation via bronchoscope, B^3 can also be cut using a stapler. The distal stump of B^3 is lifted and the back of it is peripherally denuded to move the stump away from the hilum. Lifting the stump also elevates lung tissues on both sides of it, which are cut towards the inflation–deflation line using electrocautery. Lung tissue is cut also along the V^1b and V^2c, which are preserved on the S^1 and S^2 segments, if the surgical margin is sufficient. The intersegmental plane is cut from various directions, which can facilitate simple and accurate intersegmental cutting.

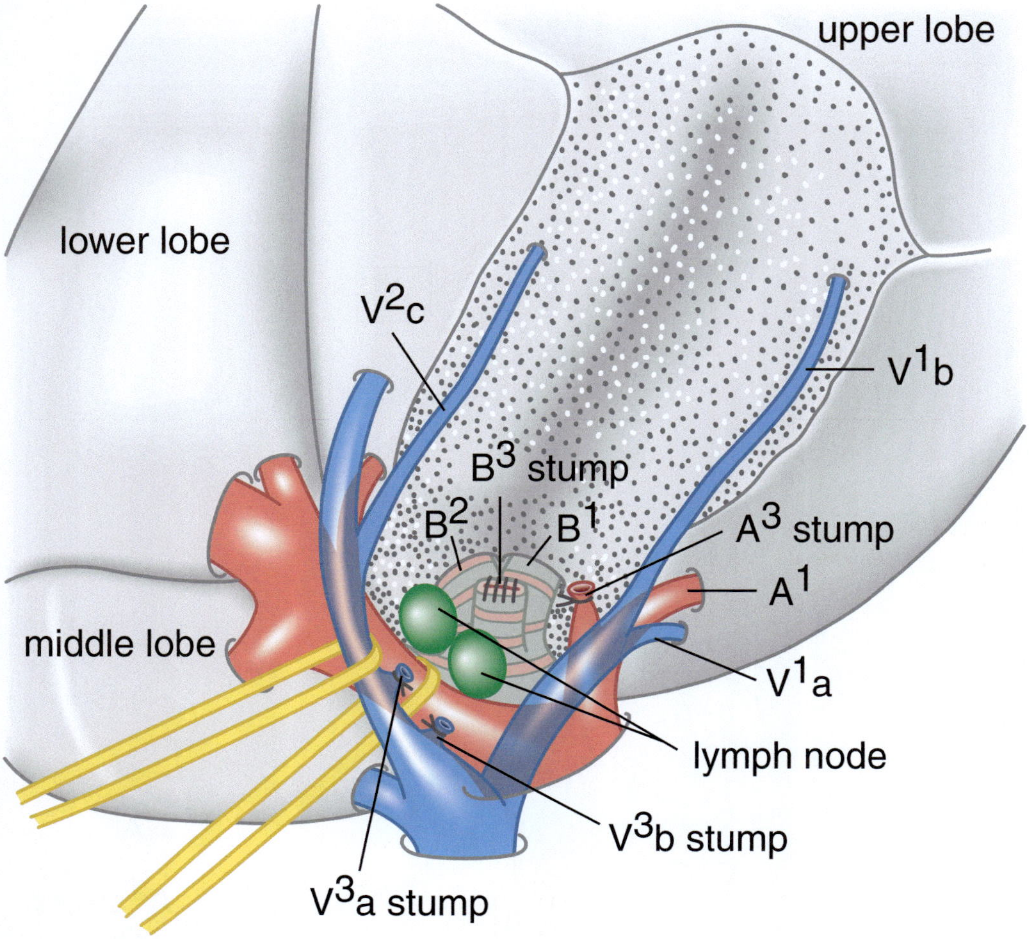

Fig. 3.3.6 V^1b and V^2c run along the intersegmental plane. Hilar lymph node dissection in the S^3-segmentectomy proceeds from the ventral side because the dorsal side of the hilum remains closed. Taping the right upper lobar bronchus, V^2, and trunks intermedius artery can expose #11s and #12 lymph nodes sufficiently, which facilitates their dissection.

3.4 Right $S^2 + S^1a$ Segmentectomy

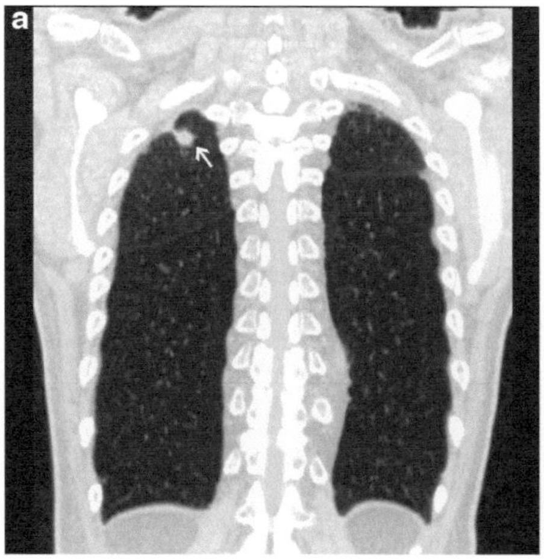

coronal view (CT scan)

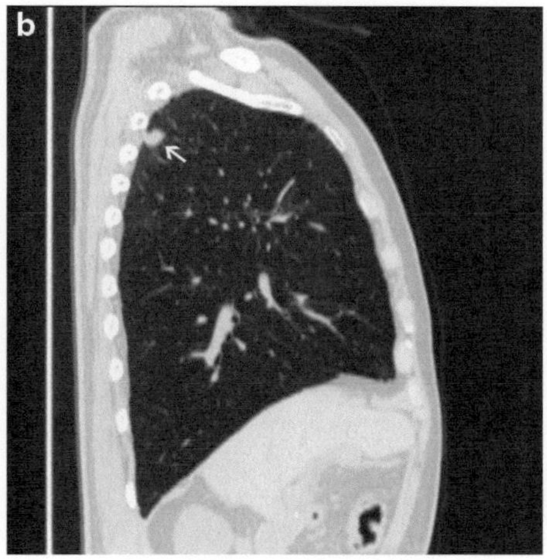

sagittal view (CT scan)

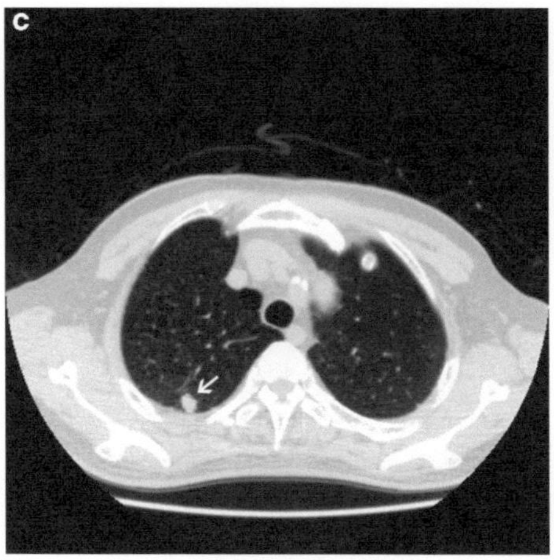

axial view (CT scan)

Chest X-ray of annual medical examination of a 61-year-old female uncovered a nodule in the right upper lobe. CT defined a 2-cm nodule with spicular formation and pleural indentation located between S^1a and S^2a. The nodule was diagnosed as adenocarcinoma from a bronchoscopic biopsy specimen. S^2+S^1a-segmentectomy was undertaken. The final pathological diagnosis was pT1aN0M0 papillary adenocarcinoma.

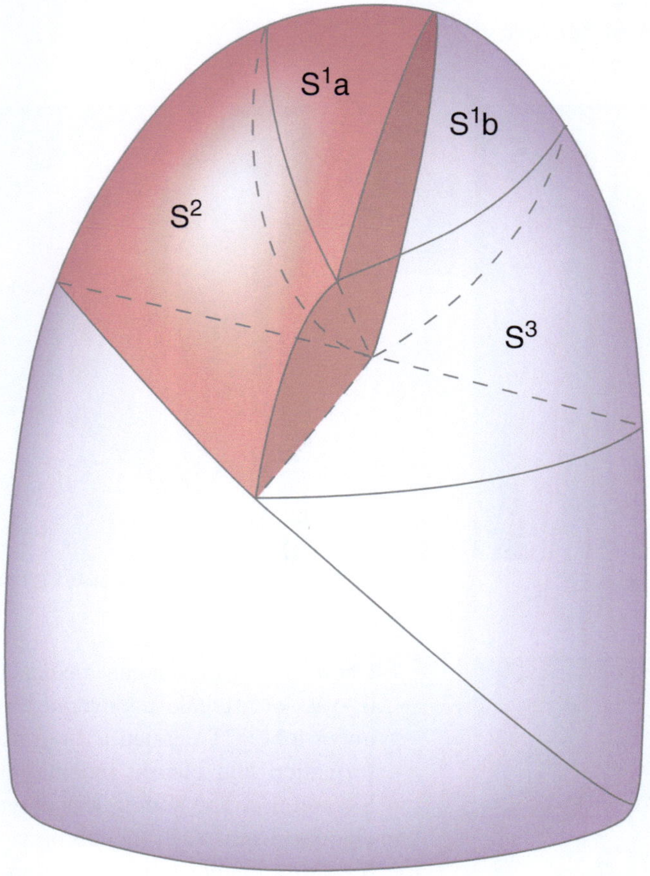

Fig. 3.4.1 The branching profile of segmental artery, vein, and bronchus branching is confirmed from axial, coronal, and sagittal HRCT views. The B^1, B^2, and B^3 branching and sizes are reconfirmed using bronchoscope after tracheal intubation. The anatomical configuration of the segmental bronchus, artery and vein in the figures of this session is the most frequent type as follows: the bronchus branches into B^1, B^2, and B^3; the artery branches into A^1, A^3 and a recurrent A^2a from the truncus superior artery; the A^2b branches as an ascending A^2; and the vein branches into apical and central veins. The optimal site for thoracotomy is generally the third intercostal space.

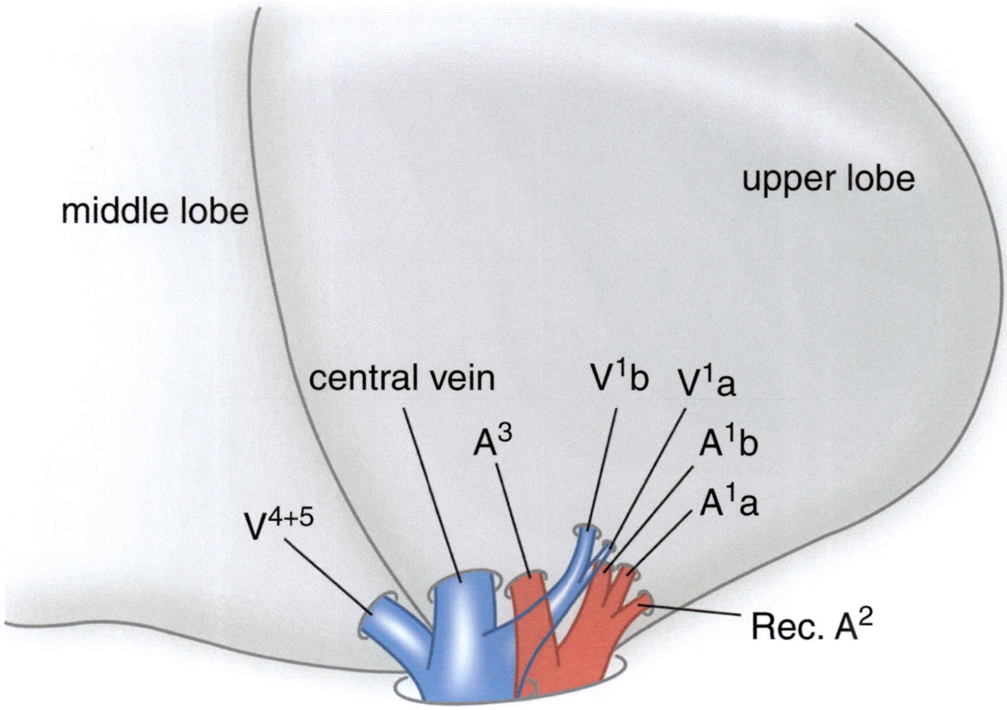

Fig. 3.4.2 The hilum of the right upper lobe is exposed from the ventral to the dorsal side to expose the superior pulmonary vein, truncus superior artery, upper lobar bronchus, and the bifurcation between the upper lobar bronchus and truncus intermedius bronchus.

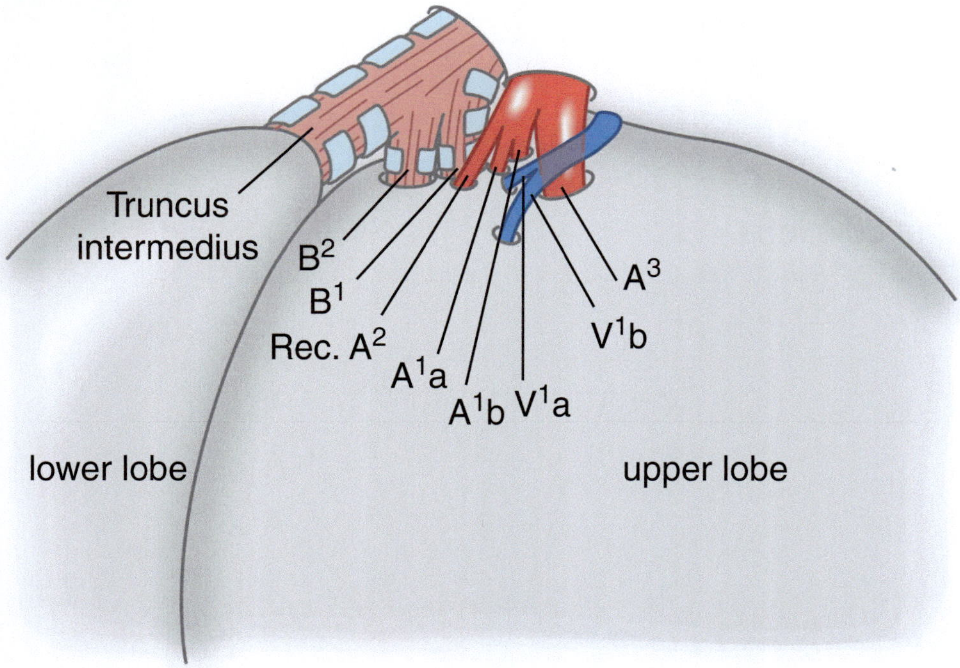

Fig. 3.4.3 The dorsal site of the upper lobar bronchus is exposed peripherally to reveal the bifurcation of B^1 and B^2, which facilitates the identification of a recurrent A^2 later. The V^1 is exposed peripherally, and then V^1a and V^1b are identified. The V^1a is the intersegmental vein between S^1a and S^1b that runs dorsally and is usually thinner than V^1b. The V^1b is the intersegmental vein between S^1 and S^3, running near the surface of the lung and towards the lung apex. A^1 is exposed peripherally to reveal A^1a and A^1b.

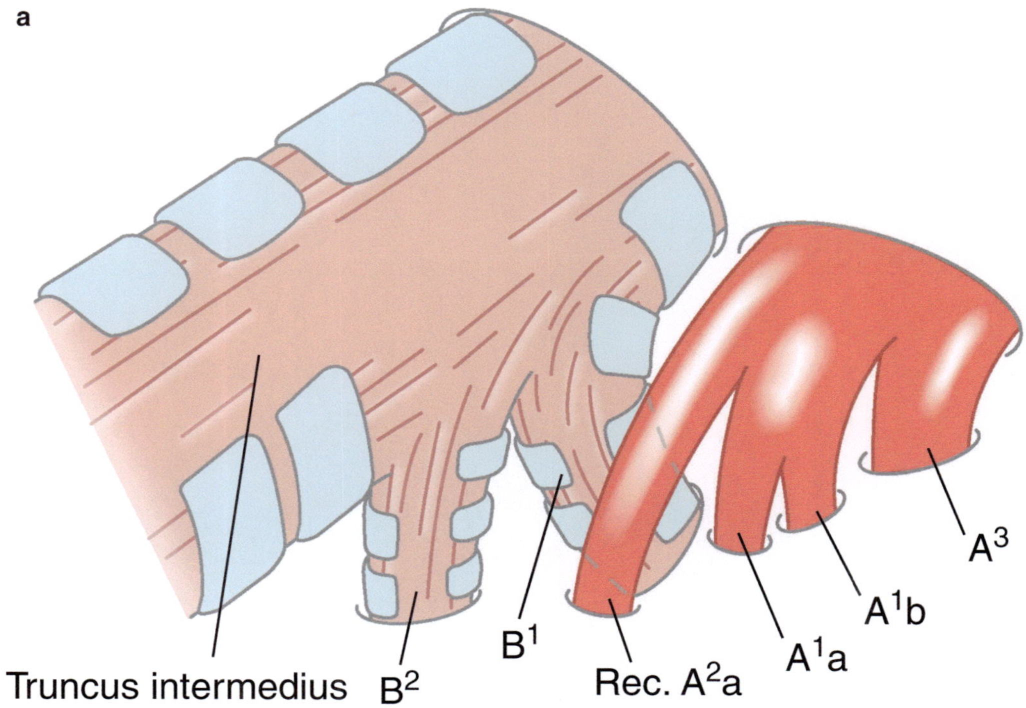

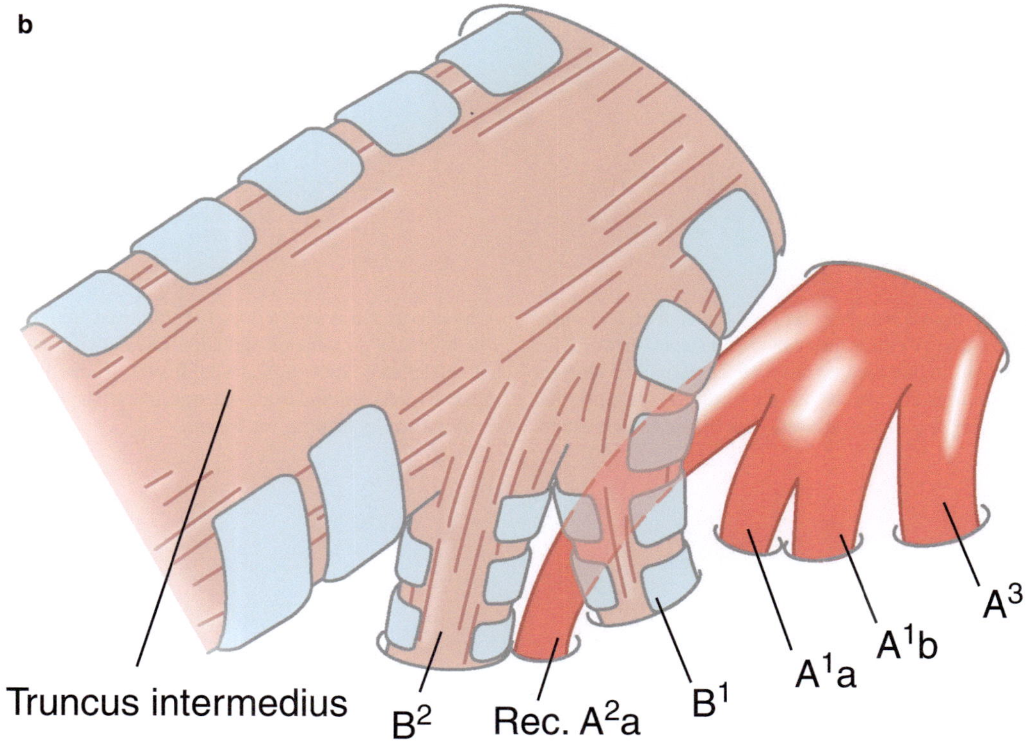

Fig. 3.4.4 There are two patterns of the recurrent A^2-route as follows: one is that a recurrent A^2 runs at the dorsal side of B^1 and then along B^2 (**a**) and another is that it runs at the ventral side of B^1 and then along B^2 (**b**). The former is more frequent than the latter and is thus presented herein.

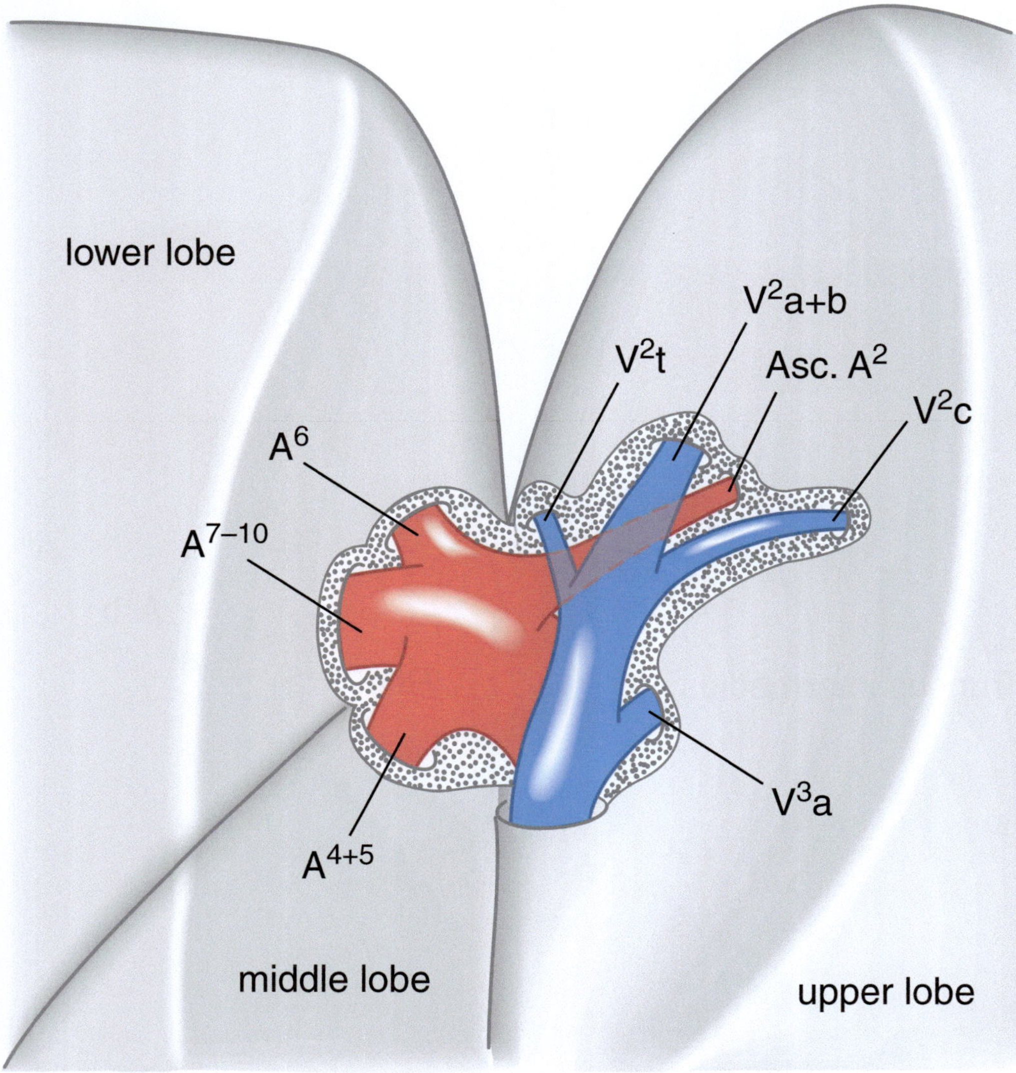

Fig. 3.4.5 The fissure between the right upper lobe and lower lobe is divided using electrocautery but not a stapler, because the staple line would impair identification of the peripheral route of V^2 and also complicate identifying the border between S^2 and S^3. The following technique facilitates the fissure-identification. A bronchoscope is inserted into B^2 followed by jet ventilation, which creates an inflation–deflation line between an inflated S^2 and a deflated lower lobe. The fissure is divided along the inflation–deflation line using electrocautery. The central vein can be visualized by dividing the fissure.

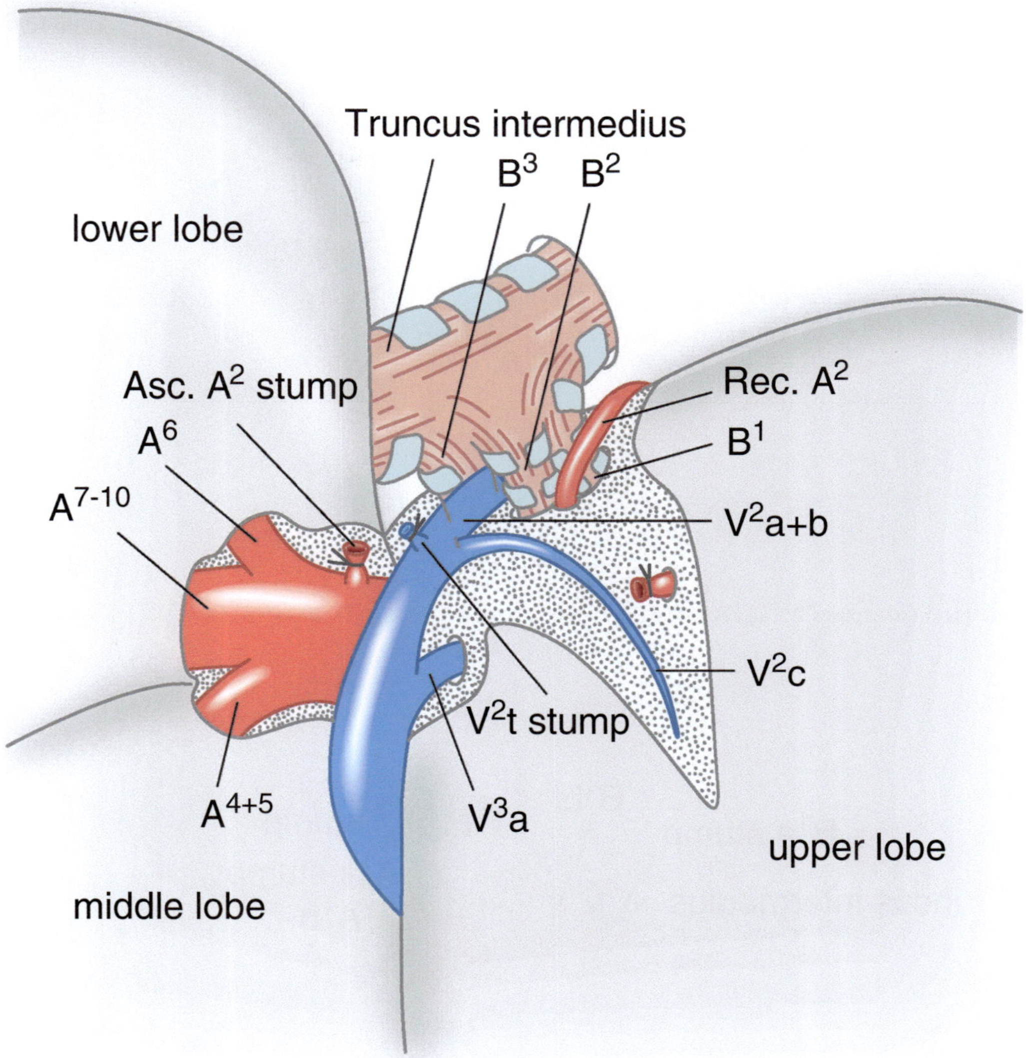

Fig. 3.4.6 V^2 is exposed and encircled with tape. V^2t runs to the dorsal direction at the fissure, which is cut. V^2c is identified and exposed peripherally. V^2c often runs alongside V^2a+b immediately after branching, where the former runs in the front and the latter runs behind in this operative view. Thereafter, V^2c runs towards the lateral side of the upper lobe near the lung surface. V^2c is exposed peripherally to clarify the border between S^2 and S^3. The ascending A^2 is identified. Because the ascending A^2 and ascending A^3a occasionally form a common truncus, the ascending artery is exposed peripherally to confirm the presence or absence of an ascending A^3a running towards the ventral side of V^2c. A confirmed ascending A^3a is preserved. The artery dorsal to the V^2c is cut because it must be the ascending A^2. After cutting the ascending A^2, B^2 is identified. B^2 runs in front, while B^3 runs behind V^2a+b in this operative view, which enables their discrimination. The upper lobar bronchus is exposed peripherally from the apical side, which enables the identification of B^1 and B^2. The B^2 is encircled with thread. Illumination from a bronchoscope can also help to reconfirm the identification of B^1, B^2, and B^3.

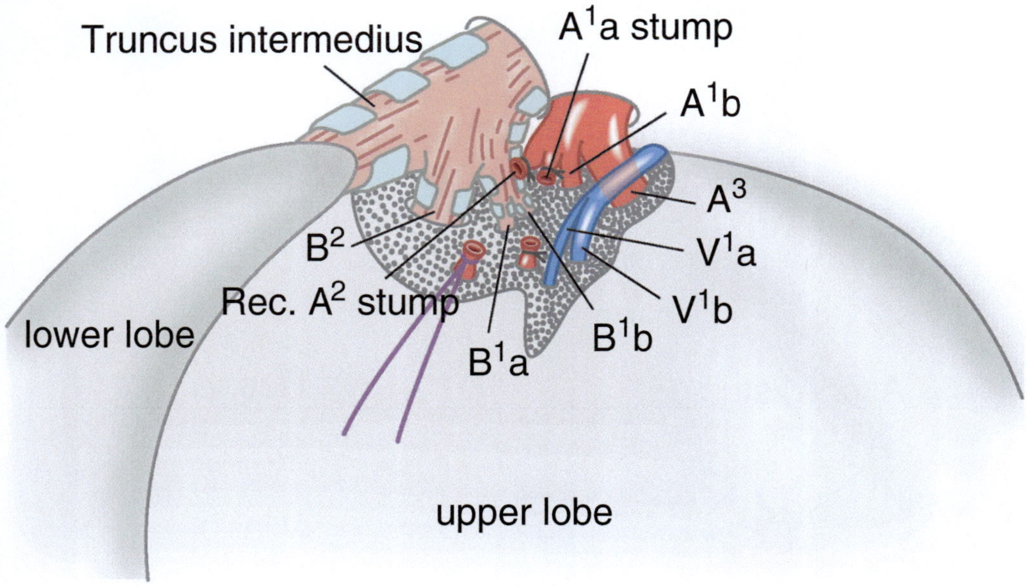

Fig. 3.4.7 A^1a is cut to exposes B^1a and B^1b. The B^1a is encircled with thread.

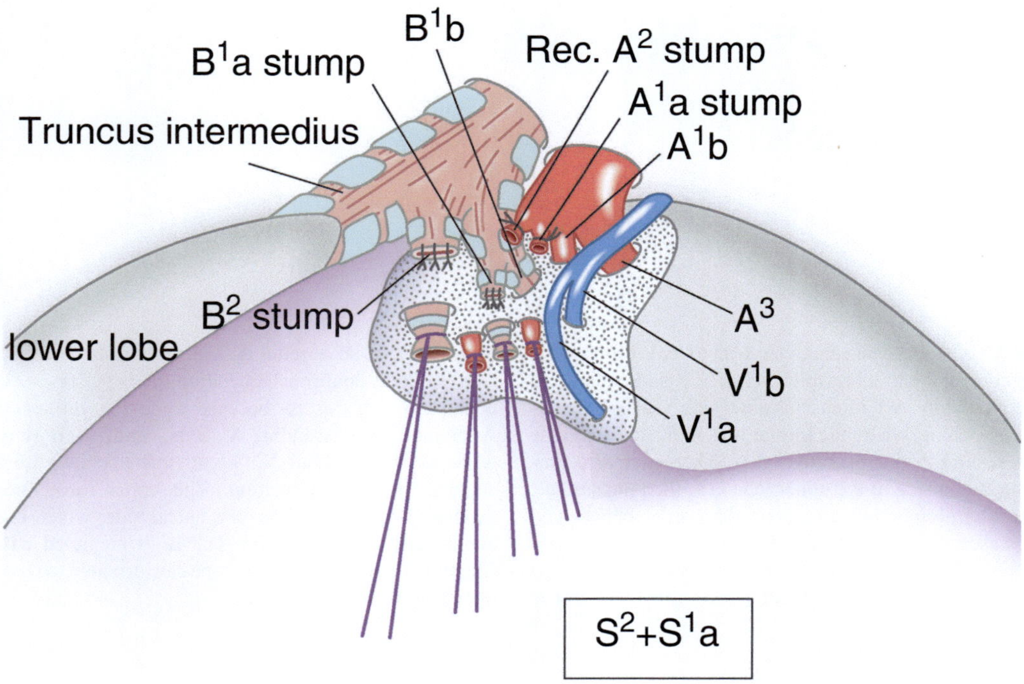

Fig. 3.4.8 S^2 and S^1a can be selectively inflated either by inserting a bronchoscope into B^2 and B^1a followed by jet ventilation, or by cutting the B^2 and B^1a and inserting a catheter into the distal stumps followed by air inflation. The distal stumps are closed to trap air within S^2 and S^1a. The proximal stumps of B^2 and B^1a are closed with suture or ligation.

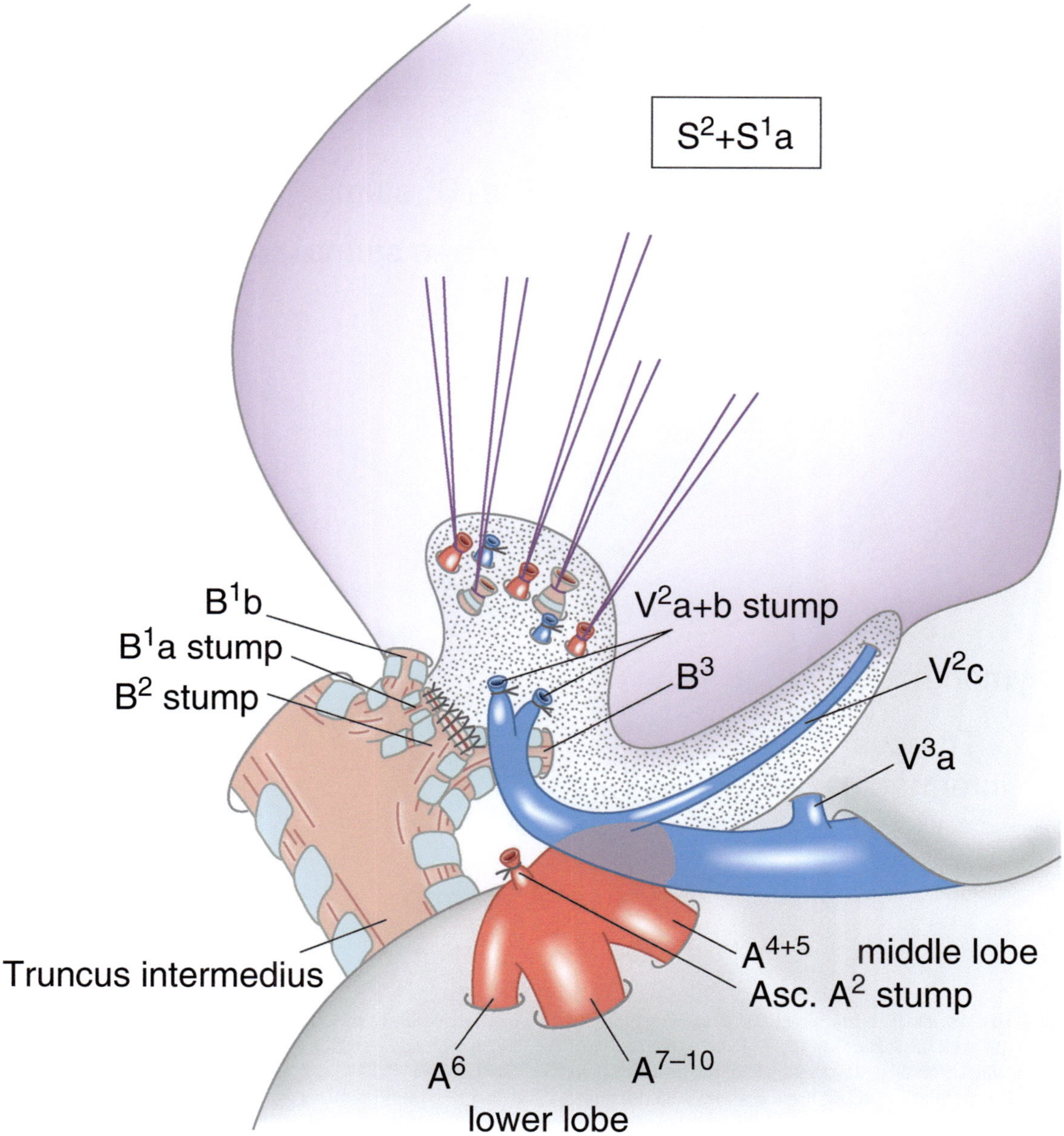

Fig. 3.4.9 The distal stumps of B^2 and B^1a are lifted, and their back side is peripherally denuded, which moves the distal B^2 and B^1a stumps away from the hilum. While V^2a+b can in principle be cut at its root, the complete central vein type has a V^1-branch along the route of the central vein, which should be taken into consideration. If so, then cutting only the vein-branches that run towards the S^2 and S^1a would be secure. Cutting the V^2a and V^2b further elevates the distal B^2 and B^1a stumps and also lifts the lung tissue on both sides of the stumps. The lung tissue on both sides of the stumps is then cut towards the inflation–deflation line using electrocautery and also along V^1a and V^2c while preserving them, if the surgical margin is sufficient. The intersegmental plane is cut from various directions to facilitate simple and accurate intersegmental cutting.

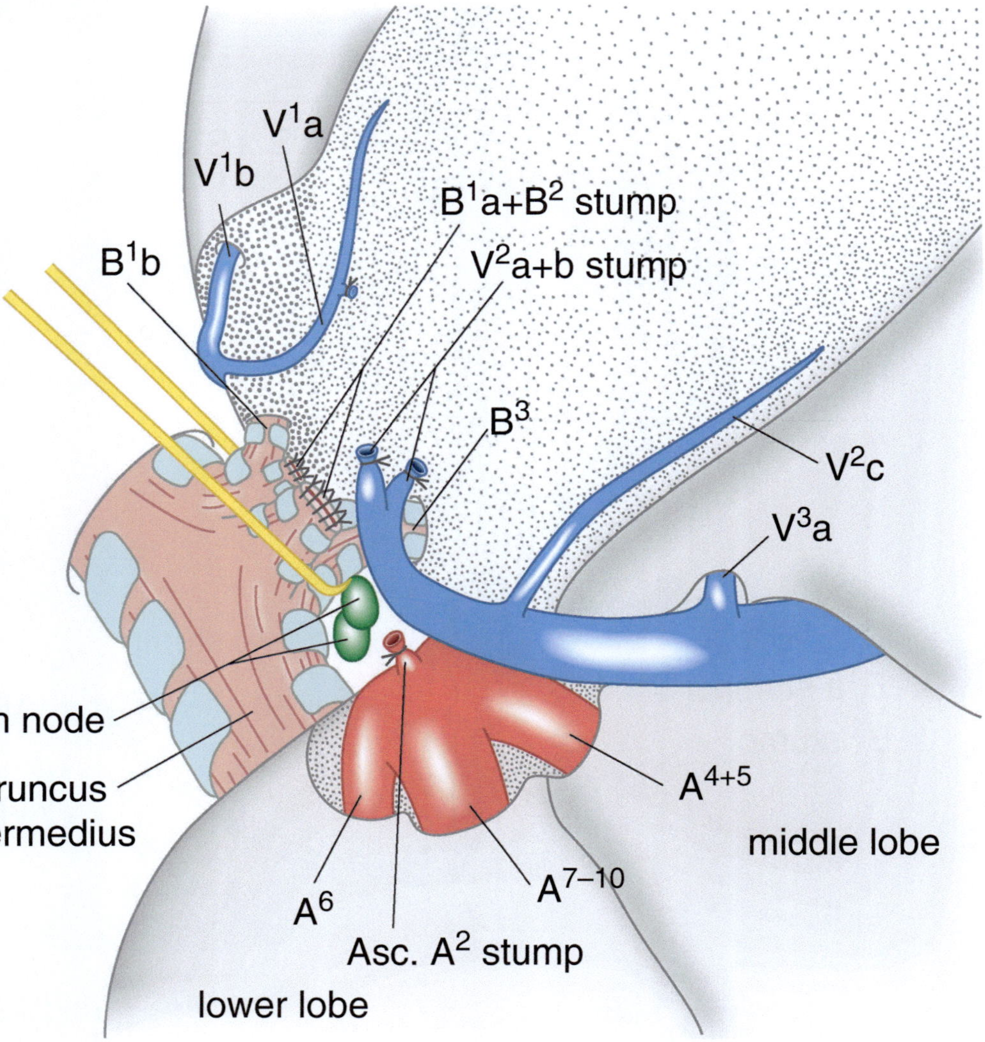

Fig. 3.4.10 V^1a and V^2c run along the intersegmental plane. Hilar lymph node dissection during S^2+S^1a-segmentectomy is relatively simple, because the dorsal site of the hilum is already opened. The right upper lobar bronchus and superior truncus pulmonary artery are encircled with tape to expose the #11s and #12 lymph nodes, which are dissected from both the caudal and cranial sides.

3.5 Right S³a + S²b Segmentectomy

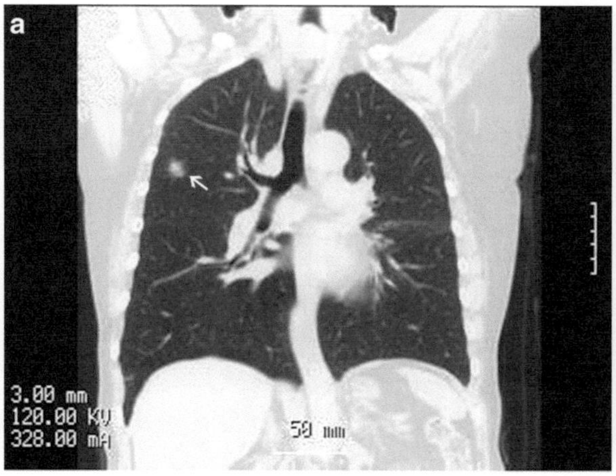

coronal view (CT scan)

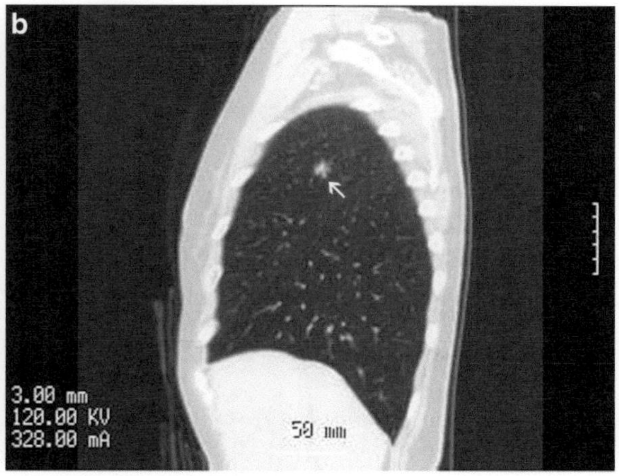

sagittal view (CT scan)

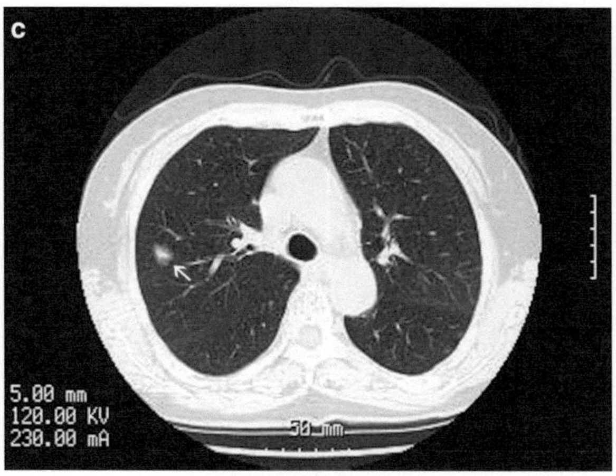

axial view (CT scan)

A 64-year-old female with symptoms of a common cold underwent an incidental CT examination. A mixed 1.4-cm GGO nodule was found and diagnosed as bronchioloalveolar carcinoma from a CT-guided needle biopsy. Segmentectomy for S^2b and S^3a was undertaken because the tumor was located deeply in the lung tissue between S^2b and S^3a. The pathological diagnosis was pT1aN0M0 adenocarcinoma with the appearance of bronchioloalveolar carcinoma in large part.

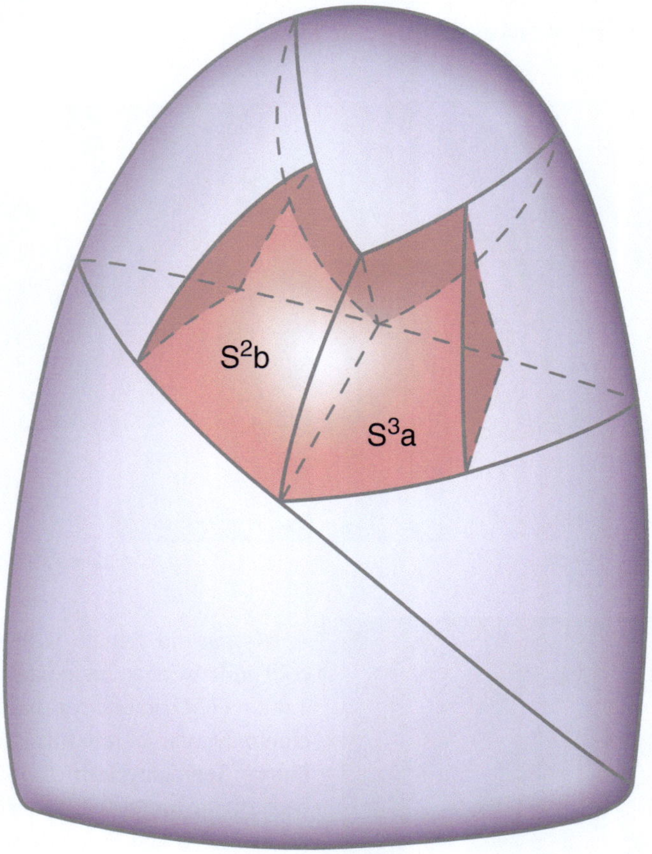

Fig. 3.5.1 S^2b+S^3a-segmentectomy is sometimes needed. For example, bronchioloalveolar carcinoma of <2 cm deeply located in the lung tissue straddling S^3a and S^2b can be curatively resected with this procedure, whereas the resection of both S^2 and S^3 results in a major decrease in the pulmonary function of the right upper lobe. Branching and sizes of B^1, B^2, and B^3 are reconfirmed using bronchoscope after tracheal intubation. In the figures of this session, the branching patterns of segmental bronchus, artery, and vein are popular ones as followings: segmental bronchus branches into three branches with B^1, B^2, and B^3; A^1 and A^3 branch from truncus superior artery; both of A^2a and A^2b branch from the ascending artery; and branching pattern of segmental vein is the most popular one, i.e. apical and central vein type. The optimal site of the thoracotomy for this procedure is usually the third intercostal space.

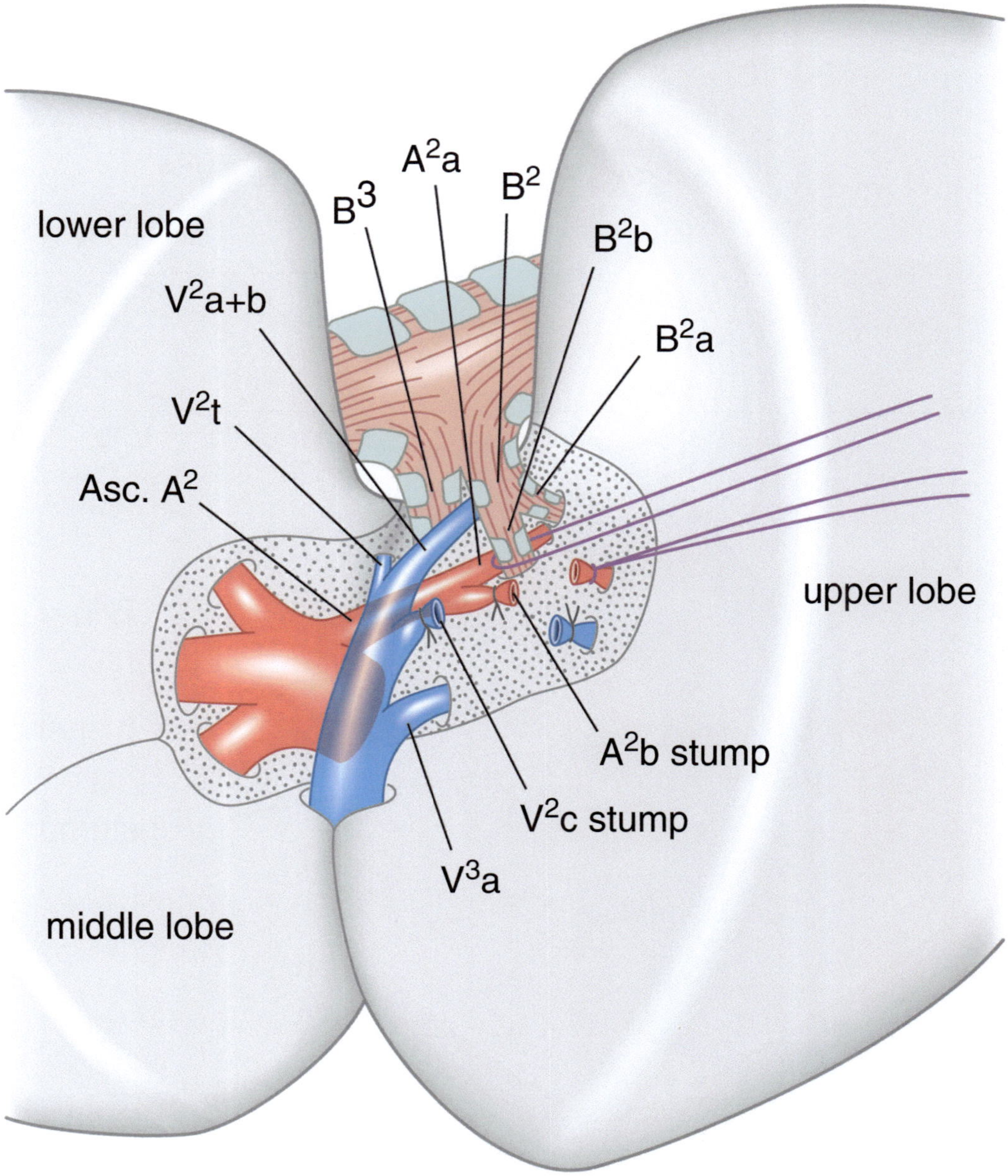

Fig. 3.5.2 The fissure between the right upper lobe and lower lobe is divided using electrocautery but not a stapler, because a staple line would impair identification of the peripheral route of V^2 and also complicate later identification of the intersegmental plane. After exposing the central vein, V^2c (between S^2b and S^3a) and V^3a (between S^3a and S^3b) are identified. V^2c often runs alongside V^2a+b immediately after branching, where the former runs in the front and the latter runs behind in this operative view. Thereafter, V^2c runs towards the lateral side of the upper lobe near the lung surface. V^3a is sometimes mistaken as V^2c, which could be differentiated each other by the followings: (1) V^2c branches at near the posterior site of the fissure and often runs side by side with V^2a+b immediately after branching; and (2) V^3a often branches almost vertically from the central vein at the center of the fissure. After V^2c is cut, V^2a+b is exposed peripherally. B^2 runs in front, while B^3 runs behind V^2a+b in this operative field. After peripherally exposing the ascending A^2, A^2b is identified and cut. By cutting the A^2b, the B^2 can be exposed. After exposing the B^2 peripherally, B^2a and B^2b are identified. B^2b is encircled with thread.

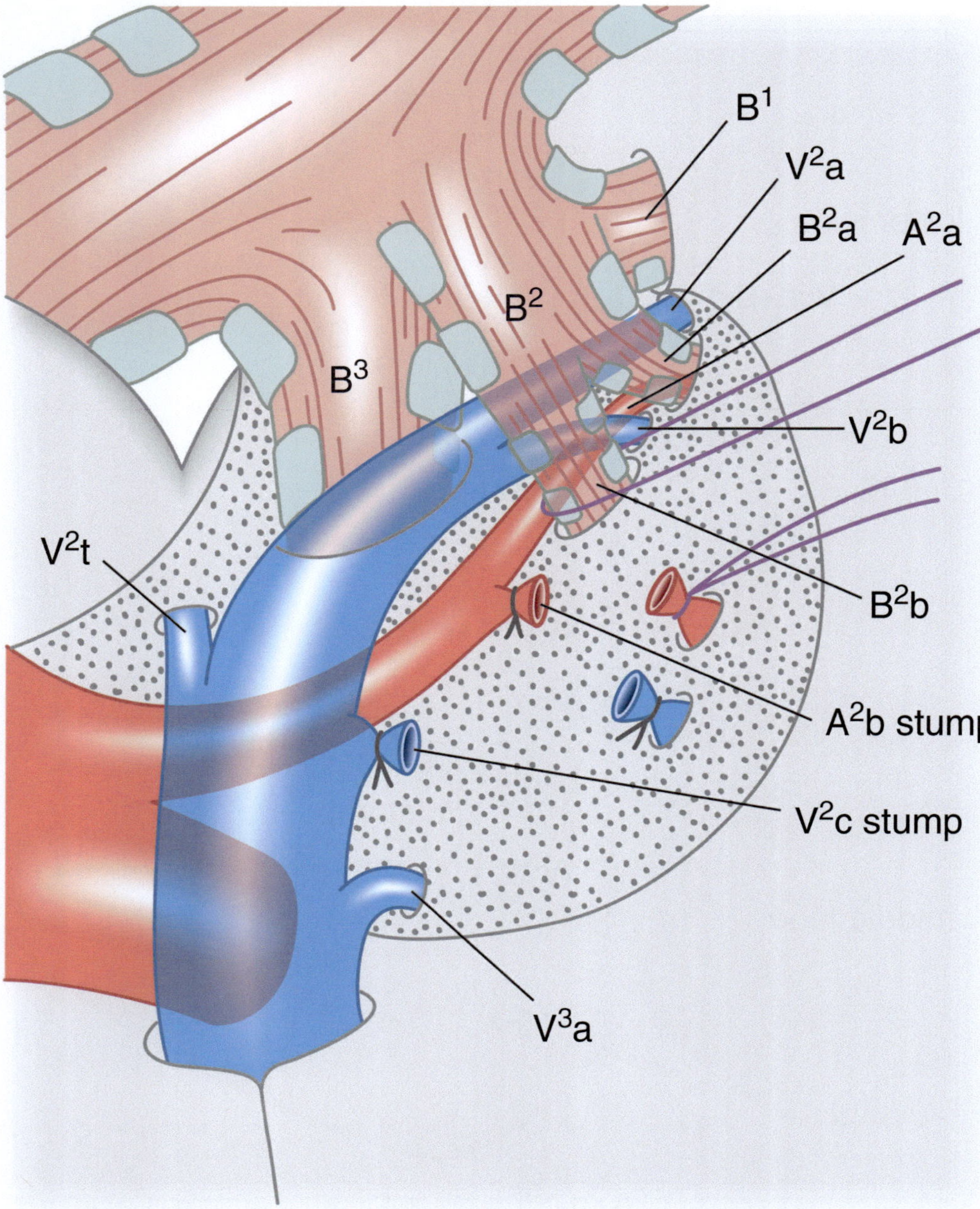

Fig. 3.5.3 This figure shows a magnified view around B^2. V^2a+b runs the backside of the B^2. V^2b branches at the back of B^2, and runs between the B^2a and B^2b. Ascending A^2a runs at the back of B^2, and runs toward the B^2a.

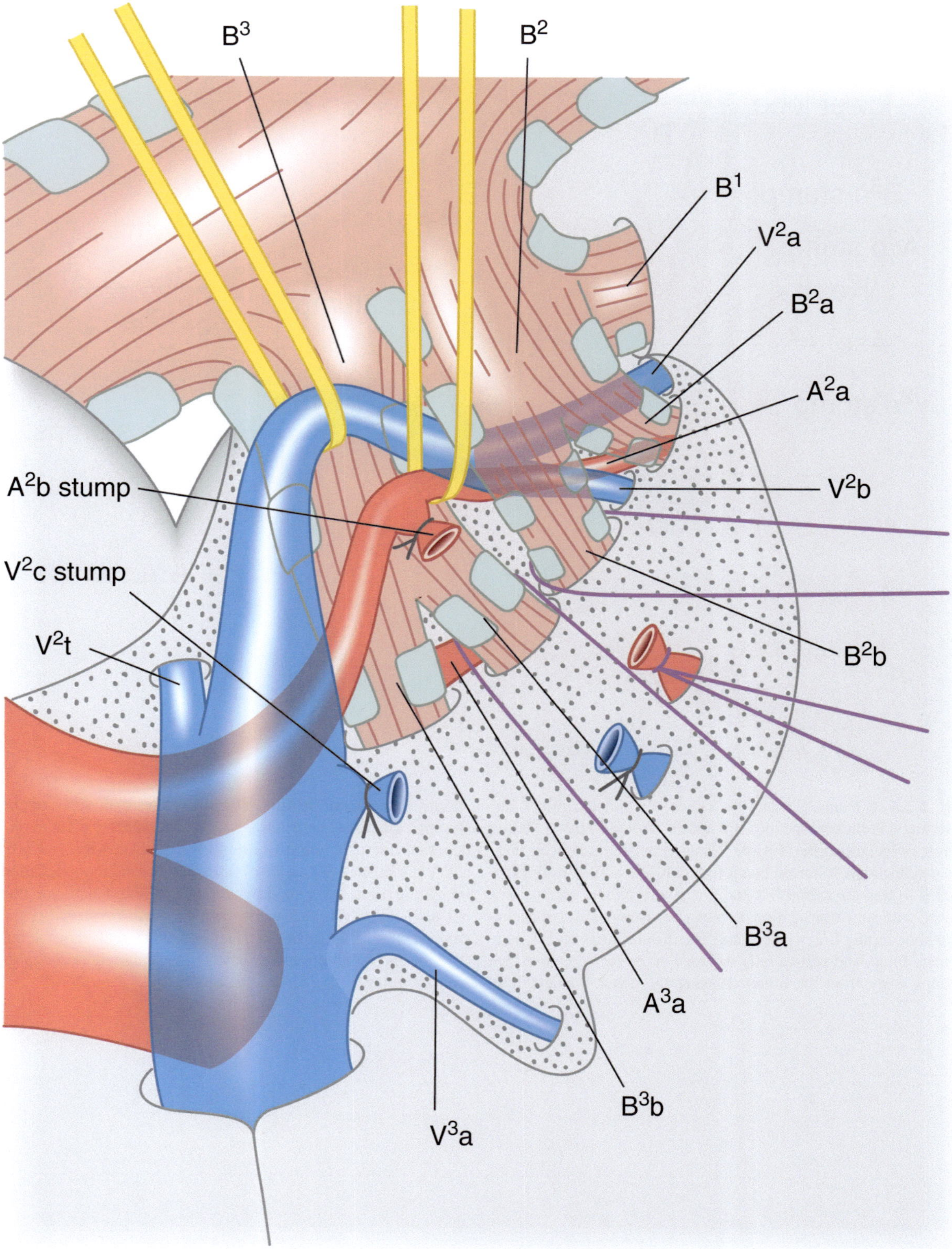

Fig. 3.5.4 After V^2a+b and ascending A^2 are encircled with tape, B^3 is exposed peripherally to reveal B^3a and B^3b running towards the lateral and ventral directions, respectively. B^3a is then encircled with thread.

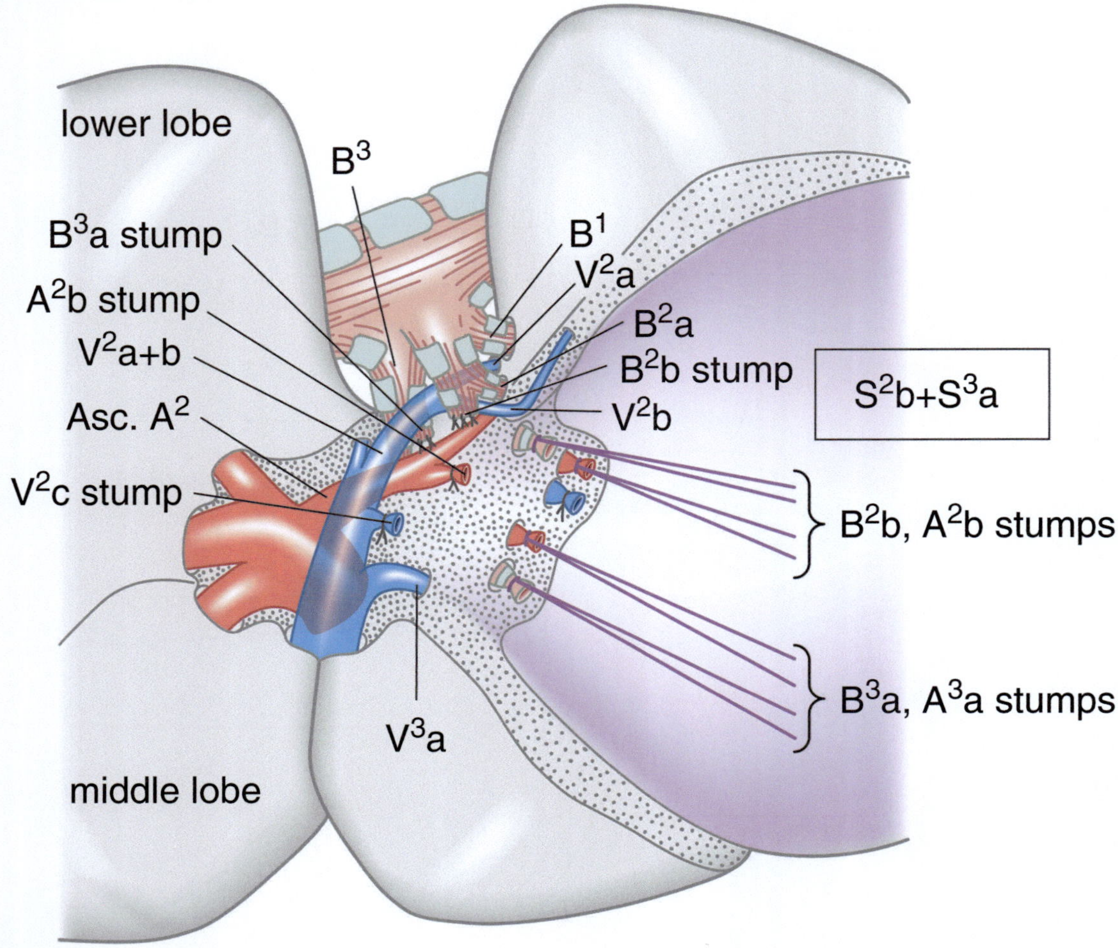

Fig. 3.5.5 S^2b and S^3a can be selectively inflated either by inserting a bronchoscope into B^2b and B^3a followed by jet ventilation, or by cutting the B^2b and B^3a and inserting a catheter into the distal stumps followed by air inflation. The distal stumps are closed to trap air within S^2b and S^3a. The proximal stumps are closed with suture or ligation. A^3b can be visualized at the backside after cutting B^3a, which is cut. The distal stumps of B^2b and B^3a are lifted, and peripherally denuded at the back to move the stumps away from the hilum. Raising the distal B^2b and B^3a stumps simultaneously lifts lung tissues on both sides of the stumps, and these lung tissues are cut towards the inflation–deflation line using electrocautery. V^2b (between S^2a and S^2b) and V^3a (between S^3a and S^3b) run along the inflation–deflation line. Lung tissue is cut not only along the inflation–deflation line but also along V^2b and V^3a, which are both preserved if the surgical margin is sufficient. The intersegmental plane is cut from various directions to facilitate simple and accurate intersegmental cutting.

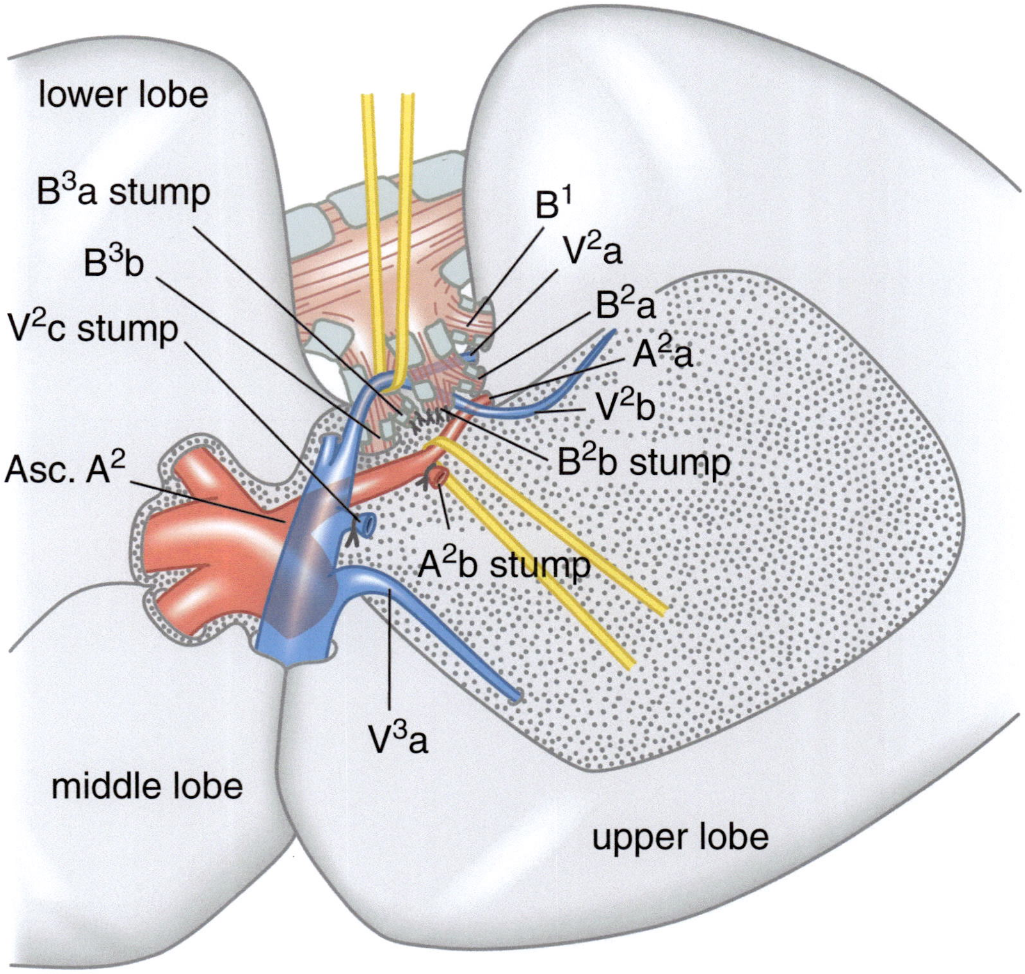

Fig. 3.5.6 V^2b and V^3a are preserved along the intersegmental plane. The hilar lymph node dissection is conducted with taping the upper lobar bronchus, V^2, ascending A^2, and truncus superior artery, which is the same way as the lymph node dissection in the S^2- or S^3-segmentectomy.

Segmentectomy of the Right Lower Lobe

4

The segmental vessels, particularly the segmental veins vary more in the lower than in the upper lobe. However, unlike the upper lobe, the segmental veins do not need to be identified for segmentectomy of the lower lobe, in which the segmental arteries are identified and cut first, followed by cutting the segmental bronchus. Next, the segmental veins running towards the segment scheduled for resection are cut, which does not require their identification. Instead, the segmental arteries should be identified accurately from both MDCT and intraoperative findings during segmentectomy of the lower lobe, without reference to the route of the segmental vein. Therefore, anatomical segmentectomy of a lower lobe depends on precise identification of the segmental arteries.

Branching profile			Frequency (%)
Bronchus	B^6	B^6a+c and B^6b	66
		B^6a+b and B^6c	28
		B^6a and B^6b and B^6c	6
	B^7	Both B^7a and B^7b run ventral to inferior pulmonary vein	64
		B^7a and B^7b straddle inferior pulmonary vein	20
		Lack of B^7	16
	B^{8-10}	B^8 and B^{9+10}	86
		B^{8+9} and B^{10}	8
		B^8 and B^9 and B^{10}	6
	B^*		4
Artery	A^6 (number of branches)	One	78
		Two	20
		Three	2
	A^7	Forms common truncus with A^8	60
		Branches from basal pulmonary artery	24
		Absent A^7	16
	A^{8-10}	A^8 and A^{9+10}	90
		A^{8+9} and A^{10}	8
		A^8 and A^9 and A^{10}	2
	A^*		4
Vein	Right inferior pulmonary vein	V^6 and common basal V	84
		V^6, superior basal V and inferior basal V	14
		V^{4+5}, V^6, and common basal V	2

H. Nomori and M. Okada, *Illustrated Anatomical Segmentectomy for Lung Cancer*,
DOI 10.1007/978-4-431-54144-8_4, © Springer Japan 2012

Branching profile			Frequency (%)
	Basal vein	V^{8+9} and V^{9+10}	30
		V^{8+9+10} and V^{10}	14
		V^{8} and V^{8+9+10}	2
		V^{8+9} and V^{10}	26
		V^{8} and V^{9+10}	18
		V^{8}, V^{9} and V^{10}	10

4.1 Right S^6 Segmentectomy

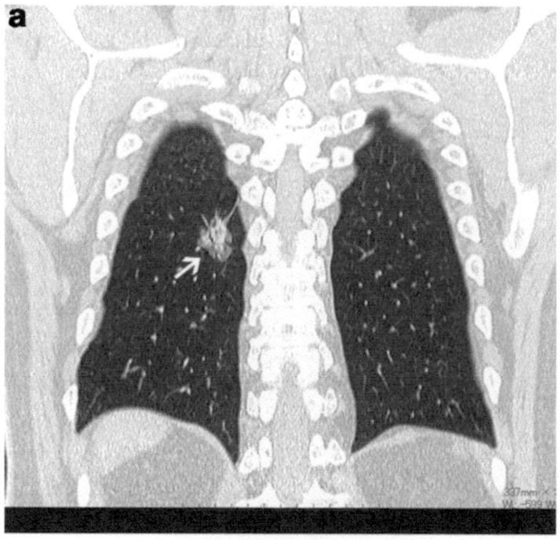

coronal view (CT scan)

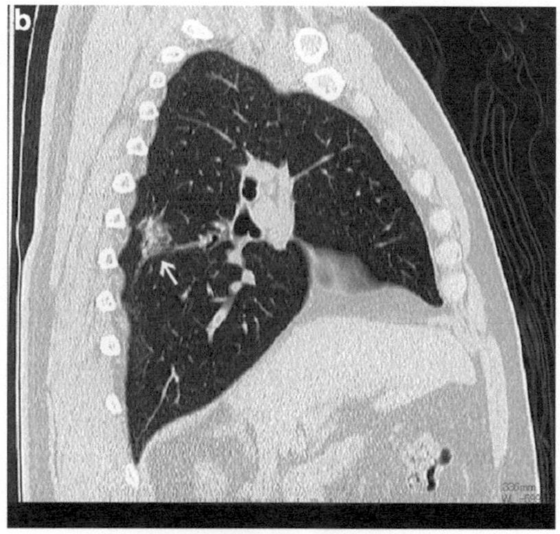

sagittal view (CT scan)

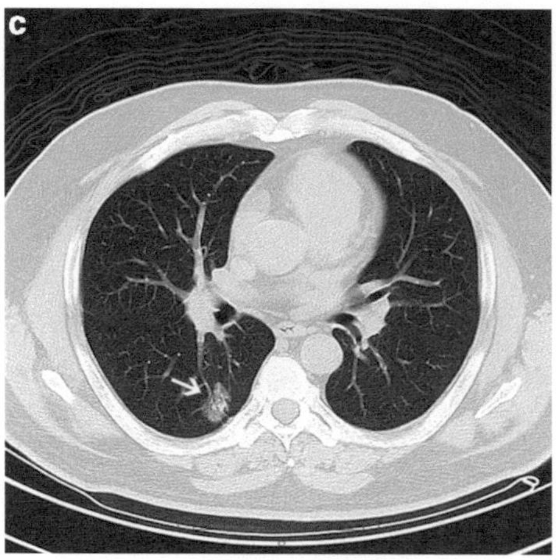

axial view (CT scan)

Routine CT medical examination of a 64-year-old male revealed a mixed 2.5-cm GGO nodule within the right S^6, which was diagnosed as bronchioloalveolar carcinoma from a CT-guided needle biopsy specimen. The final pathological diagnosis after S^6-segmentectomy was pT1bN0M0 bronchioloalveolar carcinoma.

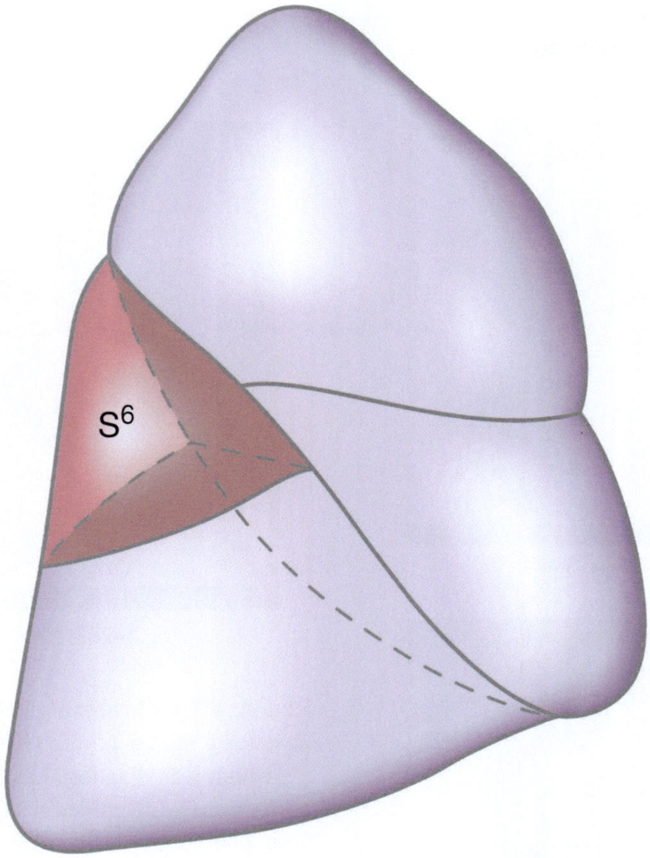

Fig. 4.1.1 The branching profiles of A^6 and V^6 are confirmed from axial, coronal, and sagittal views on HRCT. The branching and size of B^6 is further examined using bronchoscope after tracheal intubation. S^6-segmentectomy is the simplest in all types of segmentectomy, because A^6 and B^6 are easily identifiable. B^*, which branches from a basal bronchus at the caudal side of B^6 is found at a frequency of 4%, which should be checked by HRCT or by preoperative bronchoscopy. Lateral thoracotomy at the fourth intercostal space is generally appropriate for S^6-segmentectomy.

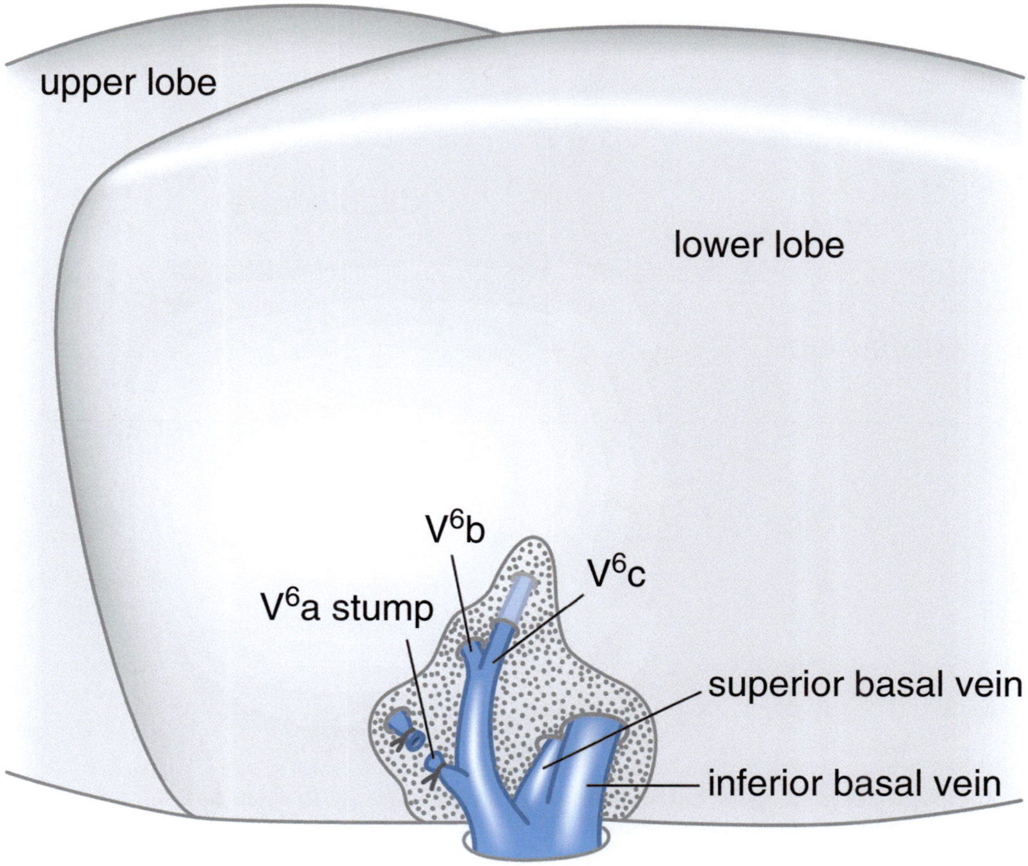

Fig. 4.1.2 The inferior pulmonary vein is exposed from the back side to identify V^6, which usually branches to V^6a and V^6b+c. The V^6a, which runs between S^6a and S^6b+c, is cut, whereas V^6b+c is preserved in principle during S^6-segmentectomy, because these veins run between S^6 and S^{8-10} and play a role not only in the venous drainage of these segments but also in guiding the intersegmental plane between S^6 and S^{8-10}. Therefore, V^6b+c is preserved on S^{8-10}. The V^6b+c is exposed peripherally, which can facilitate a later cutting between S^6 and S^{10}.

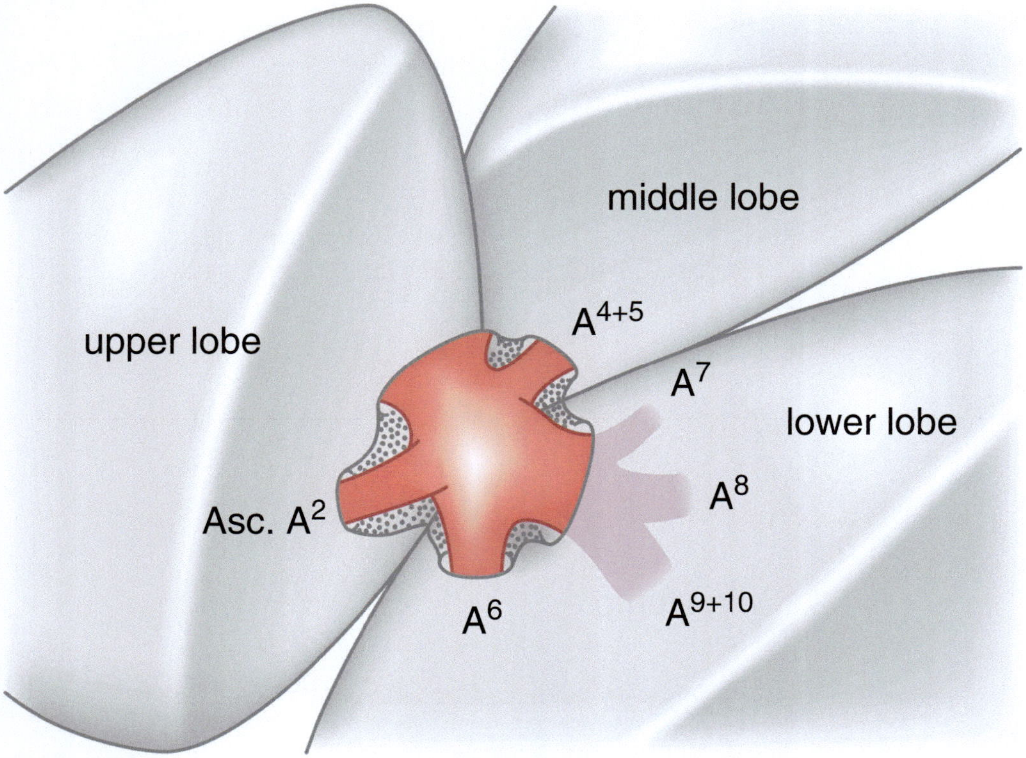

Fig. 4.1.3 The fissure between S^2 and S^6 can be cut using a stapler because the staple line usually does not interfere with S^6-segmentectomy. However, the fissure between the S^2 and S^6 generally can be simply cut using electrocautery.

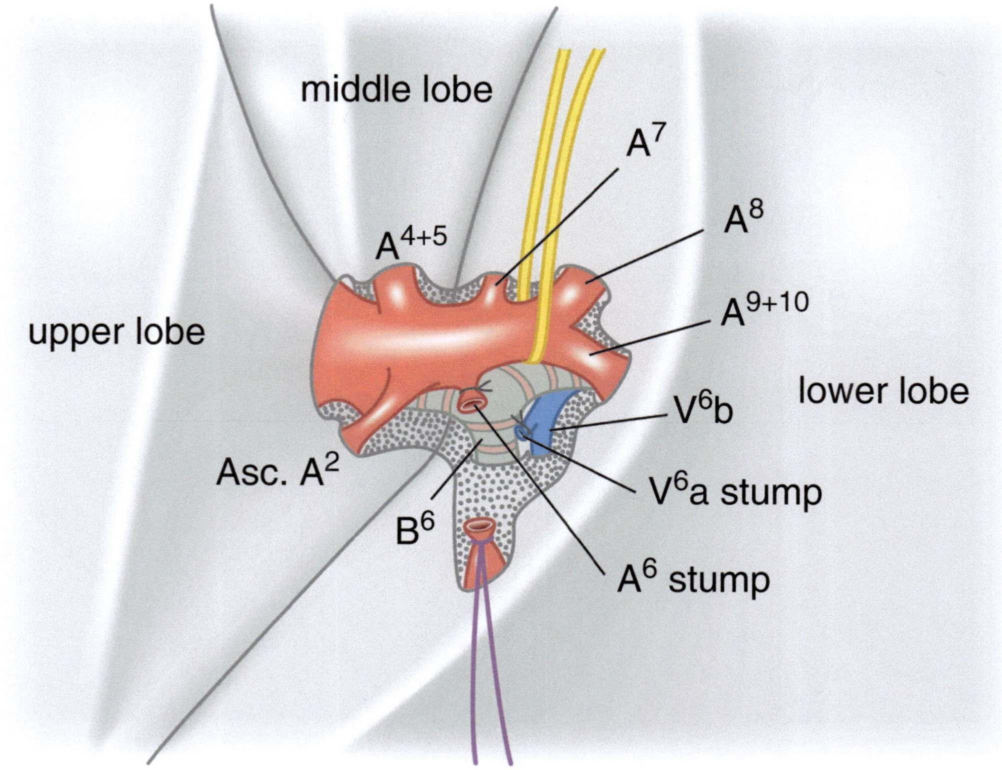

Fig. 4.1.4 A^6 is cut. The B^6 running caudally and behind the A^6 is exposed and encircled with thread, taking care to avoid damage to V^6b, which runs behind B^6.

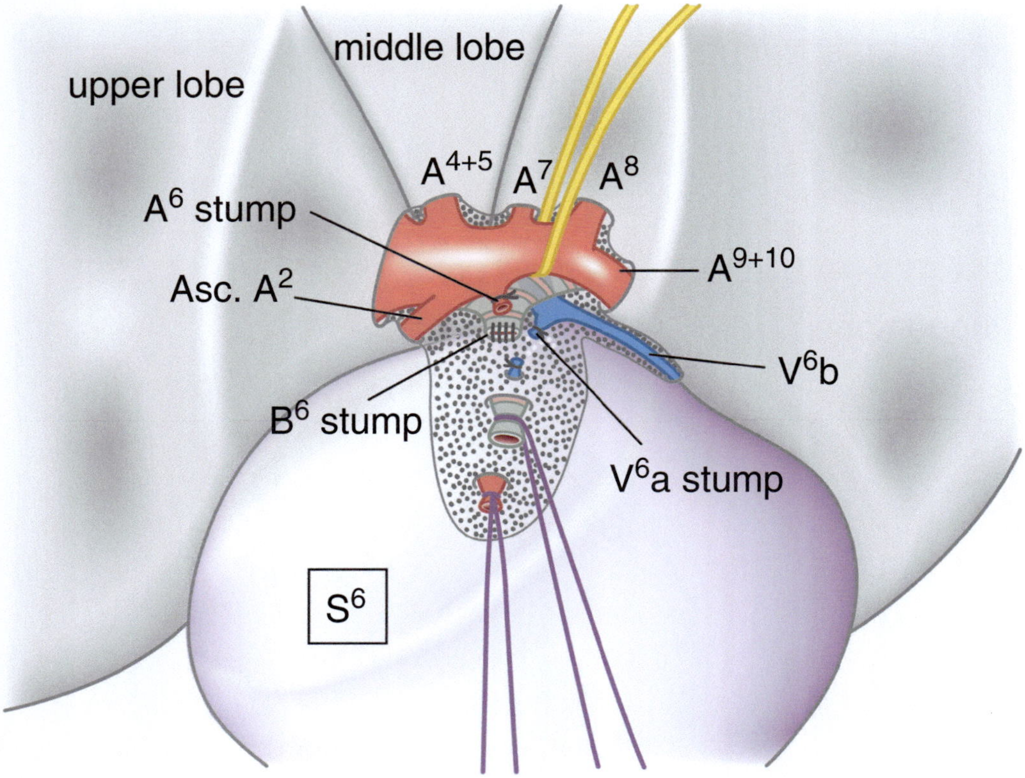

Fig. 4.1.5 S^6 is selectively inflated either by inserting a bronchoscope into B^6 followed by jet ventilation, or by cutting the B^6 and inserting a catheter into the distal stump followed by air inflation. The distal stump is closed to trap air within S^6. The proximal stump of B^6 is closed with suture or ligation. When S^6 is inflated using jet ventilation via bronchoscope, B^6 can be cut using a stapler. The distal stump of B^6 is lifted, and its back side is peripherally denuded to move the stump away from the hilum. By lifting the distal B^6-stump, the lung tissue on either sides of the stump is elevated, which is cut along the V^6b (between S^6 and S^8) and also toward the inflated–deflated line, by using an electrocautery. Cutting the lung tissue allows visualization of V^6c, which branches from V^6b+c and runs between S^6 and S^{10}. While a branch of V^6b running between S^6b and S^6c is cut, the remaining V^6b and V^6c are preserved on S^8 and S^{10}, respectively, because they not only guide the boundary between S^6 and S^{8-10} but also have a role for venous return from S^{8-10}.

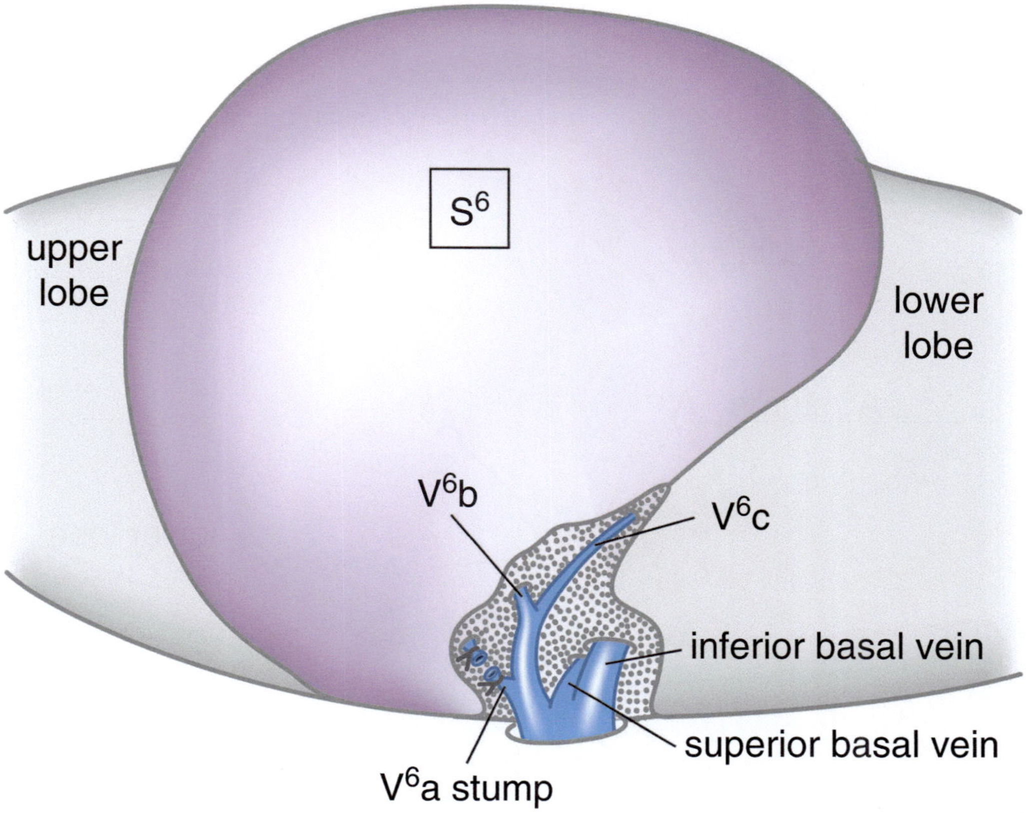

Fig. 4.1.6 The lung tissue is cut from the back along the V^6b+c and also along the inflation–deflation line, which completes the S^6-segmentectomy. The intersegmental plane is cut from various directions to facilitate simple and accurate segmentectomy.

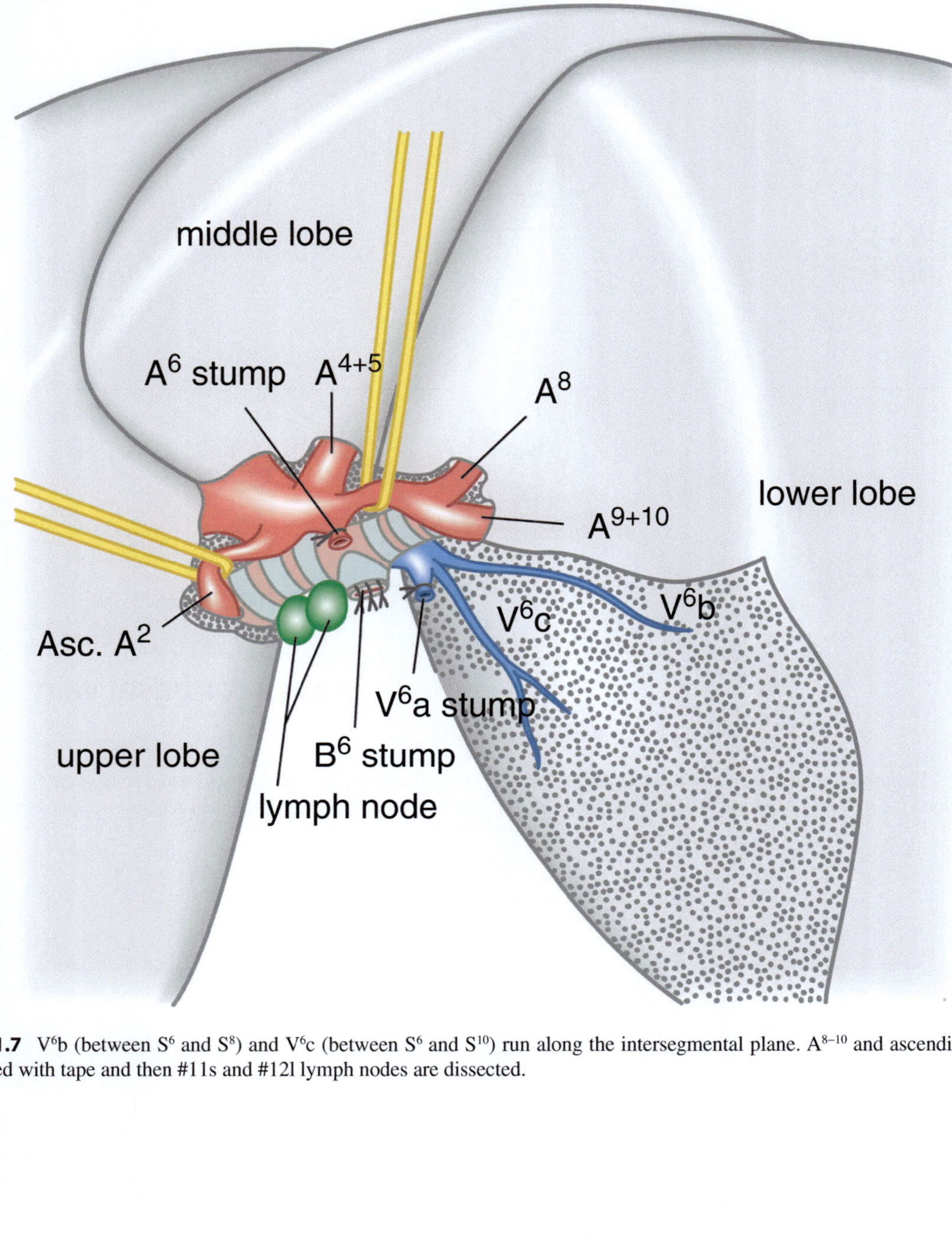

Fig. 4.1.7 V^6b (between S^6 and S^8) and V^6c (between S^6 and S^{10}) run along the intersegmental plane. A^{8-10} and ascending A^2 are encircled with tape and then #11s and #12l lymph nodes are dissected.

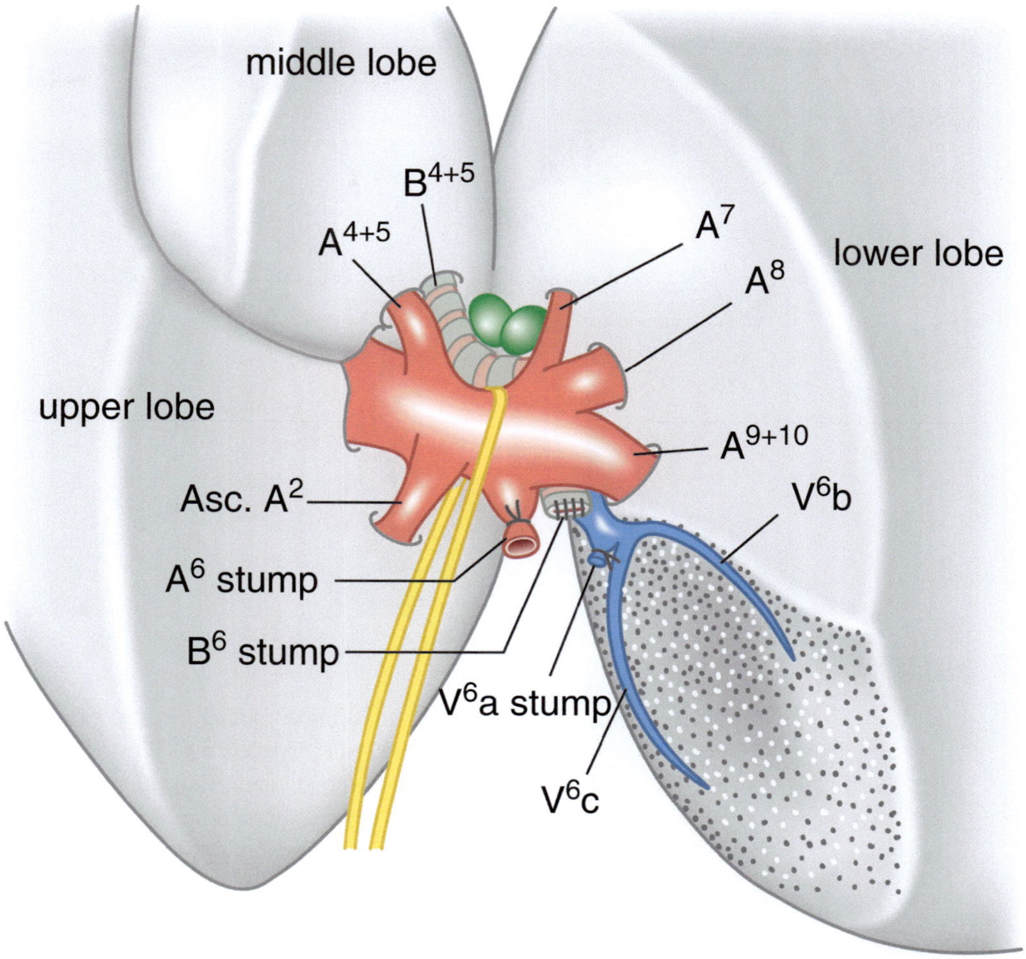

Fig. 4.1.8 The #11i and anterior #12l nodes are dissected from the ventral side after taping the inferior pulmonary artery.

4.2 Right S^8 Segmentectomy

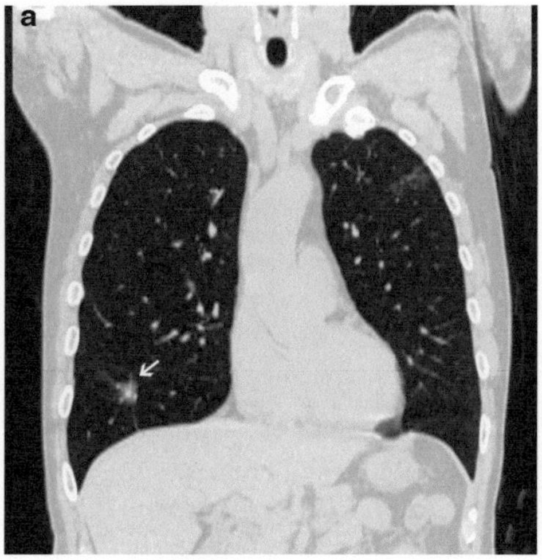

coronal view (CT scan)

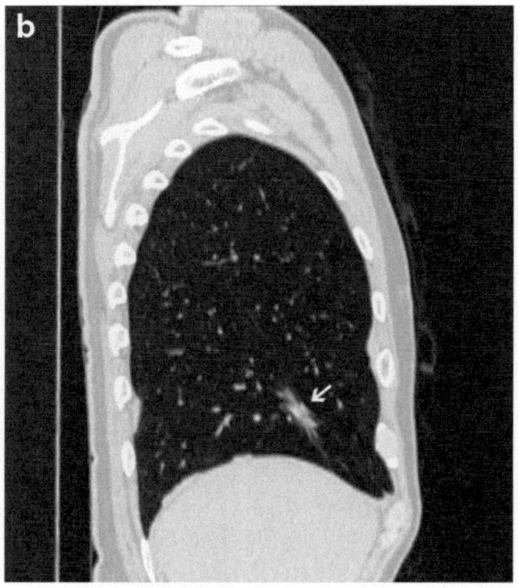

sagittal view (CT scan)

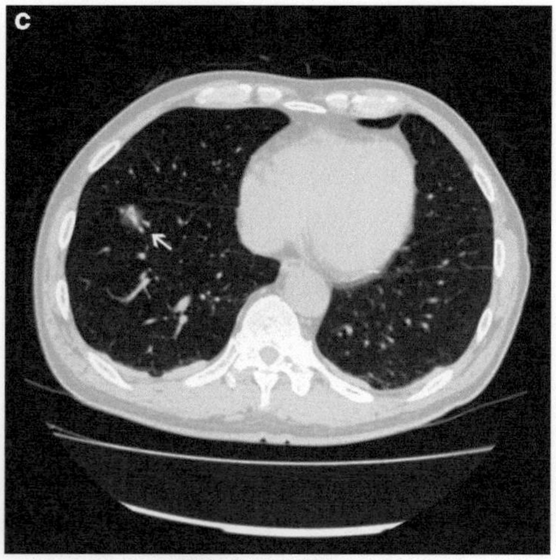

axial view (CT scan)

A CT scan during a routine medical examination of a 63-year-old male revealed a GGO nodule in the right lower lobe that had been followed up for 5 years. The lesion had increased and transformed into a solid tumor. Computed tomography imaging revealed a 1.8-cm mixed GGO lesion with spicular formation and pleural indentation at the right S^8a and also a 1-cm mixed GGO lesion in the right S^1. Both lesions were diagnosed as adenocarcinoma from CT-guided needle biopsy specimens. S^1- and S^8-segmentectomies were proceeded. The pathological diagnoses of both lesions were pT1aN0M0 adenocarcinoma.

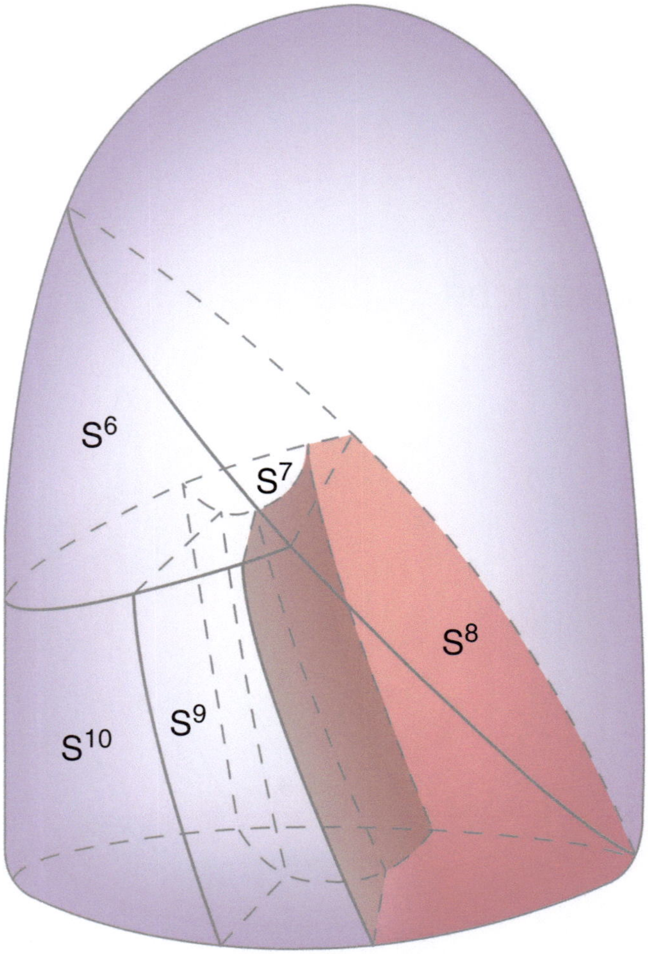

Fig. 4.2.1 The segmental arteries (A^{7-10}) and bronchi (B^{7-10}) are identified from axial, coronal, and sagittal HRCT images. The branching profiles and size of B^7, B^8, B^9, and B^{10} are further identified by bronchoscopy after tracheal intubation. The optimal site of thoracotomy is generally a lateral thoracotomy at the fifth intercostal space for S^8-segmentectomy. Bronchial and arterial branching in the figures of this session is of the most frequent type, i.e. B^8 and B^{9+10}, and A^8 and A^{9+10}.

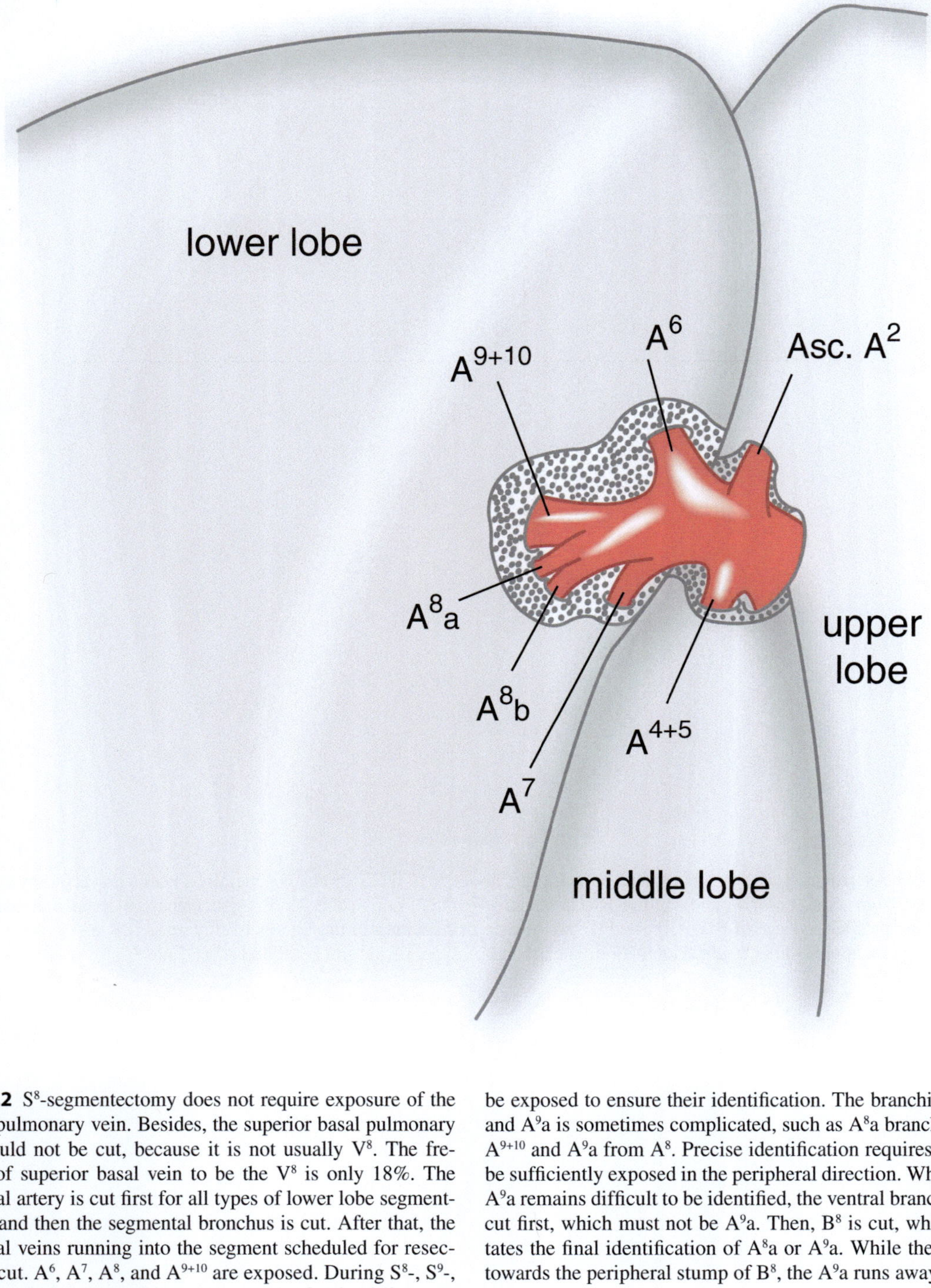

Fig. 4.2.2 S^8-segmentectomy does not require exposure of the inferior pulmonary vein. Besides, the superior basal pulmonary vein should not be cut, because it is not usually V^8. The frequency of superior basal vein to be the V^8 is only 18%. The segmental artery is cut first for all types of lower lobe segmentectomy, and then the segmental bronchus is cut. After that, the segmental veins running into the segment scheduled for resection are cut. A^6, A^7, A^8, and A^{9+10} are exposed. During S^8-, S^9-, and S^{10}-segmentectomy, all branches of A^6, A^7, A^8, A^{9+10} should be exposed to ensure their identification. The branching of A^8a and A^9a is sometimes complicated, such as A^8a branching from A^{9+10} and A^9a from A^8. Precise identification requires the A^8 to be sufficiently exposed in the peripheral direction. When A^8a or A^9a remains difficult to be identified, the ventral branch of A^8 is cut first, which must not be A^9a. Then, B^8 is cut, which facilitates the final identification of A^8a or A^9a. While the A^8a runs towards the peripheral stump of B^8, the A^9a runs away from it.

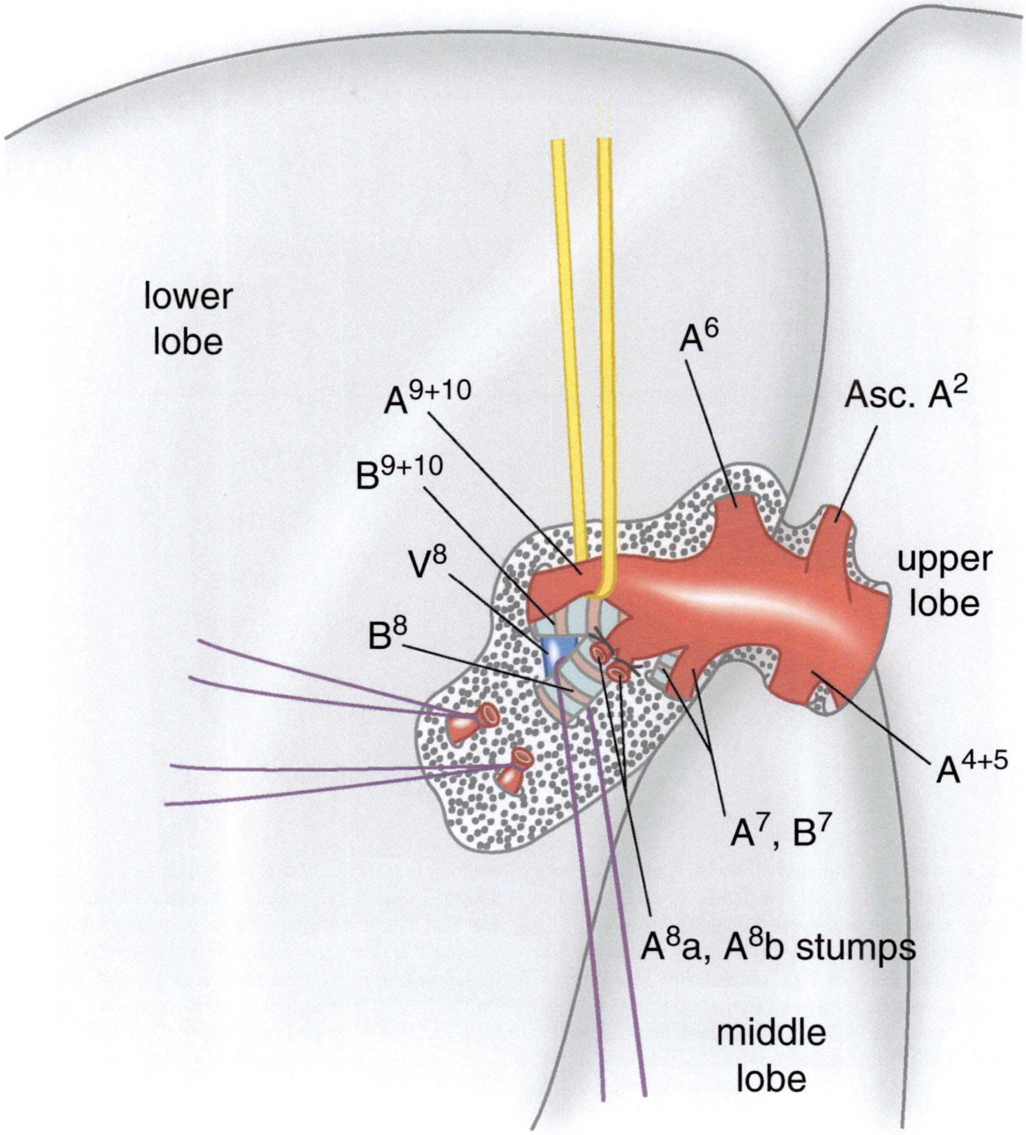

Fig. 4.2.3 B^8 runs behind the A^8. The B^8 is carefully encircled with thread to avoid damage to V^8 running behind it. When B^8 cannot be identified with certainty, the bronchoscope is inserted into B^8, B^9, and B^{10}, of which illumination can help the identification of B^8.

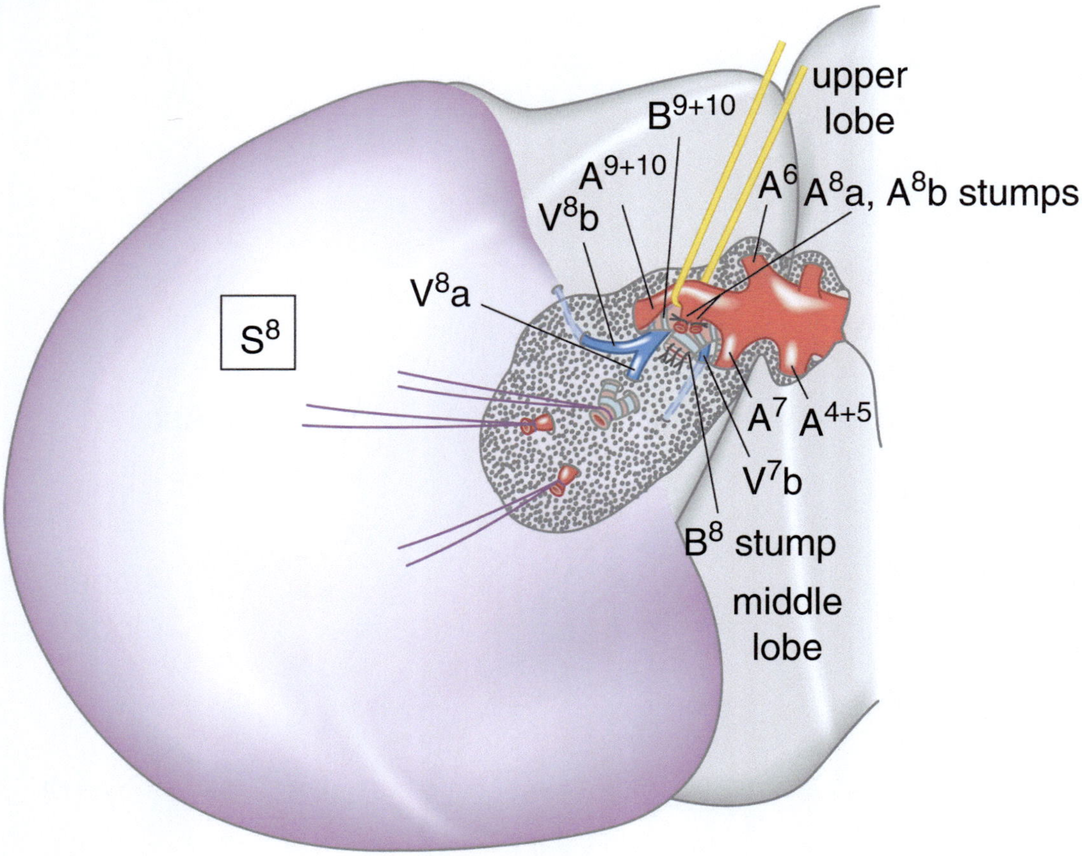

Fig. 4.2.4 S^8 is selectively inflated either by inserting a bronchoscope into B^8 followed by jet ventilation, or by cutting the B^8 and inserting a catheter into the distal stump followed by air inflation. The distal stump is closed to trap air within S^8. The proximal stump of B^8 is closed with suture or ligation. When S^8 is inflated using jet ventilation via bronchoscope, B^8 can be cut using a stapler. The distal stump of B^8 is lifted, and the back is denuded peripherally to move the stump away from the hilum. Lifting the distal stump reveals V^8a (between S^8a and S^8b) running into the S^8. V^8a is cut, which further elevates the distal stump. Lung tissue around the distal stump of B^8 is further elevated by cutting V^8a, which is cut along V^8b (between S^8 and S^9) and V^7b (between S^7 and S^8) and also towards the inflation–deflation line using electrocautery. V^7b and V^8b are preserved on the S^7 and S^9 for their venous return and also for use as a landmark for the segmental cutting plane, if the surgical margin is sufficient. The intersegmental plane is cut from various directions to facilitate simple and accurate intersegmental cutting.

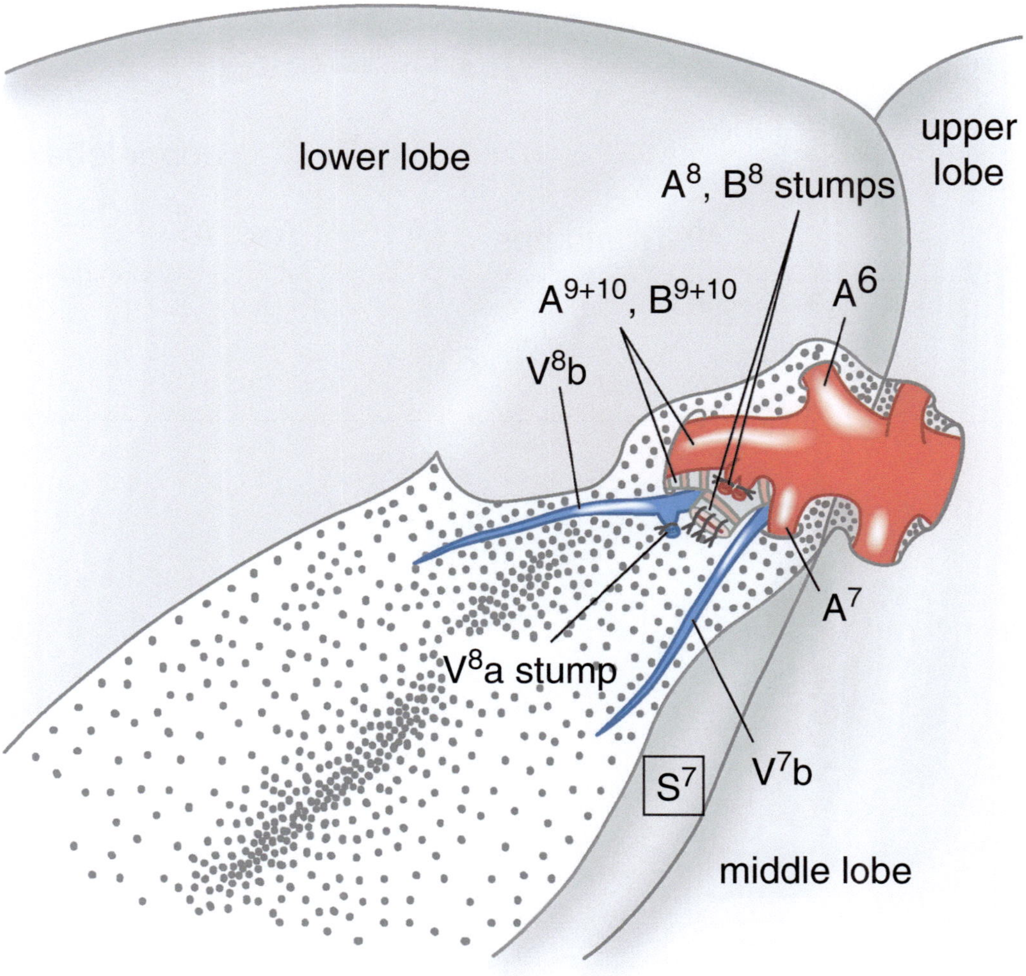

Fig. 4.2.5 After resection of S^8, V^7b (between S^7 and S^8) and V^8b (between S^8 and S^9) are revealed on the S^7 and S^9, respectively.

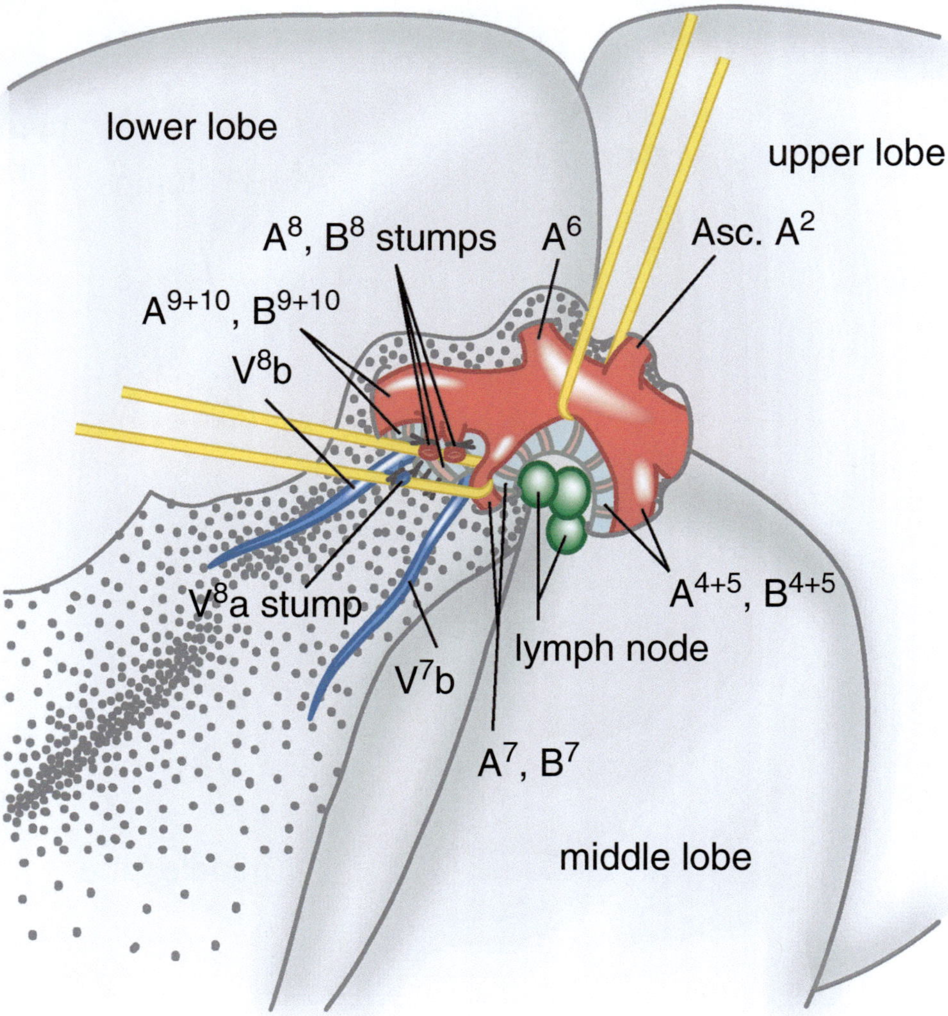

Fig. 4.2.6 The truncus intermedius artery and A^7 are encircled with tape. The #11i and anterior #12l hilar lymph nodes between the right middle and lower lobar bronchus are dissected. The posterior #12l and #13 (around B^6) lymph nodes are dissected with taping A^6, which is important because they lie along the lymphatic chain from S^8 towards the #7 node.

4.3 Right S^9 Segmentectomy

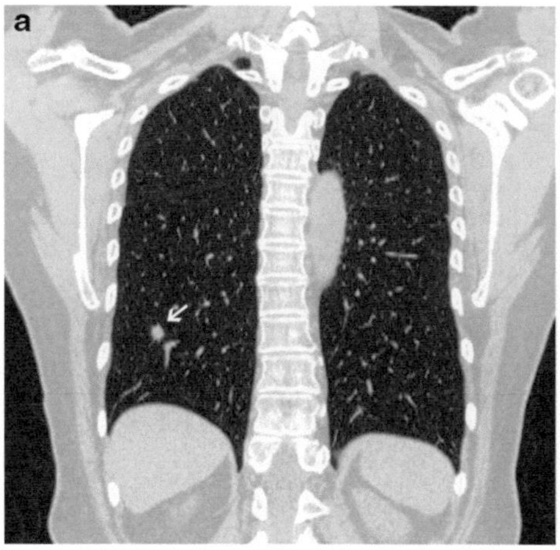

coronal view (CT scan)

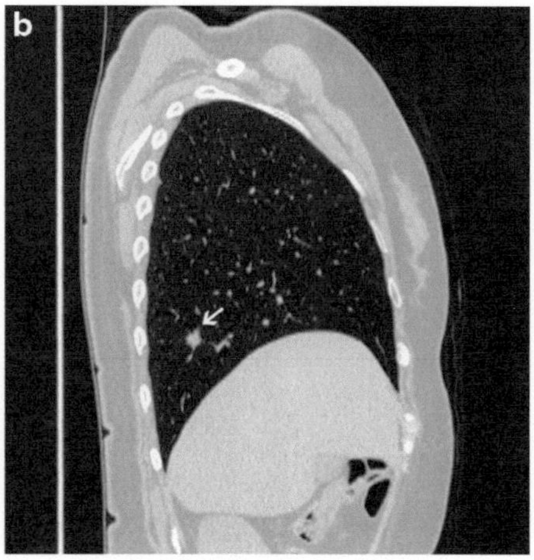

sagittal view (CT scan)

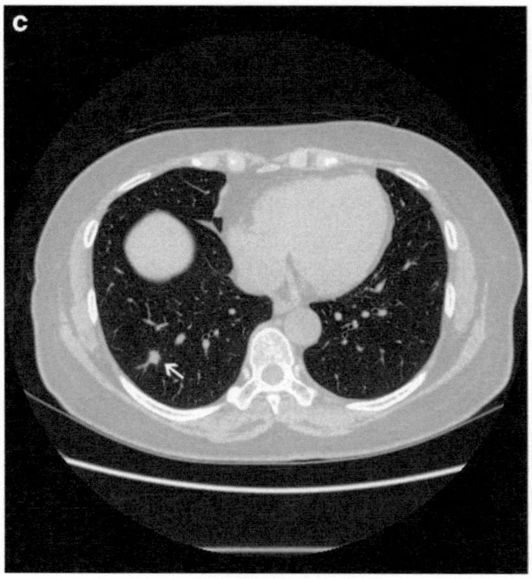

axial view (CT scan)

A CT scan of a 66-year-old female revealed a 1.0-cm nodule with spicular formation at the right S^9 that was diagnosed as adenocarcinoma from a CT-guided needle biopsy specimen. S^9-segmentectomy was undertaken because the tumor was located apart from both the V^8b (between S^8 and S^9) and V^9b (between S^9 and S^{10}). The final pathological diagnosis after S^9-segmentectomy was pT1aN0M0 papillary adenocarcinoma.

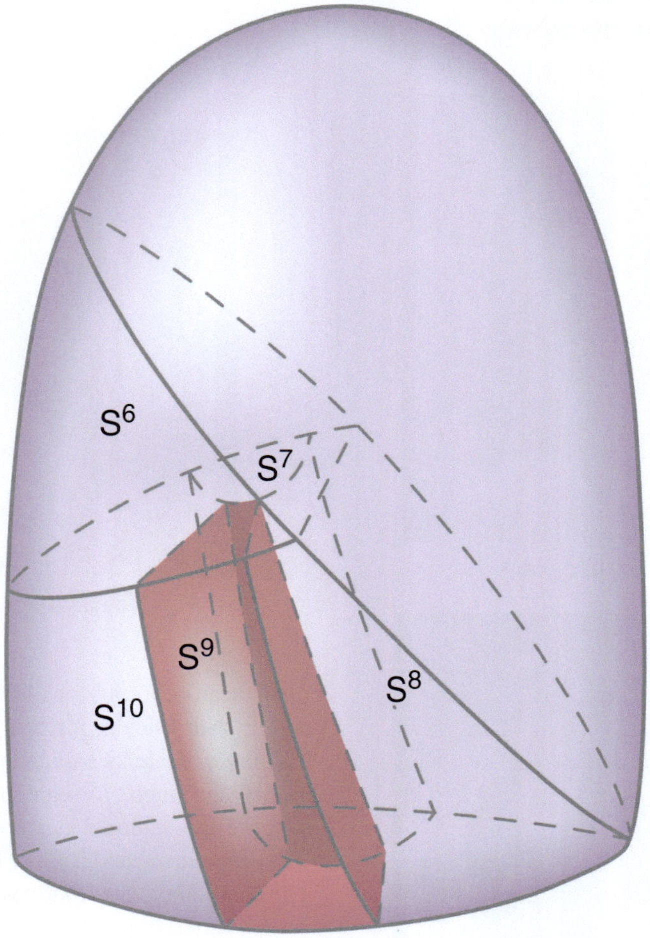

Fig. 4.3.1 The segmental arteries (A^{7-10}) and bronchi (B^{7-10}) are identified from axial, coronal, and sagittal HRCT images. The branching profiles and sizes of B^7, B^8, B^9, and B^{10} are further determined by bronchoscopy after tracheal intubation. The anatomical configuration of bronchial and arterial branching in the figures of this session is of the most frequent type, namely B^8 and B^{9+10}, and A^8 and A^{9+10}. Lateral thoracotomy at the fifth intercostal space is generally appropriate for S^9-segmentectomy.

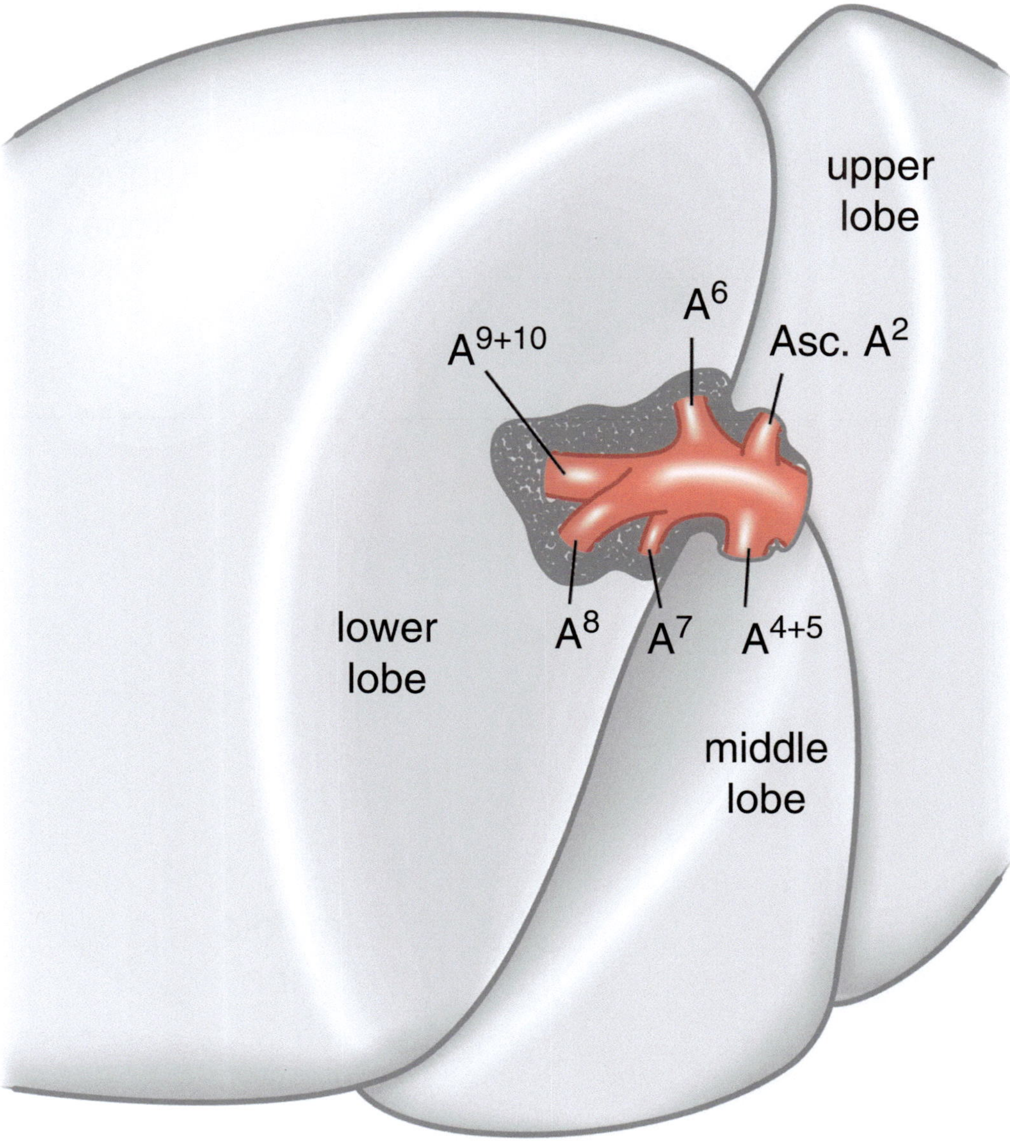

Fig. 4.3.2 The interlobar pulmonary artery is exposed, followed by exposing A^6, A^7, A^8, and A^{9+10}. The inferior pulmonary vein does not need to be exposed for S^9-segmentectomy, because V^9 is usually impossible to identify from the root of the inferior pulmonary vein. In all kinds of the lower lobe segmentectomy, a segmental artery is cut first, followed by cutting segmental bronchus. Finally, segmental veins running into the segment scheduled for resection are cut.

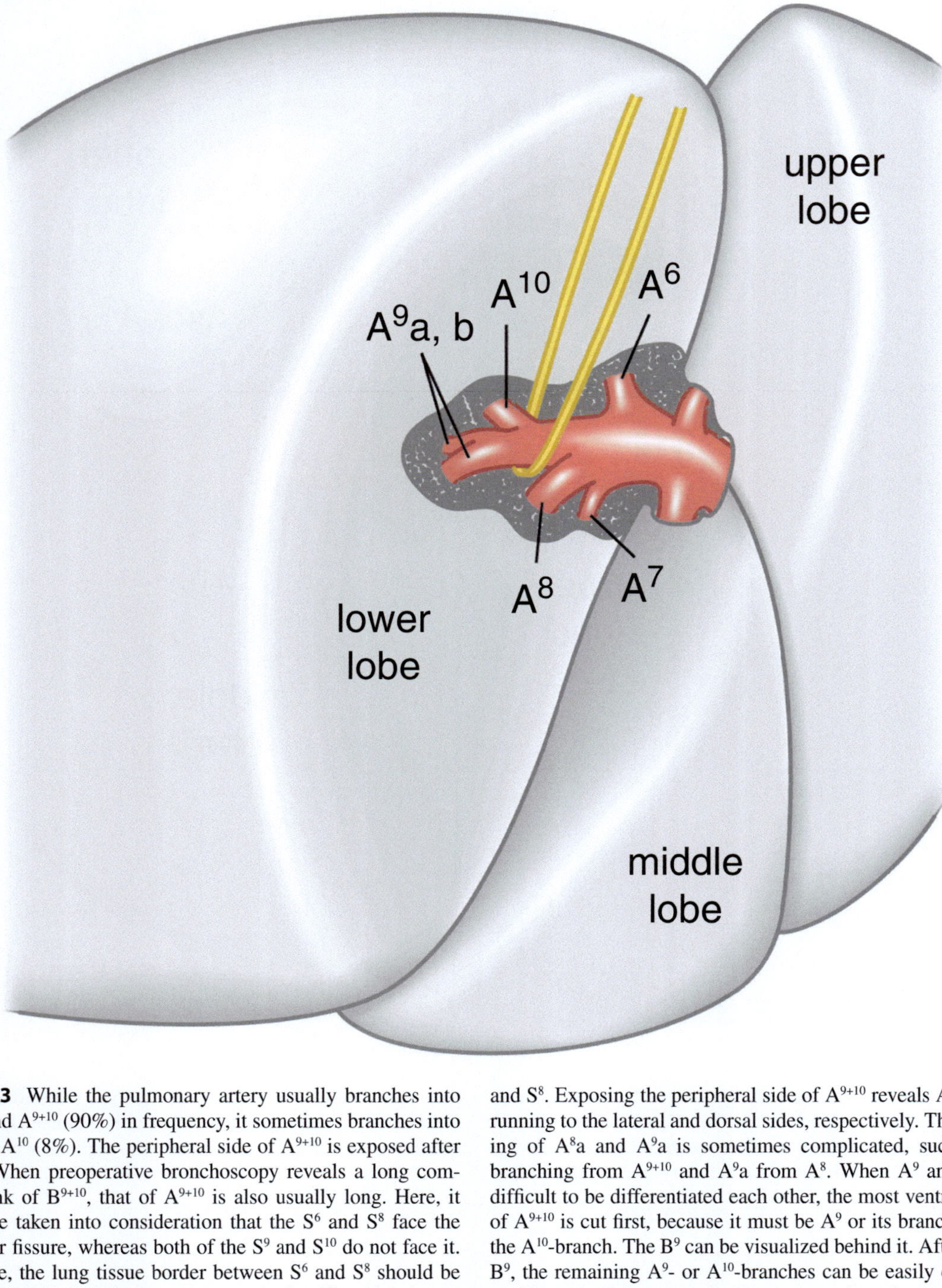

Fig. 4.3.3 While the pulmonary artery usually branches into the A^8 and A^{9+10} (90%) in frequency, it sometimes branches into A^{8+9} and A^{10} (8%). The peripheral side of A^{9+10} is exposed after taping. When preoperative bronchoscopy reveals a long common trunk of B^{9+10}, that of A^{9+10} is also usually long. Here, it should be taken into consideration that the S^6 and S^8 face the interlobar fissure, whereas both of the S^9 and S^{10} do not face it. Therefore, the lung tissue border between S^6 and S^8 should be cut from the interlobar fissure to reach the S^9, which is not always easy because there is no landmark of border between S^6 and S^8. Exposing the peripheral side of A^{9+10} reveals A^9 and A^{10} running to the lateral and dorsal sides, respectively. The branching of A^8a and A^9a is sometimes complicated, such as A^8a branching from A^{9+10} and A^9a from A^8. When A^9 and A^{10} are difficult to be differentiated each other, the most ventral branch of A^{9+10} is cut first, because it must be A^9 or its branch, but not the A^{10}-branch. The B^9 can be visualized behind it. After cutting B^9, the remaining A^9- or A^{10}-branches can be easily differentiated because they, respectively, run towards and away from the S^9 scheduled for resection.

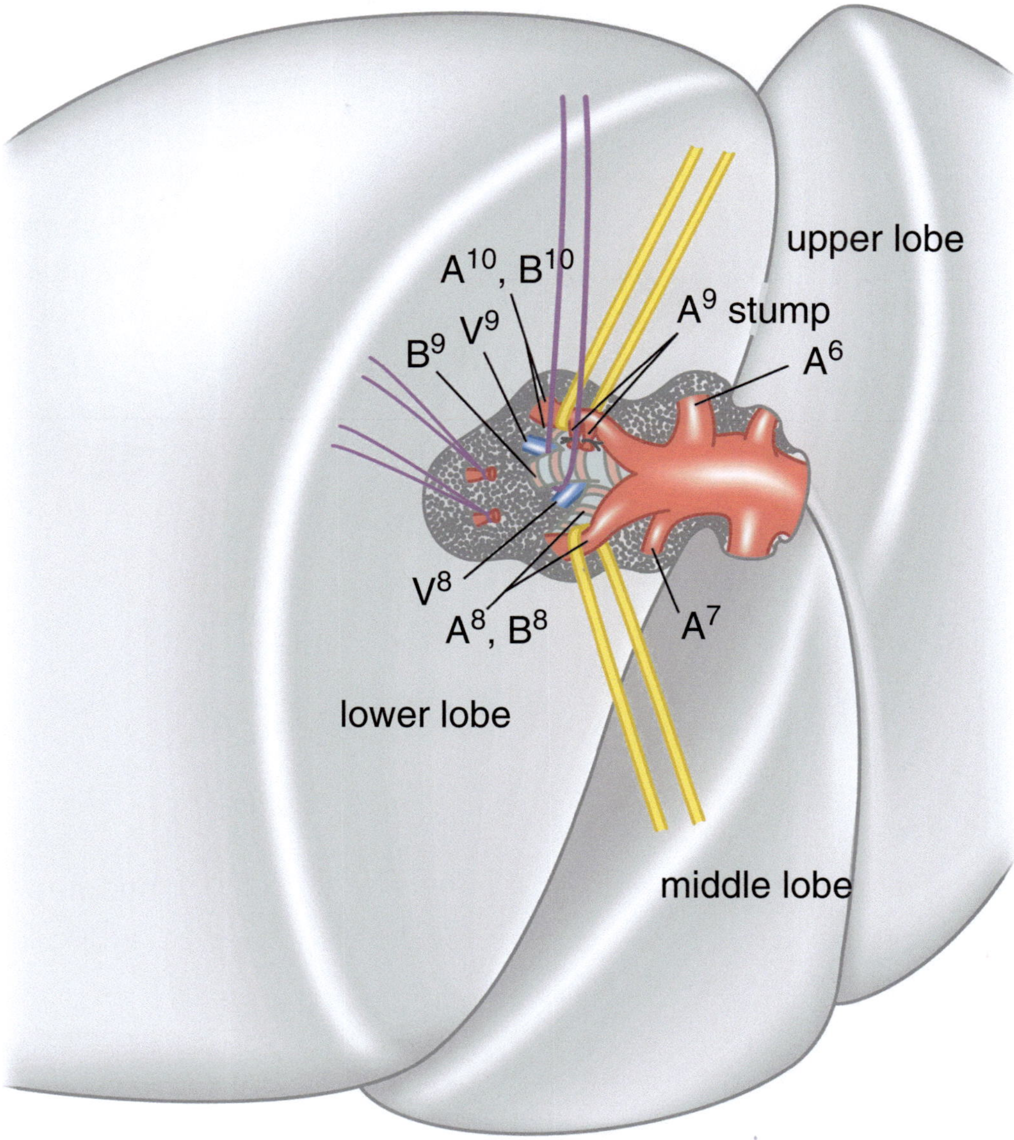

Fig. 4.3.4 B^9 is carefully encircled with thread because V^9 runs behind it. The identification of B^9 and B^{10} can be confirmed by illumination from a bronchoscope inserted into each of them.

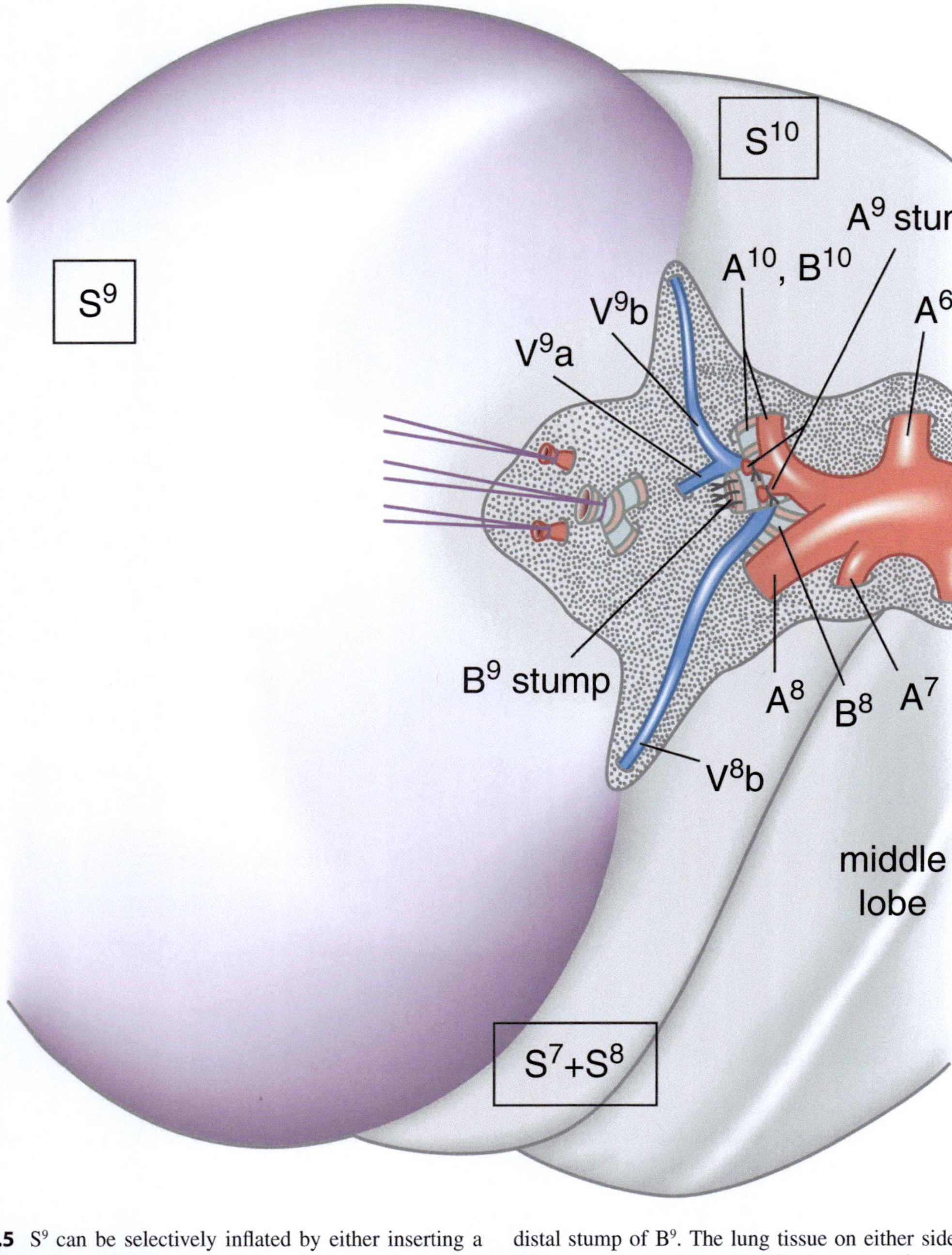

Fig. 4.3.5 S^9 can be selectively inflated by either inserting a bronchoscope into it followed by a jet ventilation, or by cutting the B^9 and inserting a catheter into the distal stump followed by air inflation. The distal stump is closed to trap air within S^9. The proximal stump of B^9 is closed with suture or ligation. The distal stump of B^9 is lifted and denuded peripherally at the back to move it away from the hilum. Lifting the distal stump of B^9 reveals V^9a (between S^9a and S^9b) running into the S^9 scheduled for resection, which is cut. Cutting the V^9a further elevates the distal stump of B^9. The lung tissue on either side of the distal B^9-stump is cut along the V^8b (between S^8 and S^9) and V^9b (between S^9 and S^{10}) and also toward the inflation–deflation line using electrocautery. V^8b and V^9b are preserved on S^8 and S^{10}, respectively, because they not only guide the intersegmental plane but also preserve venous return from S^8 and S^{10}. The intersegmental plane is cut from various directions to facilitate simple and accurate intersegmental cutting.

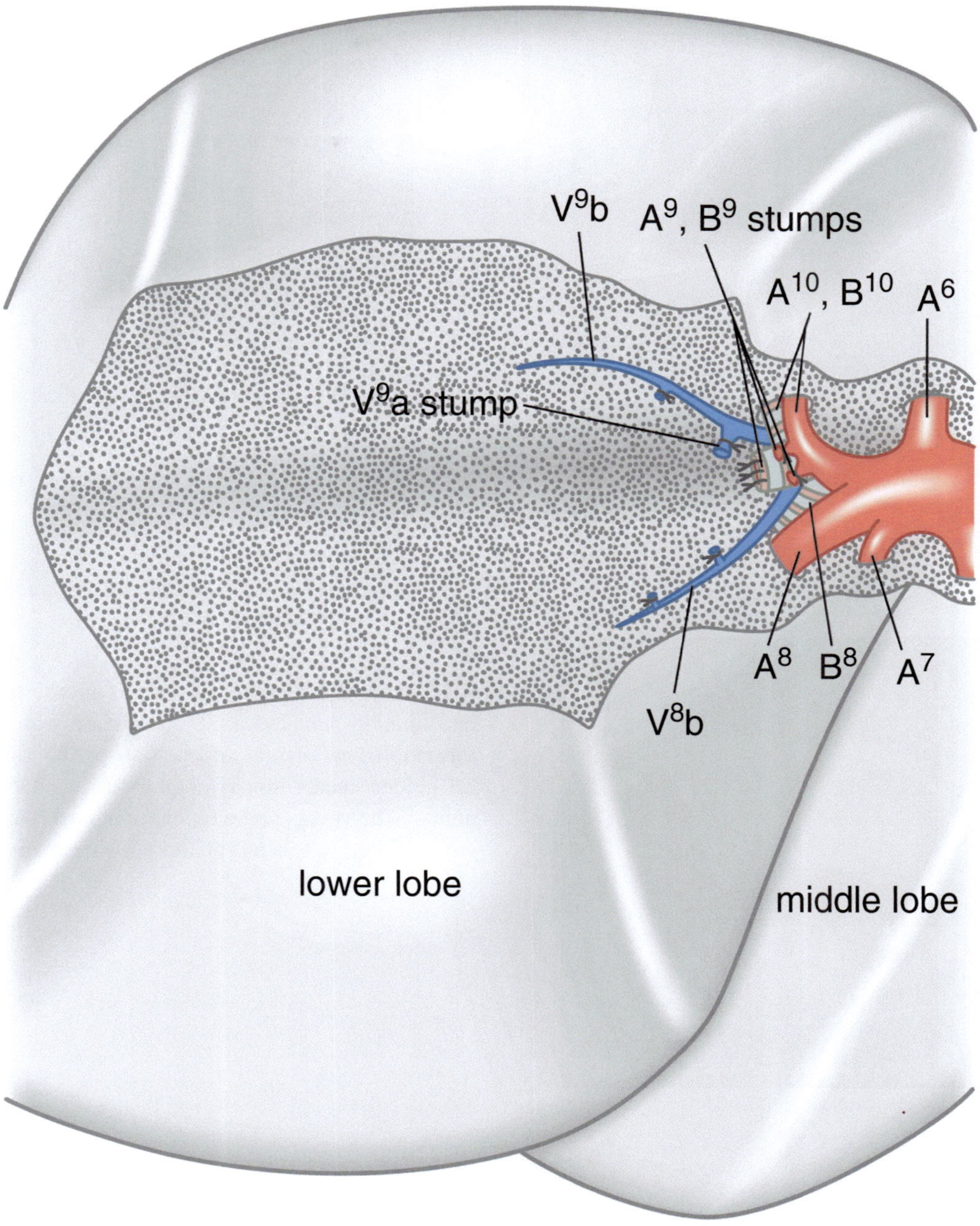

Fig. 4.3.6 V^8b and V^9b are preserved on the intersegmental plane. The B^6, A^6, and A^{8-10} are encircled with tape to allow dissection of the posterior #12l and #13 (around B^6) as well as #11i and anterior #12l that lies between the right middle and lower lobar bronchus. The dissection of #12l and #13 (around B^6) is important, because these nodes lie along the lymphatic chain from S^9 towards the #7 node.

4.4 Right S^{10} Segmentectomy

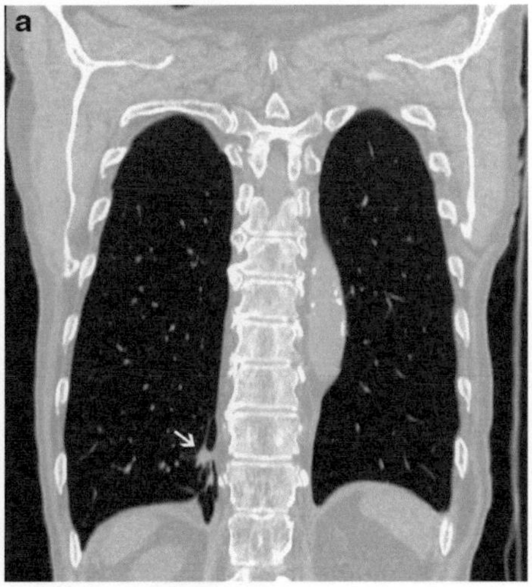

coronal view (CT scan)

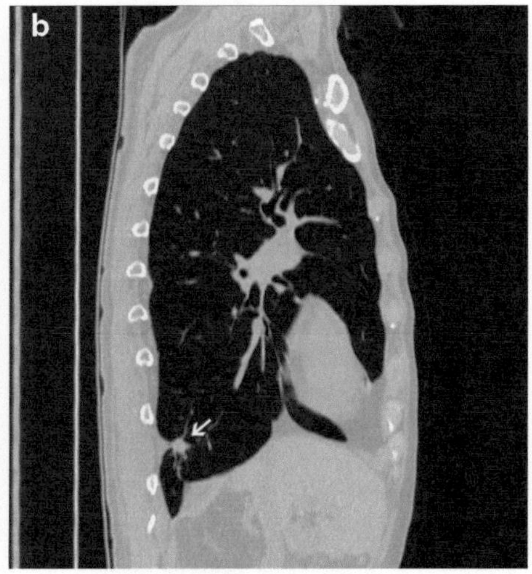

sagittal view (CT scan)

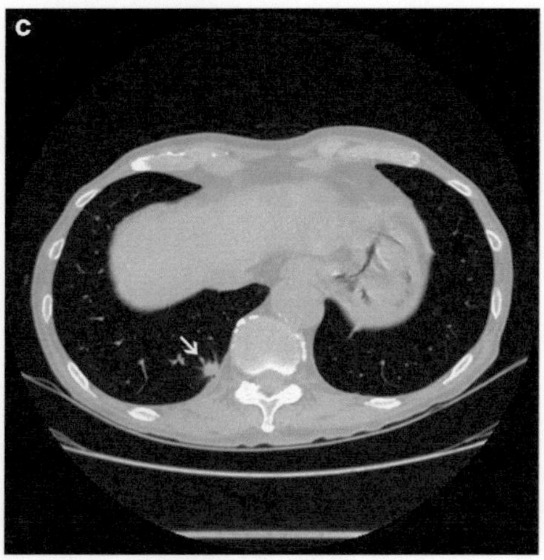

axial view (CT scan)

A CT scan of a 70-year-old male at a routine medical examination revealed a 1.0-cm nodule with spicular formation and pleural indentation at the right S^{10}c. CT-guided needle biopsy diagnosed it as adenocarcinoma. The final pathological diagnosis after S^{10}-segmentecotmy was pT1aN0M0 adenocarcinoma.

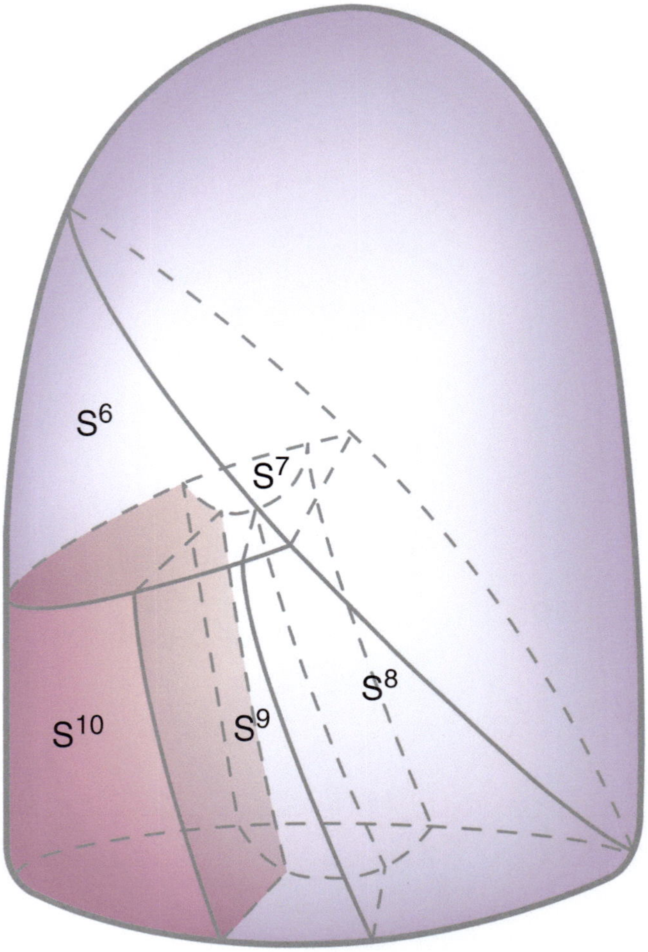

Fig. 4.4.1 S^{10}-segmentectomy is one of the most difficult procedures in segmentectomy, because S^{10} does not face the interlobar fissure. In addition, the border between S^6 and S^8 should be cut from the interlobar fissure to reach the S^{10}, which is not always easy because there is no landmark of the border between them. Furthermore, A^{10} is difficult to be identified and exposed due to branching from A^{9+10} in the dorsal direction, which is far away from the lateral thoracotomy. The segmental arteries (A^{7-10}) and bronchi (B^{7-10}) are identified from axial, coronal, and sagittal views on HRCT. The branching and size of B^7, B^8, B^9, and B^{10} are further confirmed by bronchoscopy after tracheal intubation. The branching patterns of segmental bronchus are B^8 and B^{9+10} in the frequency of 86%, B^{8+9} and B^{10} in 8%, and B^8, B^9, and B^{10} in 6%. When S^* is present (4% in frequency), care should be taken to differentiate between $A^{10}a$ and A^*, and between $B^{10}a$ and B^*. While the usual thoracotomy site is at the fifth or sixth intercostal space, the sixth intercostal space is preferable for reaching the A^9 and A^{10} branches, which is the point of S^{10}-segmentectomy.

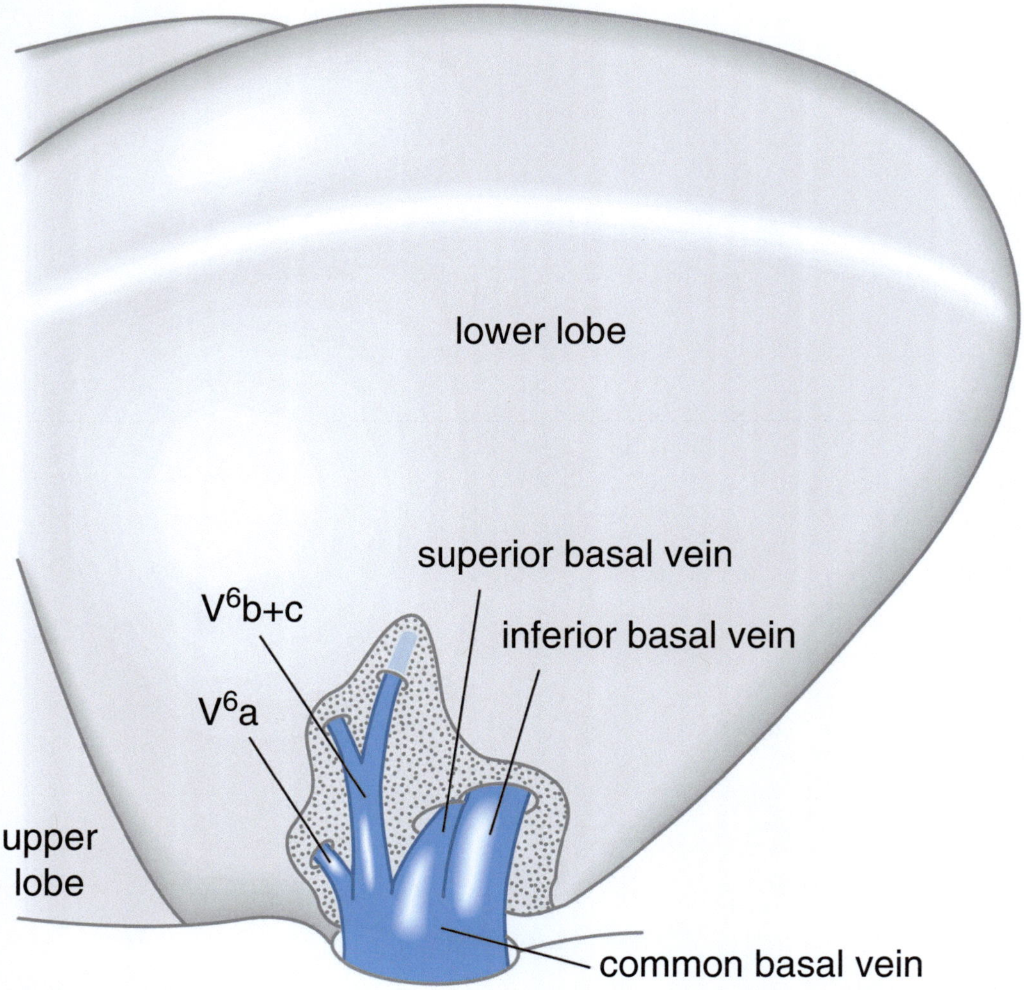

Fig. 4.4.2 The inferior pulmonary ligament is divided and then the inferior pulmonary vein is exposed. While exposure of the inferior pulmonary vein is not needed for S^8- or S^9-segmentectomy, it is necessary for S^{10}-segmentectomy, because S^{10} generally faces the inferior pulmonary vein. V^6b+c is exposed peripherally to clarify the border between S^6 and S^{10}. The V^6b+c is exposed peripherally, which will become a landmark for a later cutting between S^6 and S^{10}.

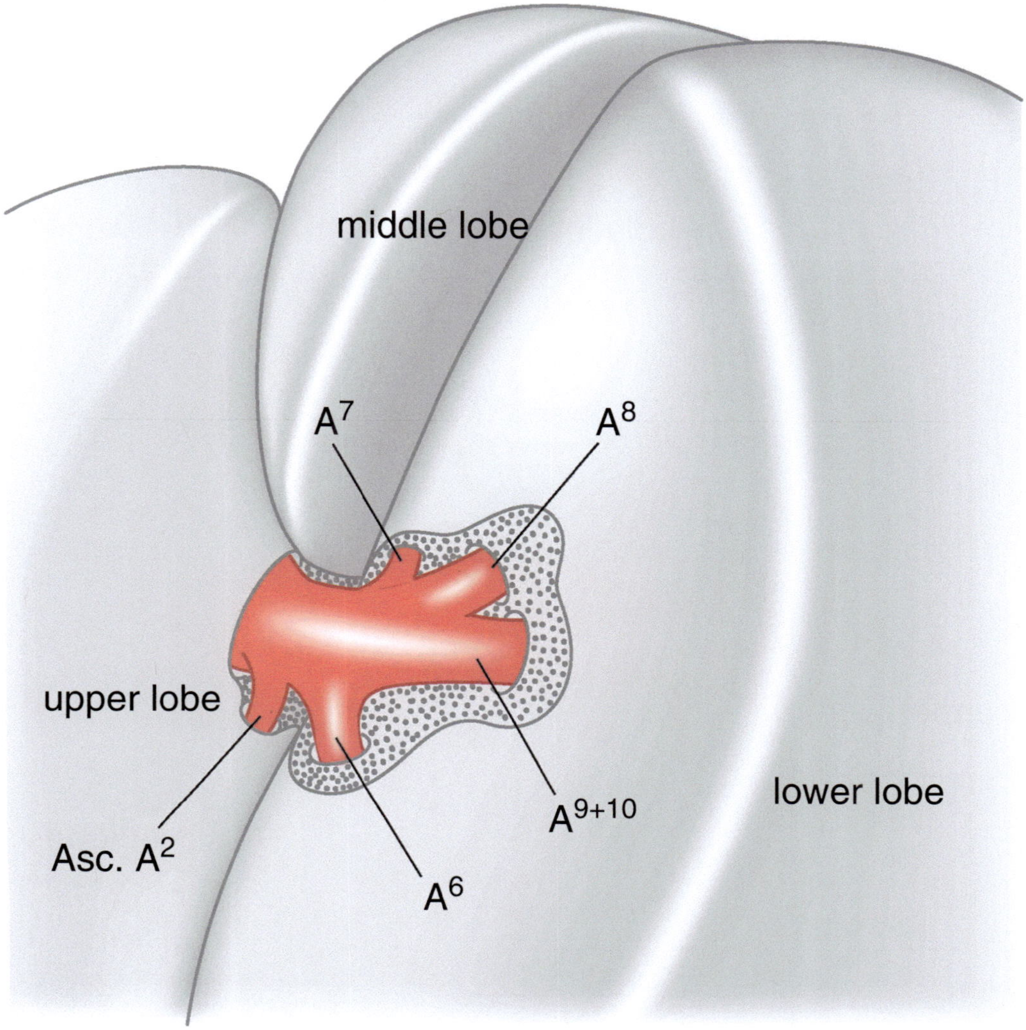

Fig. 4.4.3 The operator stands at the dorsal side of the patient, because A^{10} can be more easily visualized from that position than from the ventral side. The anatomical configuration of bronchial and arterial branching in the figures of this session is of the most frequent type, namely B^8 and B^{9+10}, and A^8 and A^{9+10}. The A^6, A^7, A^8, and A^{9+10} are exposed sufficiently. A^{9+10} is encircled with tape and exposed peripherally. When bronchoscopy shows that the trunk of B^{9+10} is long, that of A^{9+10} will also be long.

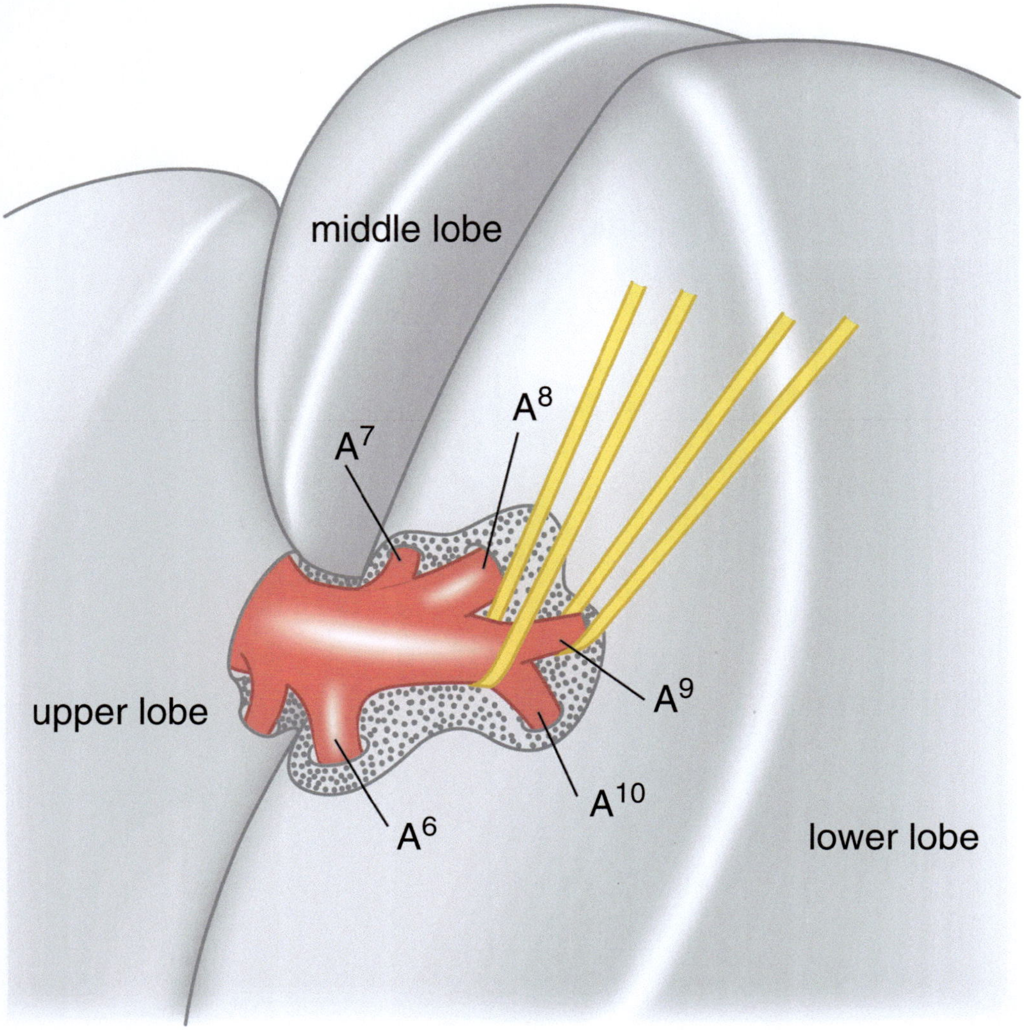

Fig. 4.4.4 A^9 and A^{10}, respectively, run in the lateral and dorsal directions. When A^{10} is difficult to be identified, the most dorsal branch is cut first, because it must be A^{10} or its branch but not the A^9-branch. Cutting the most dorsal branch reveals B^{10} behind it. The remaining arterial branches can be easily identified after cutting B^{10}, because the A^{10} and A^9 branches run, respectively, towards and away from the S^{10} scheduled for resection. Because there are fewer variations in bronchial branching than in arterial one, the latter can be identified from the former.

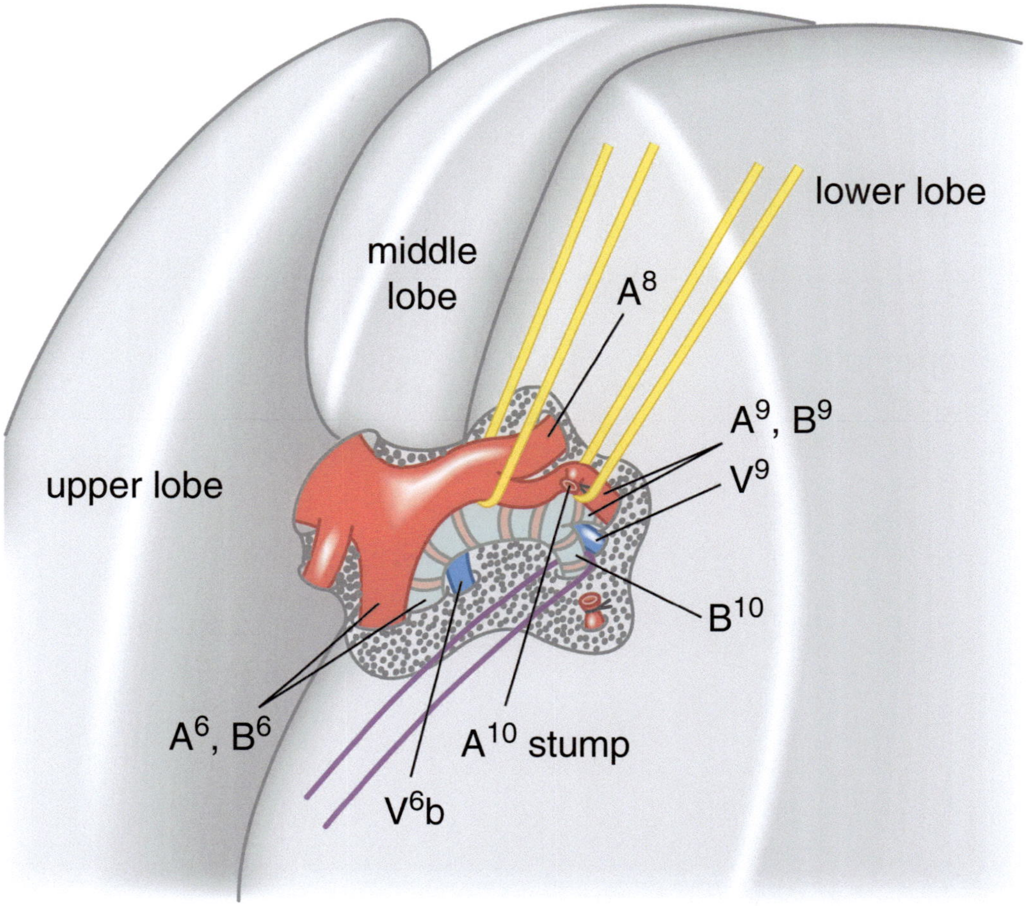

Fig. 4.4.5 B^{10} is carefully encircled with thread to avoid damaging V^{9} and V^{10} running behind it. B^{10} is confirmed by illumination from a bronchoscope inserted into B^{9} and B^{10}.

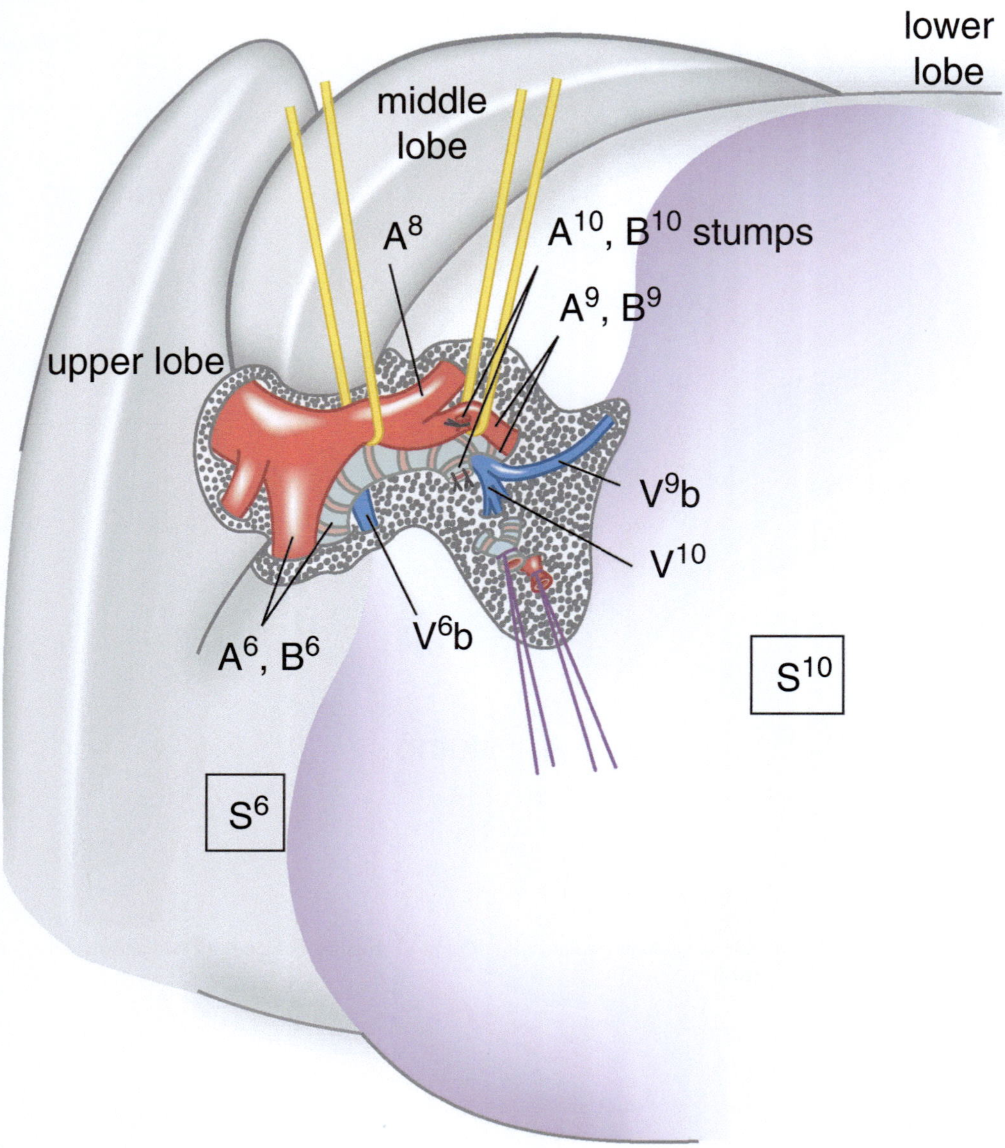

Fig. 4.4.6 S^{10} is selectively inflated either by inserting a bronchoscope into B^{10} followed by jet ventilation, or by cutting the B^{10} and inserting a catheter into the distal stump followed by air inflation. The distal stump is closed to trap air within S^{10}. The proximal stump of B^{10} is closed with suture or ligation. The distal stump of B^{10} is lifted and denuded peripherally at the back to move it away from the hilum. Lifting the distal B^{10}-stump exposes the V^{10} branches that run into the S^{10} segment scheduled for resection. Cutting V^{10} further elevates the distal stump of B^{10} together with the lung tissues on both sides of it, which are cut along the V^9b (between S^9 and S^{10}) and V^6c (between S^6 and S^{10}) and also towards the inflation–deflation line using electrocautery.

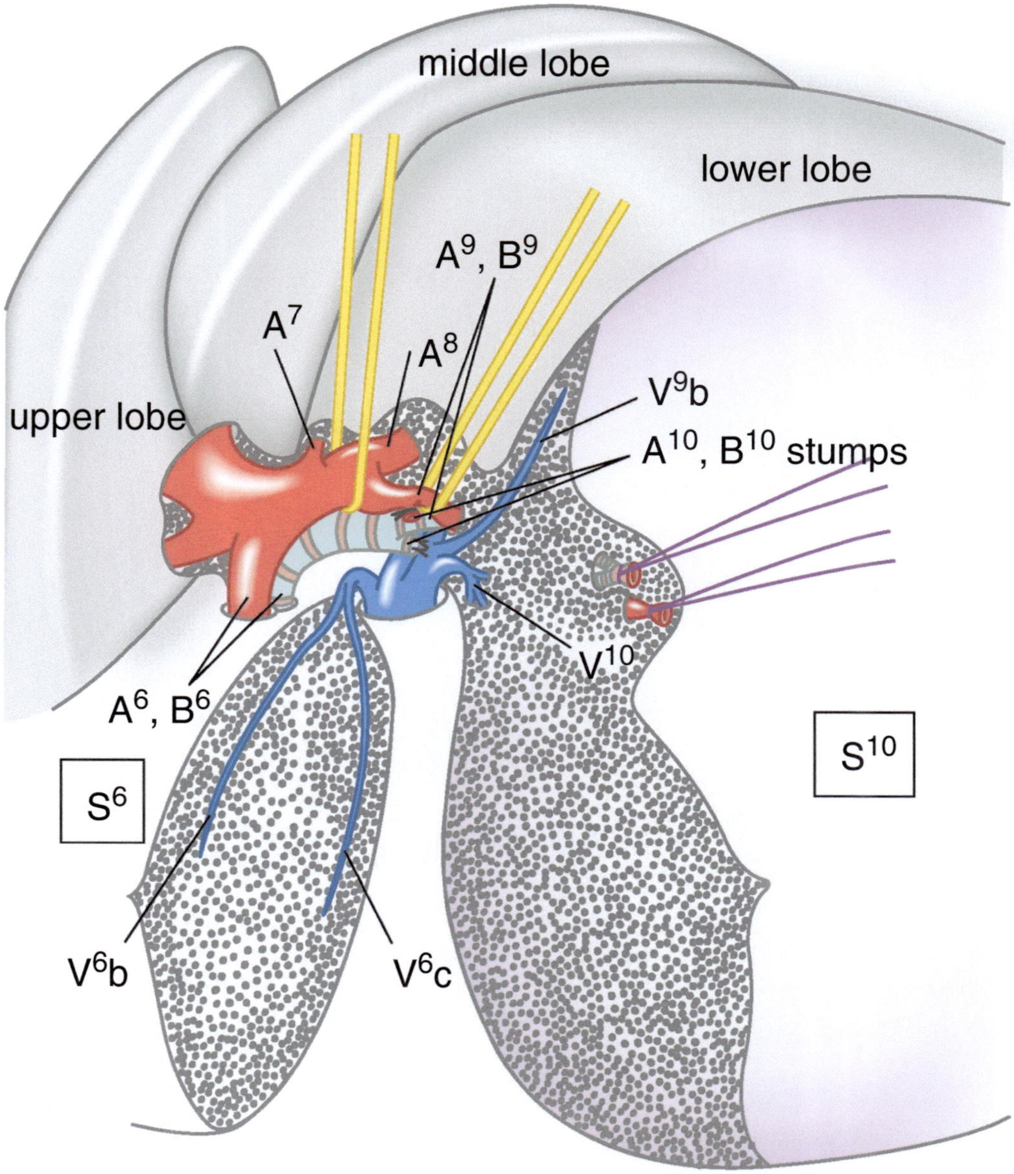

Fig. 4.4.7 When cutting lung tissue, the border between S^6 and S^{10} had better be cut first, because V^9 can be easily seen by dividing S^6 and S^{10}. V^6b and V^6c are preserved on the intersegmental plane of S^6. Because S^6 is finally divided from the basal segment, V^6b and V^6c is preserved on S^6 for S^6-venous return. V^9b runs along the inflation–deflation line between S^9 and S^{10}. Lung tissue is then cut along V^9b and also along the inflation–deflation line using electrocautery. V^9b is preserved on S^9 if the surgical margin is sufficient.

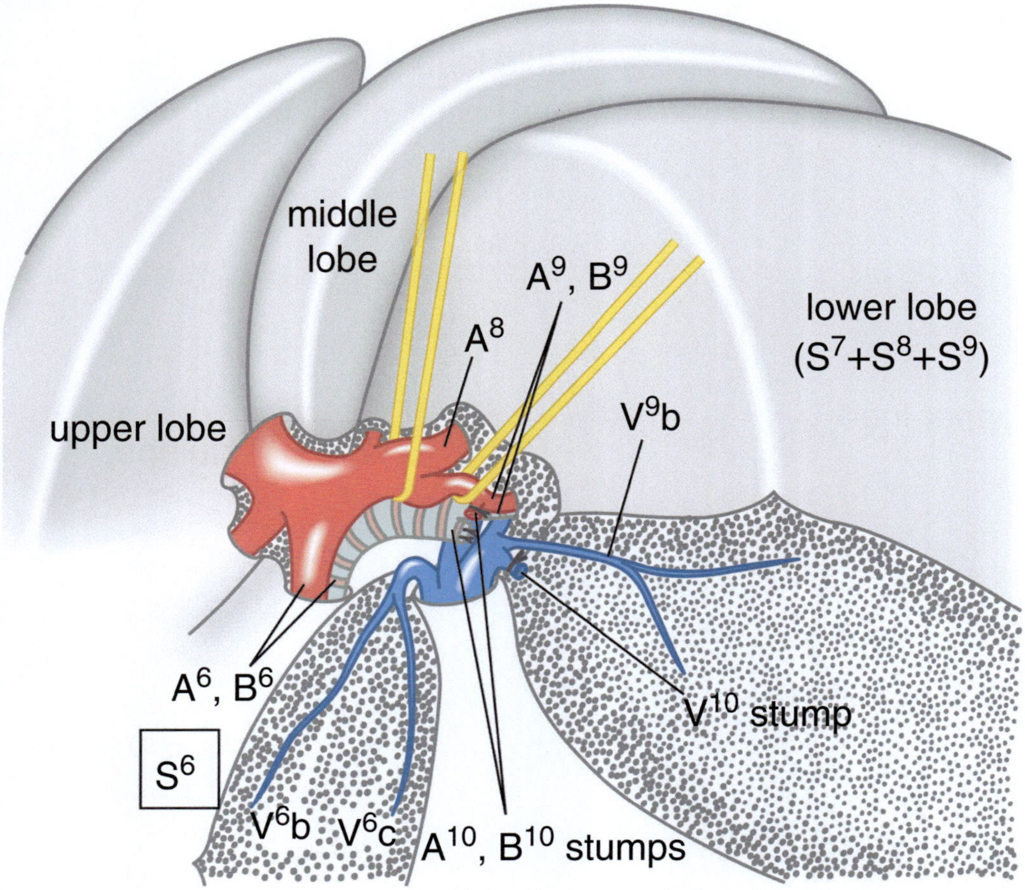

Fig. 4.4.8 S^6 and S^7+S^8+S^9 are completely separated after S^{10}-segmentectomy. The B^6, A^6 and A^{8-10} are encircled with tape. The posterior #12l and #13 (around B^6) lymph nodes, which lie along the lymphatic chain from S^{10} towards the #7 node, are dissected. The #11i and anterior #12l nodes located between the right middle and lower lobar bronchus, are also dissected.

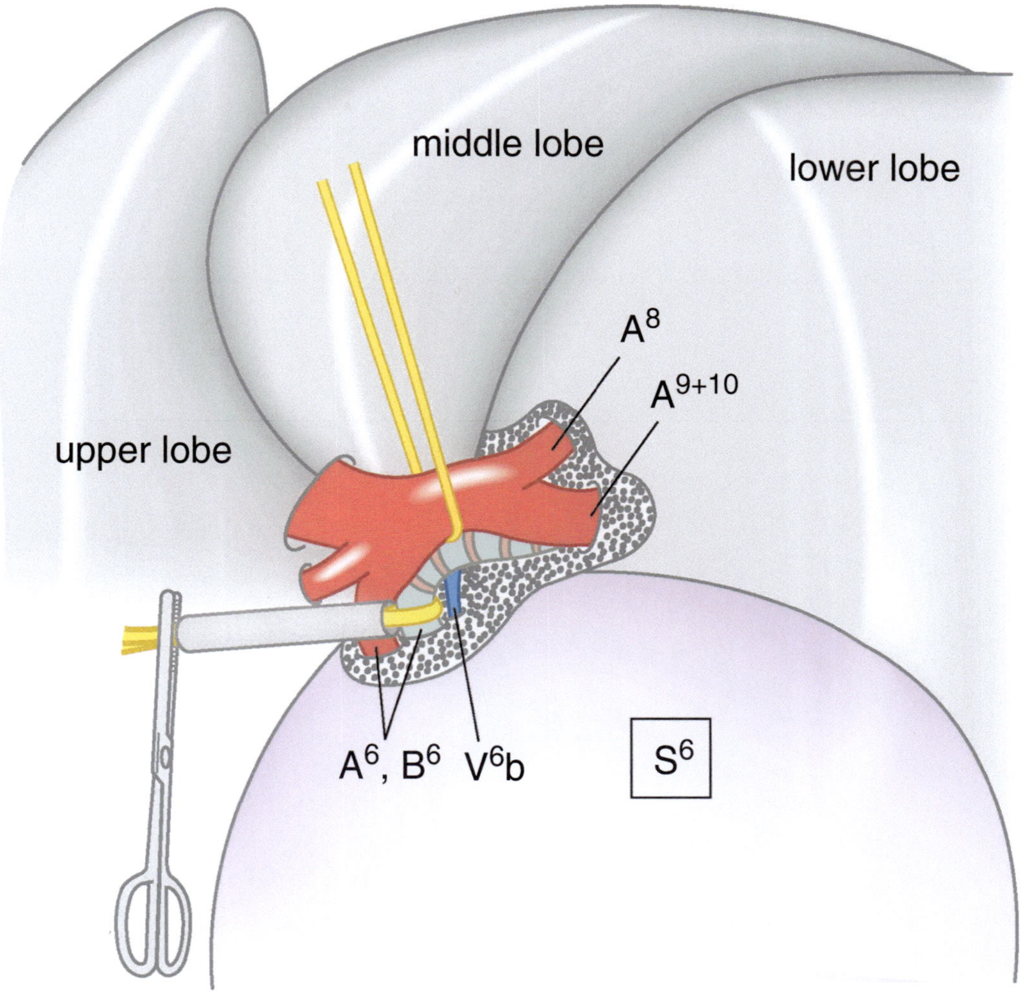

Fig. 4.4.9 Figures 4.4.9 and 4.4.10 show another approach to S^{10}-segmentectomy. The main difficulties encountered with S^{10}-segmentectomy arise from exposing and discriminating A^{10} from the interlobar artery. The approach only from the fissure can be complicated as described at the Fig. 4.4.3 of this session. Therefore, for another method to expose A^{10}, the procedure which divides S^6 and S^{10} at first is shown here. The concept of this approach is as follows: because S^6 and S^{10} are finally divided, the intersegmental plane between S^6 and S^{10} is cut at first, which facilitates exposing A^{10}. To do it, A^6 and B^6 are exposed first, and then B^6 is encircled with tape. B^6 is jet-ventilated and clamped using a tourniquet to create an inflation–deflation line between S^6 and S^{10} and also between S^6 and S^8.

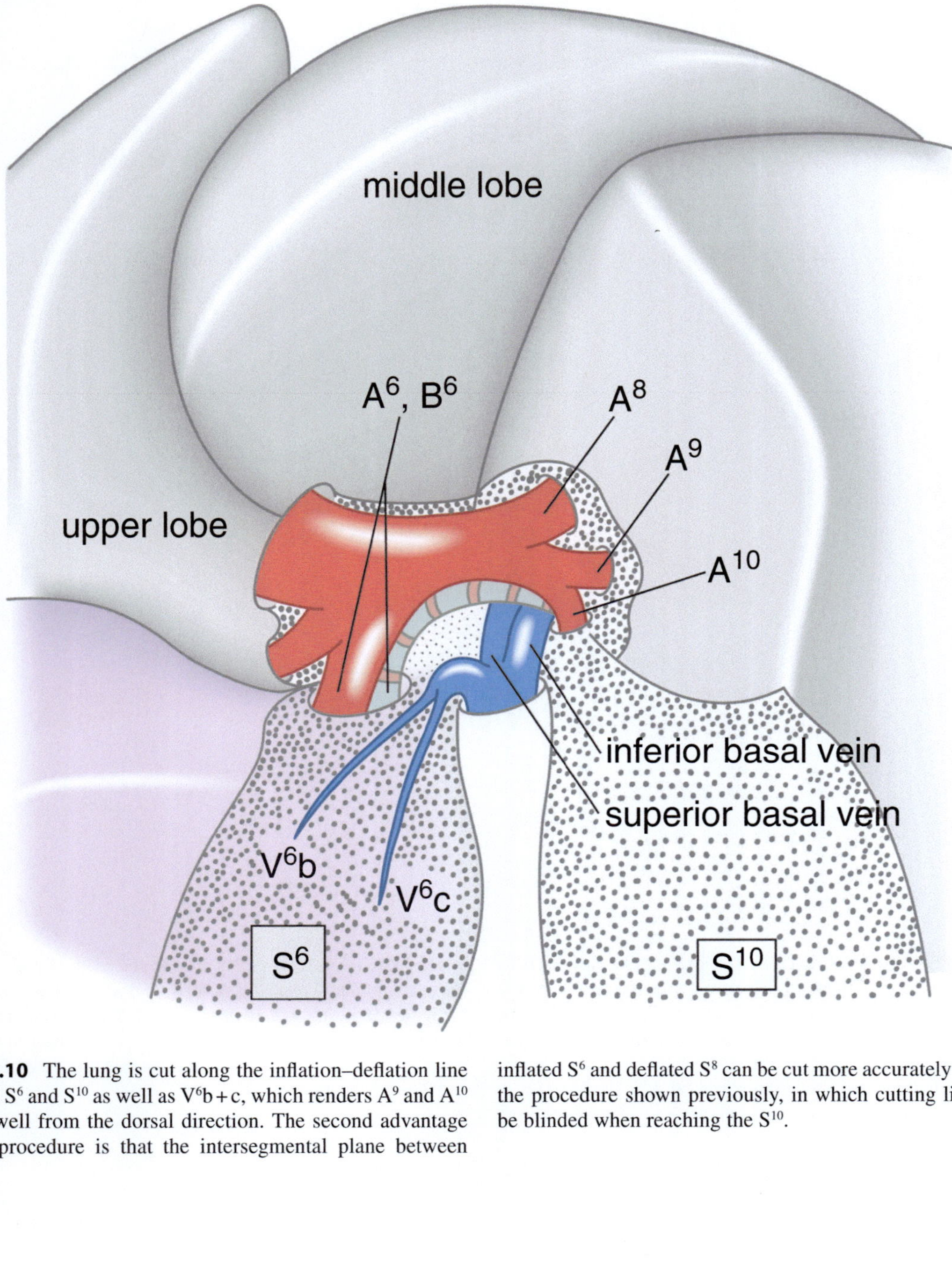

Fig. 4.4.10 The lung is cut along the inflation–deflation line between S^6 and S^{10} as well as V^6b+c, which renders A^9 and A^{10} visible well from the dorsal direction. The second advantage of this procedure is that the intersegmental plane between inflated S^6 and deflated S^8 can be cut more accurately than with the procedure shown previously, in which cutting line would be blinded when reaching the S^{10}.

4.5 Right S^9+S^{10} Segmentectomy

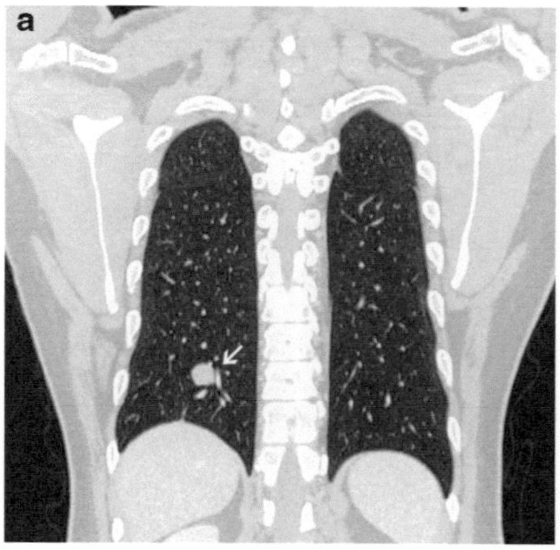

coronal view (CT scan)

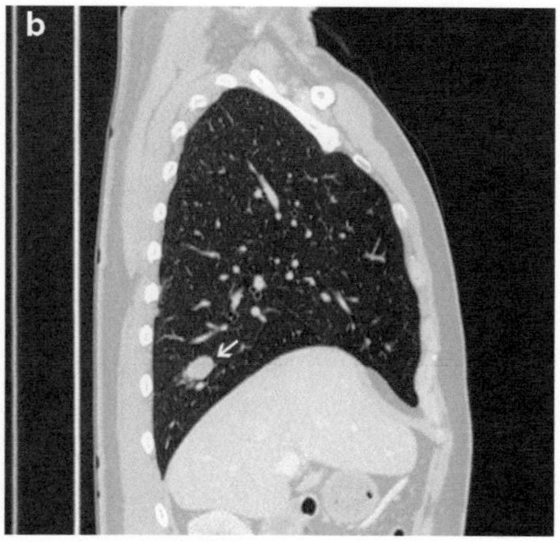

sagittal view (CT scan)

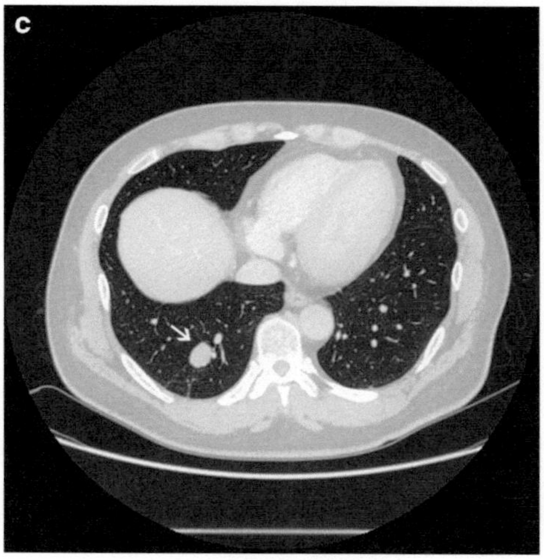

axial view (CT scan)

A CT scan of a 46-year-old male at a routine medical examination revealed a 2-cm round nodule at the border between the right S^9 and S^{10} that was diagnosed as carcinoid from a CT-guided needle biopsy specimen. Segmentectomy for right S^{9+10} was proceeded, and the final pathological diagnosis was a pT1aN0M0 carcinoid.

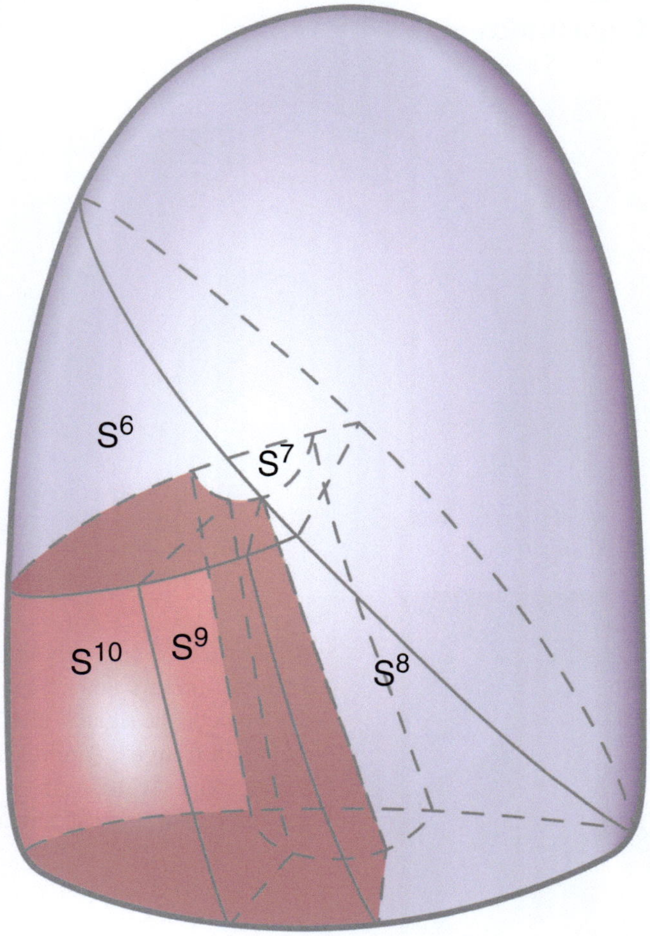

Fig. 4.5.1 The segmental arteries (A^{7-10}) and bronchi (B^{7-10}) are identified from axial, coronal, and sagittal views on HRCT. After tracheal intubation, the branching and diameter of each B^7, B^8, B^9, and B^{10} are further confirmed by bronchoscopy. The branching patterns of B^{8-10} are as follows: two branches with B^8 and B^{9+10} (86% in frequency), B^{8+9} and B^{10} (8%), and three with B^8, B^9, and B^{10} (6%). The segmental bronchus and artery in the figures of this session branch into the most frequent type, i.e. B^8 and B^{9+10}, and A^8 and A^{9+10}, respectively.

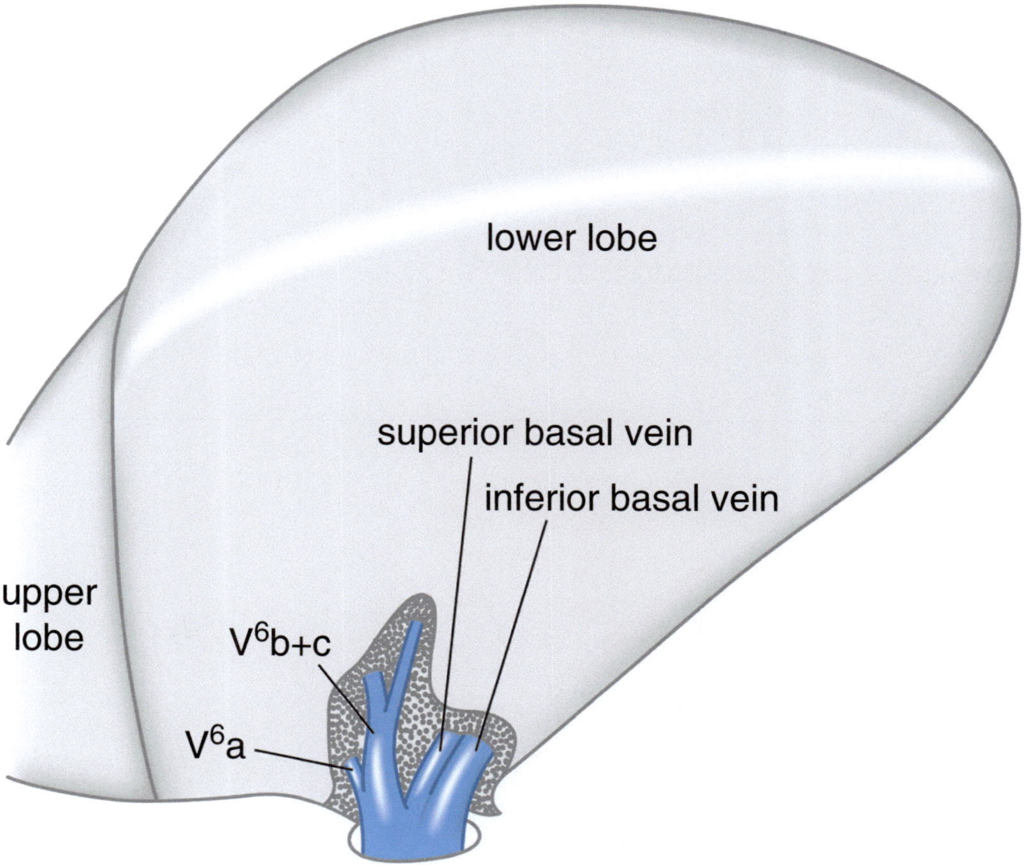

Fig. 4.5.2 The inferior pulmonary ligament is divided to expose the inferior pulmonary vein, V^6, and the common basal pulmonary vein. The inferior basal pulmonary vein should not be cut at this point, because the frequency of V^{9+10} being the inferior basal pulmonary vein is only 18%.

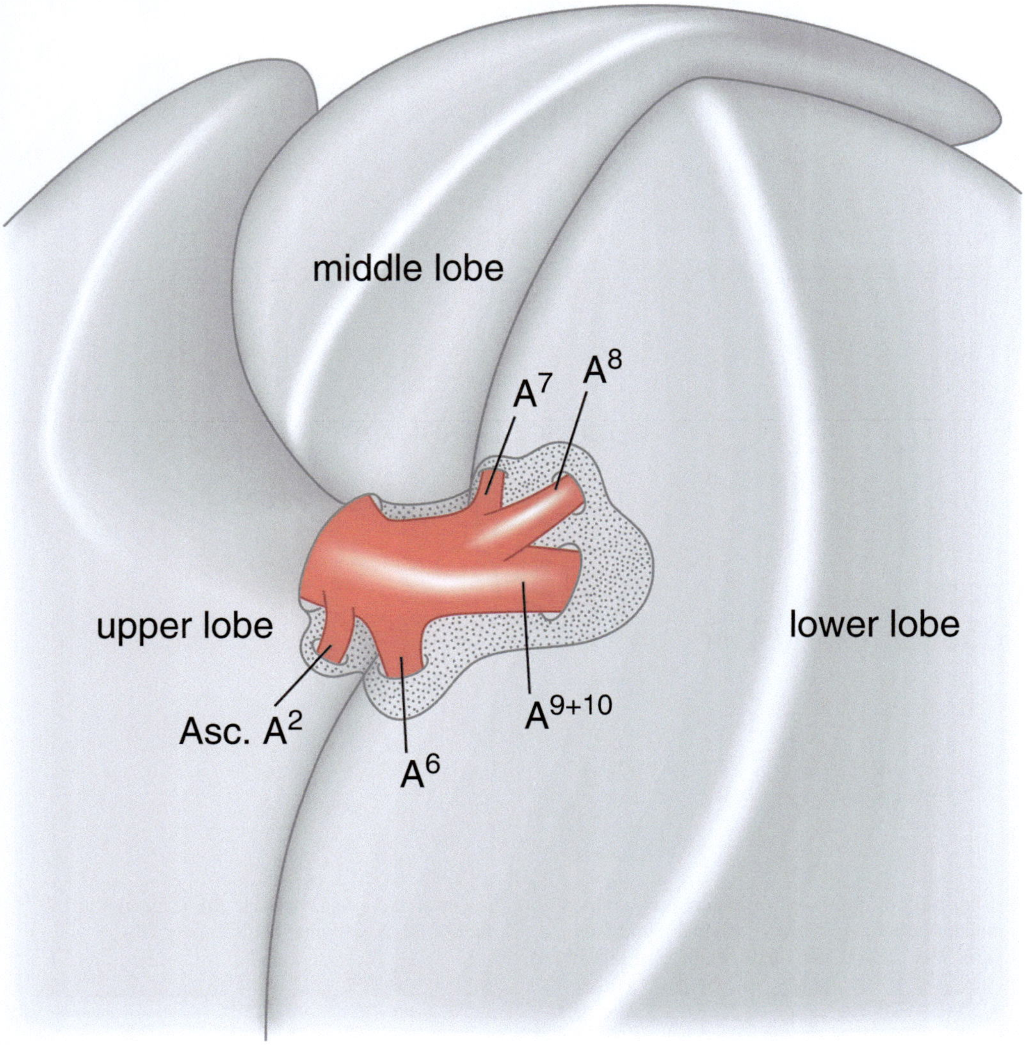

Fig. 4.5.3 The operator stands at the dorsal side of the patient. The branches of A^6, A^7, A^8, and A^{9+10} are exposed and confirmed, which is critically important during segmentectomy of the lower lobe. A^{9+10} is encircled with tape and exposed peripherally. The branching of A^8a and A^9a is sometimes complicated, such as A^8a branching from A^9 and A^9a from A^8.

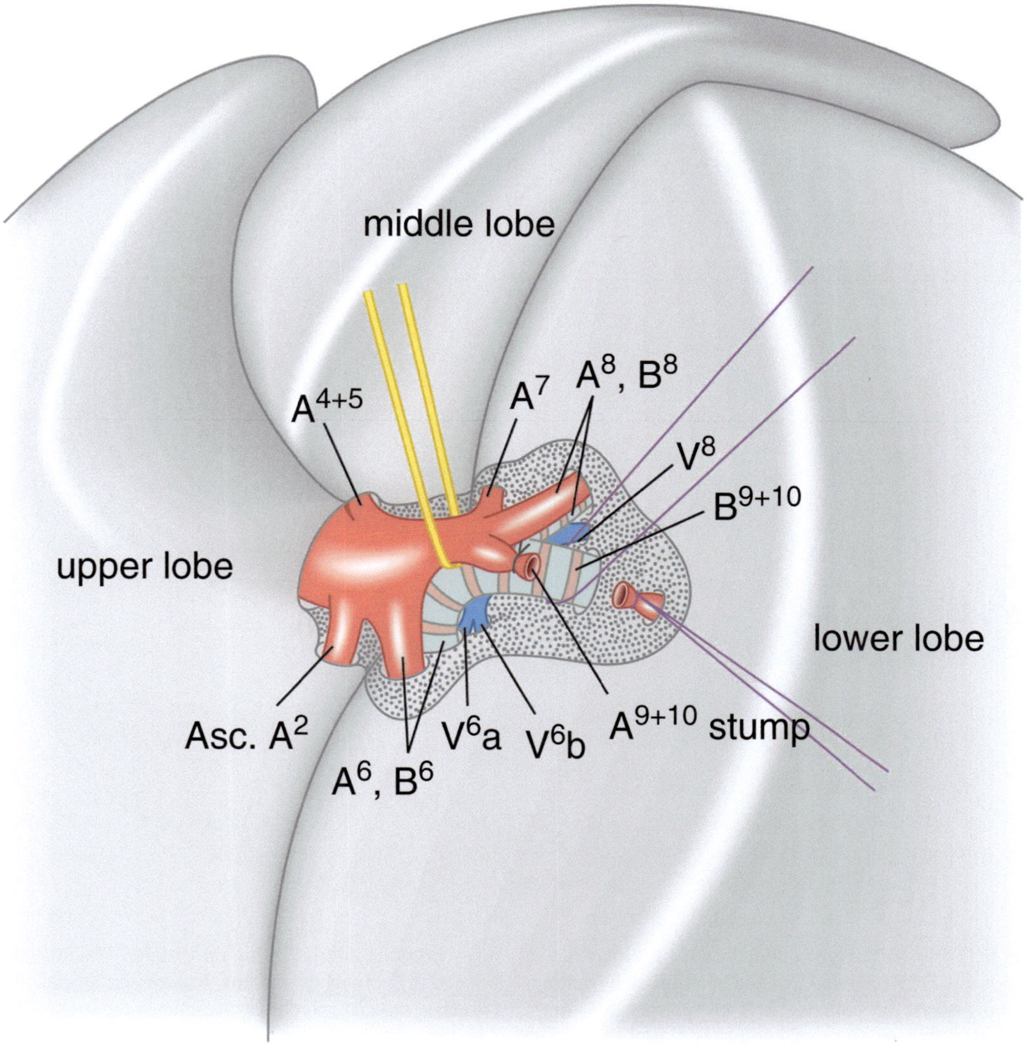

Fig. 4.5.4 After cutting A^{9+10}, B^{9+10} is visualized behind it. The B^{9+10} is carefully encircled with thread to avoid damage to V^8 which runs behind it. B^{9+10} can be also confirmed by illumination from a bronchoscope inserted into B^8, B^9 and B^{10}.

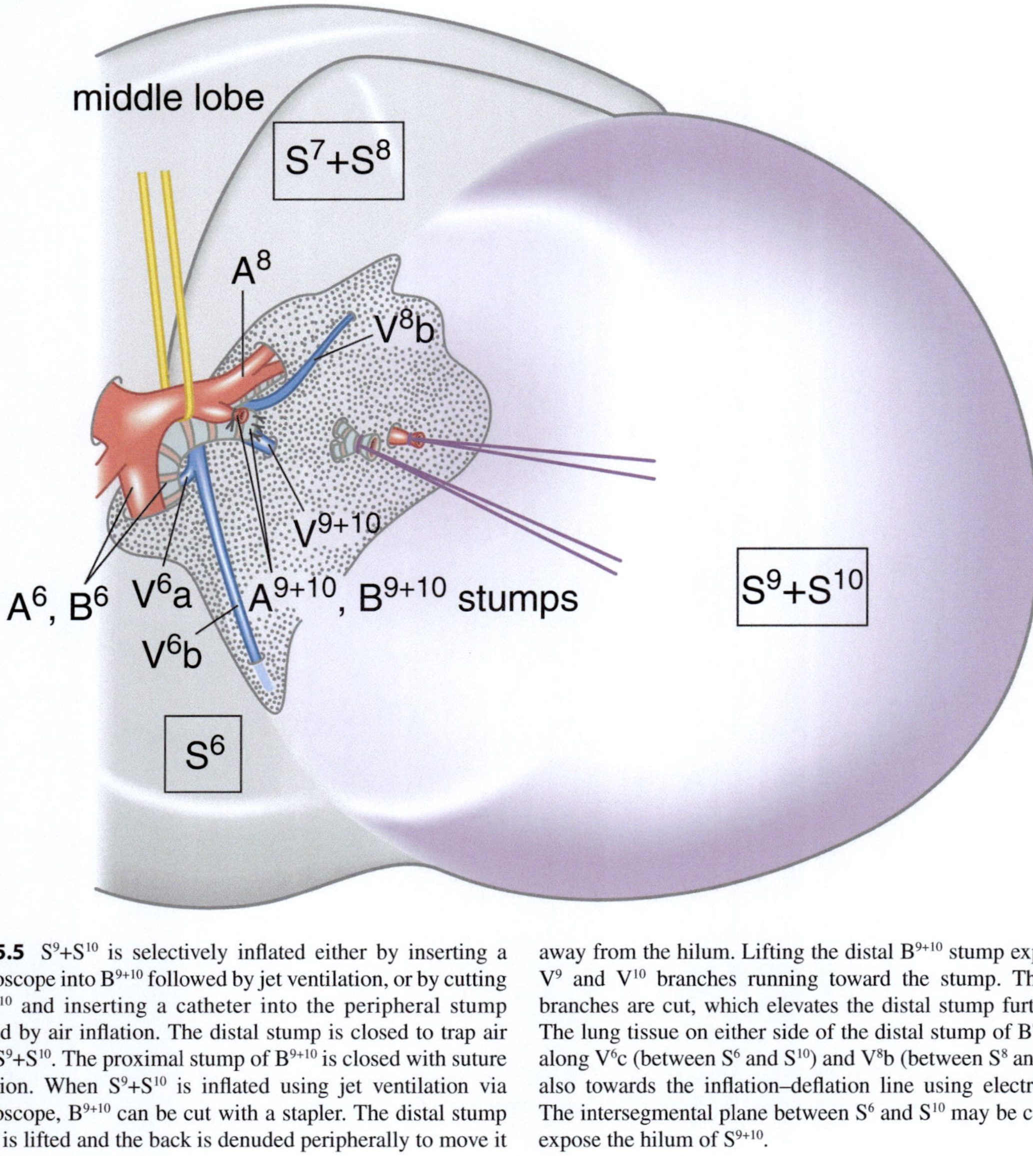

Fig. 4.5.5 S^9+S^{10} is selectively inflated either by inserting a bronchoscope into B^{9+10} followed by jet ventilation, or by cutting the B^{9+10} and inserting a catheter into the peripheral stump followed by air inflation. The distal stump is closed to trap air within S^9+S^{10}. The proximal stump of B^{9+10} is closed with suture or ligation. When S^9+S^{10} is inflated using jet ventilation via bronchoscope, B^{9+10} can be cut with a stapler. The distal stump of B^{9+10} is lifted and the back is denuded peripherally to move it away from the hilum. Lifting the distal B^{9+10} stump exposes the V^9 and V^{10} branches running toward the stump. These vein branches are cut, which elevates the distal stump furthermore. The lung tissue on either side of the distal stump of B^{9+10} is cut along V^6c (between S^6 and S^{10}) and V^8b (between S^8 and S^9) and also towards the inflation–deflation line using electrocautery. The intersegmental plane between S^6 and S^{10} may be cut first to expose the hilum of S^{9+10}.

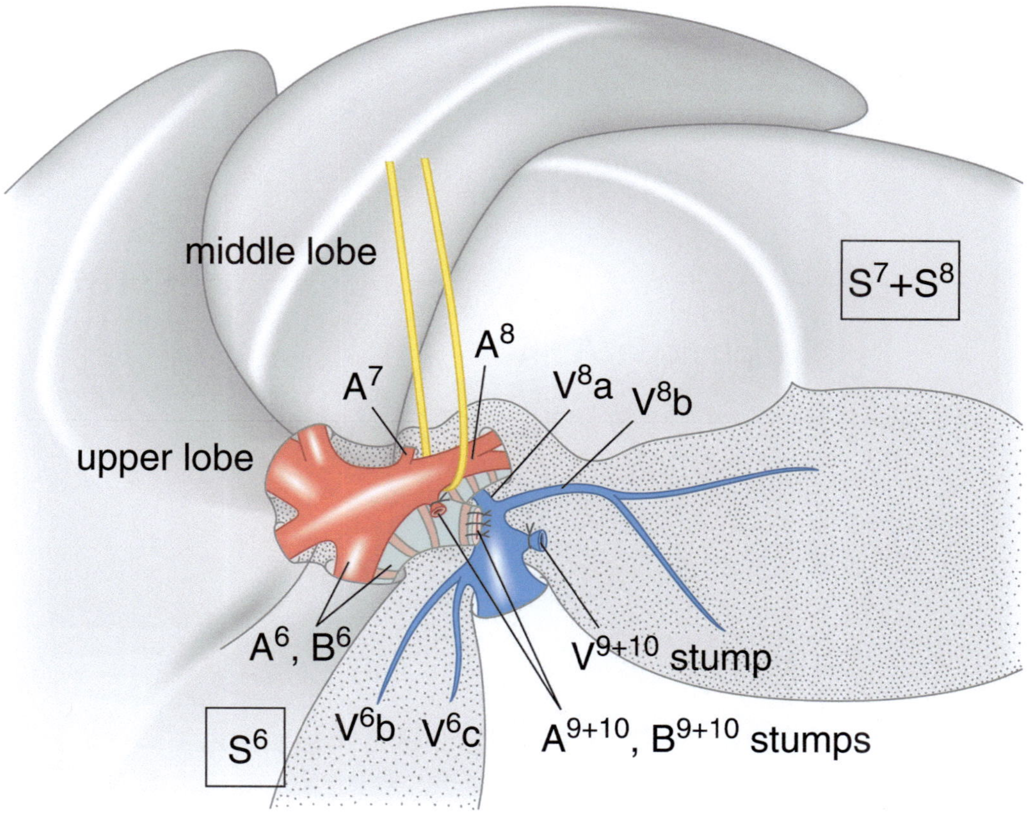

Fig. 4.5.6 S^9+S^{10}-segmentectomy completely divide the S^6 and S^7+S^8. V^6b and V^6c are preserved on S^6 and V^8b is preserved on S^8. If the surgical margin is sufficient, these segmental veins are preserved to maintain the venous return from S^6 and S^8.

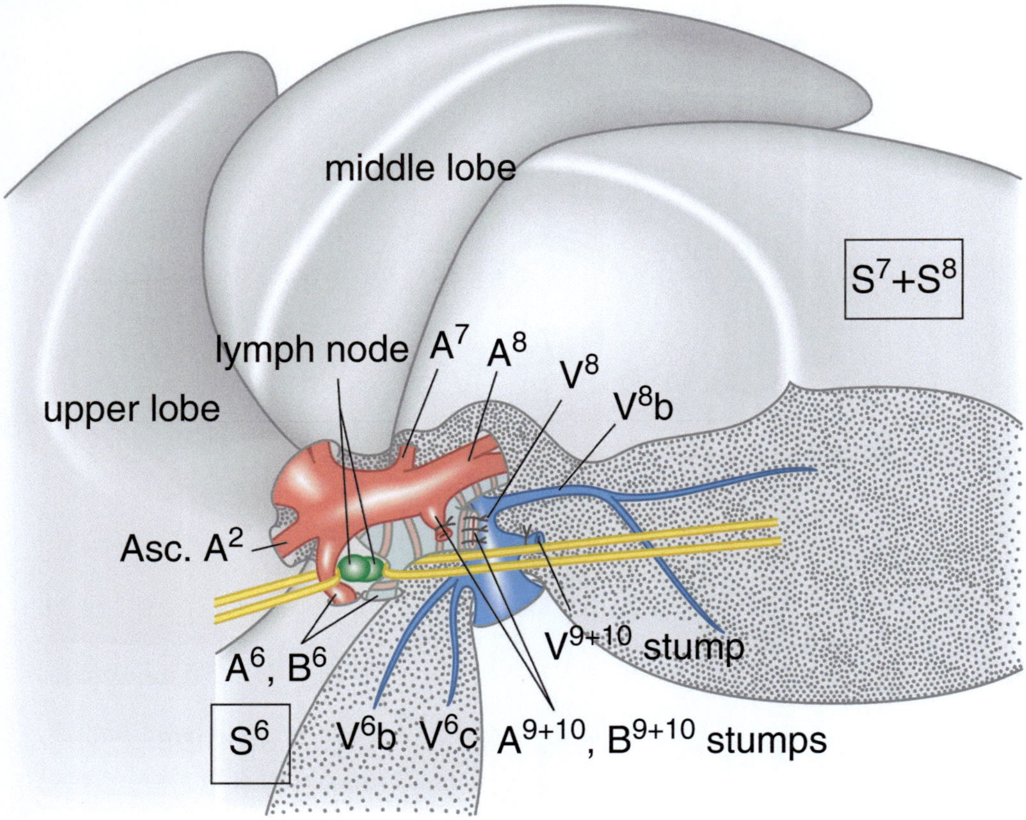

Fig. 4.5.7 B^6, A^6, and A^{8-10} are encircled with tape for dissection of the hilar lymph nodes. The posterior #12l and #13 (around B^6) nodes, which lie along the lymphatic chain from S^9 and S^{10} towards the #7 node, are dissected.

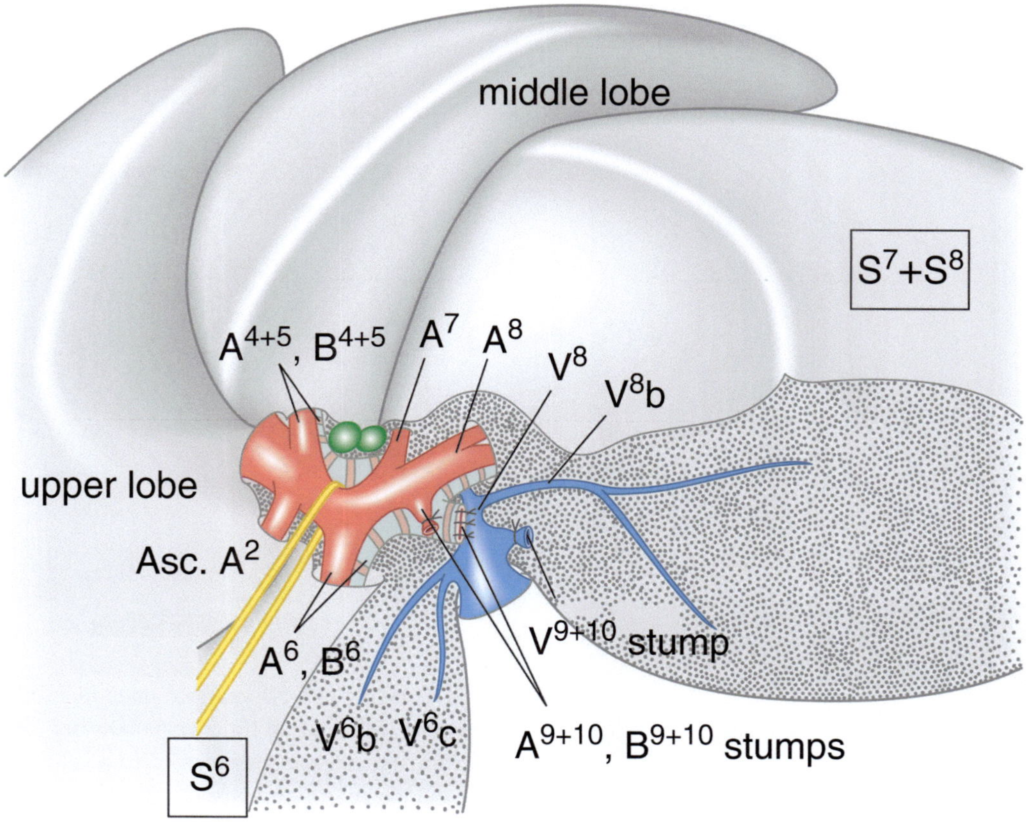

Fig. 4.5.8 A^{6-10} is encircled with tape for dissecting the anterior #12l and #11i nodes which lie between the right middle and lower lobar bronchus.

4.6 Right $S^6 + S^8a$ Segmentectomy

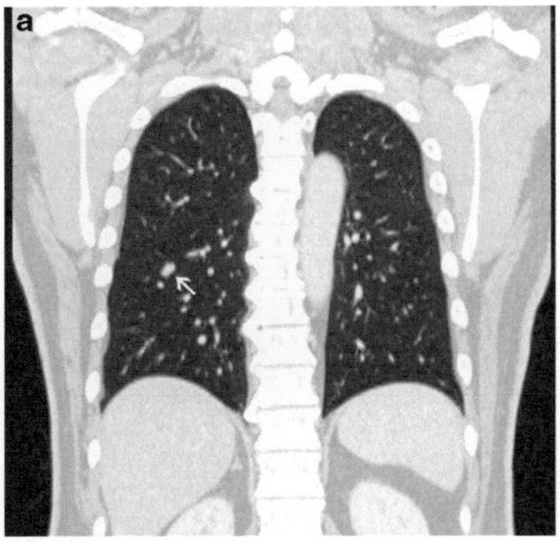

coronal view (CT scan)

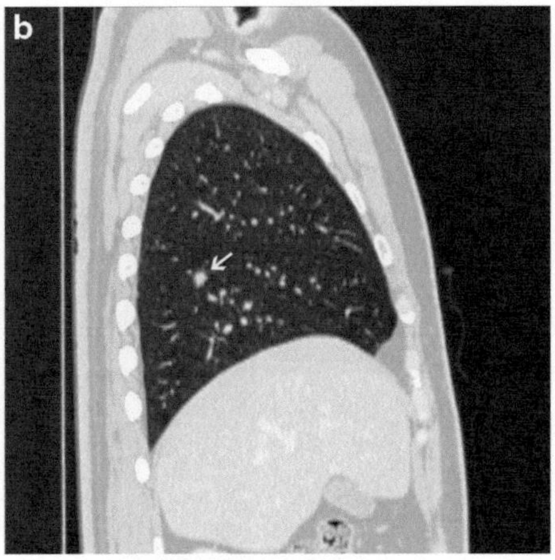

sagittal view (CT scan)

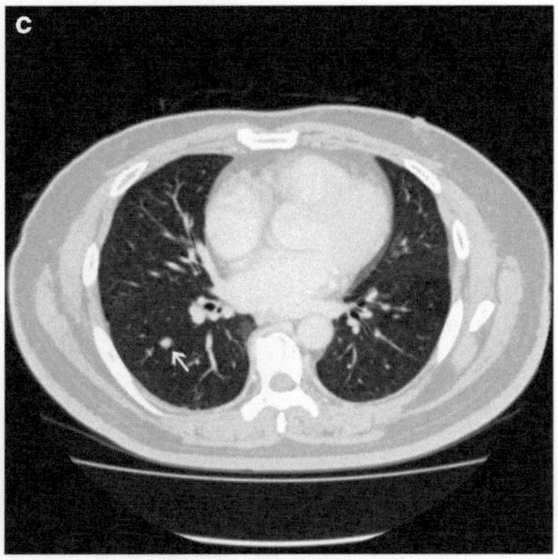

axial view (CT scan)

A GGO lesion in a 58-year-old male identified on CT had been followed up for 5 years. During that period, it had increased and transformed to a solid tumor that was diagnosed as adenocarcinoma from a CT-guided needle biopsy specimen. The tumor was localized within S^6 and close to V^6b, which runs between S^6 and S^8a. Therefore, the S^6+S^8a-segmentectomy was proceeded. The final pathological diagnosis was pT1aN0M0 papillary adenocarcinoma.

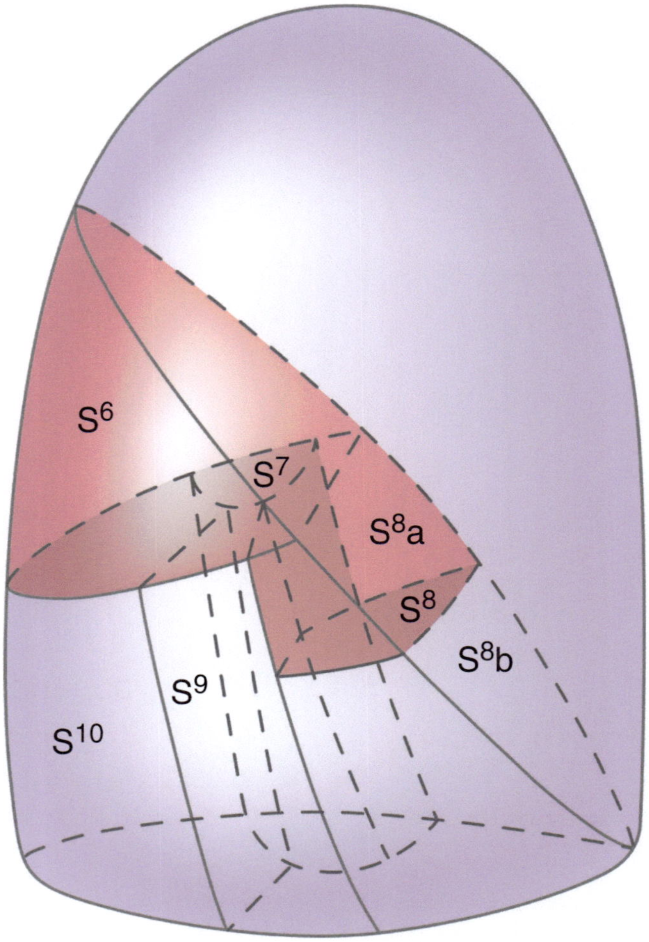

Fig. 4.6.1 This procedure is for a tumor in S^6b that is located near S^8a. The segmental arteries (A^{7-10}) and bronchi (B^{7-10}) are identified from axial, coronal, and sagittal views on HRCT. The branching and size of B^7, B^8, B^9, and B^{10} are further checked by bronchoscope after tracheal intubation. The branching patterns of bronchus are as follows: two branches into B^8 and B^{9+10} (86% in frequency), B^{8+9} and B^{10} (8%), and three into B^8, B^9, and B^{10} (6%). The optimal site of the thoracotomy is usually a lateral thoracotomy at the fifth intercostal space.

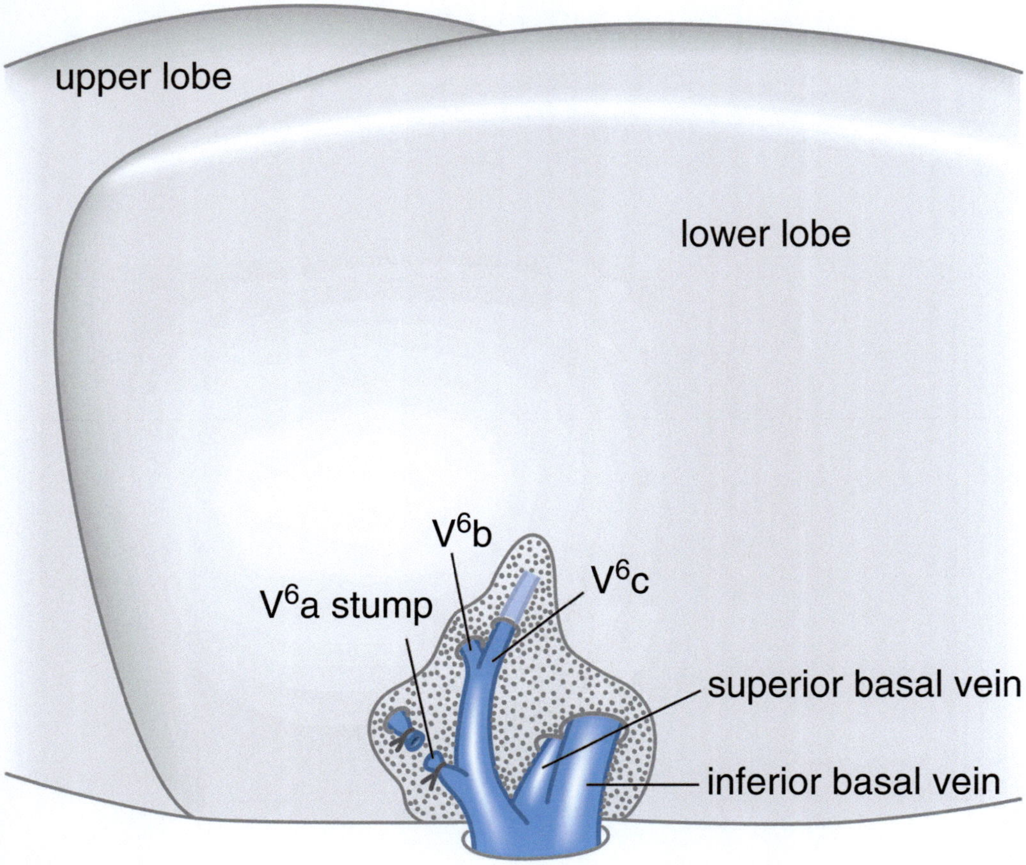

Fig. 4.6.2 The inferior pulmonary vein is exposed to identify V^6, which frequently branches into V^6a and V^6b+c. V^6a (between S^6a and S^6b+c) is cut. V^6b and V^6c are sometimes difficult to identify at this point, because they branch deeply into lung tissue. V^6b+c is exposed peripherally, which can be used as a landmark for later cutting between S^6 and S^{10}.

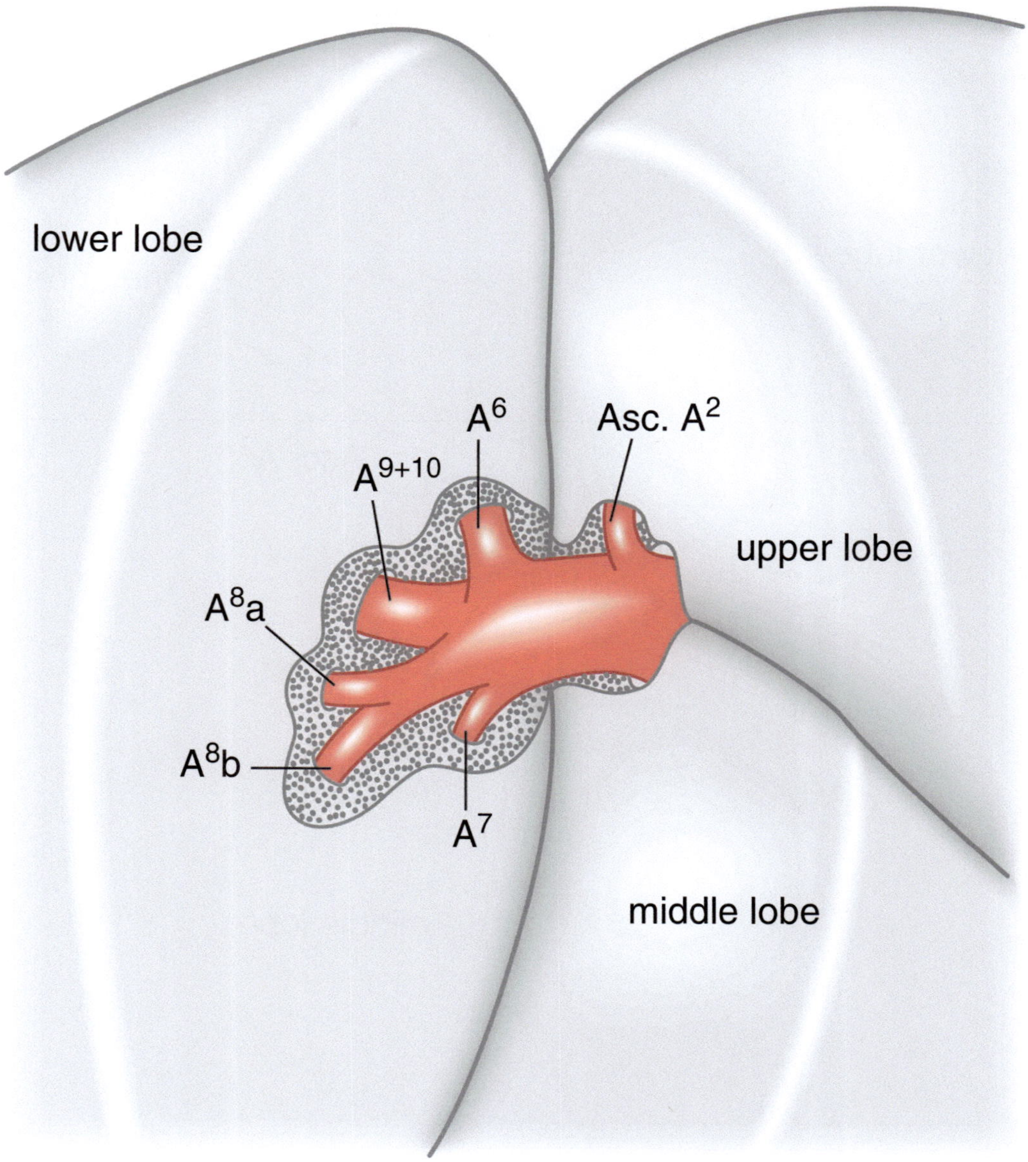

Fig. 4.6.3 In the figures of this session, the operator is positioned at the ventral side of the patient. The branches of A^6, A^7, A^8, and A^{9+10} are exposed. Because segmental artery branching in the lower lobe widely varies, all branches should be exposed for identification.

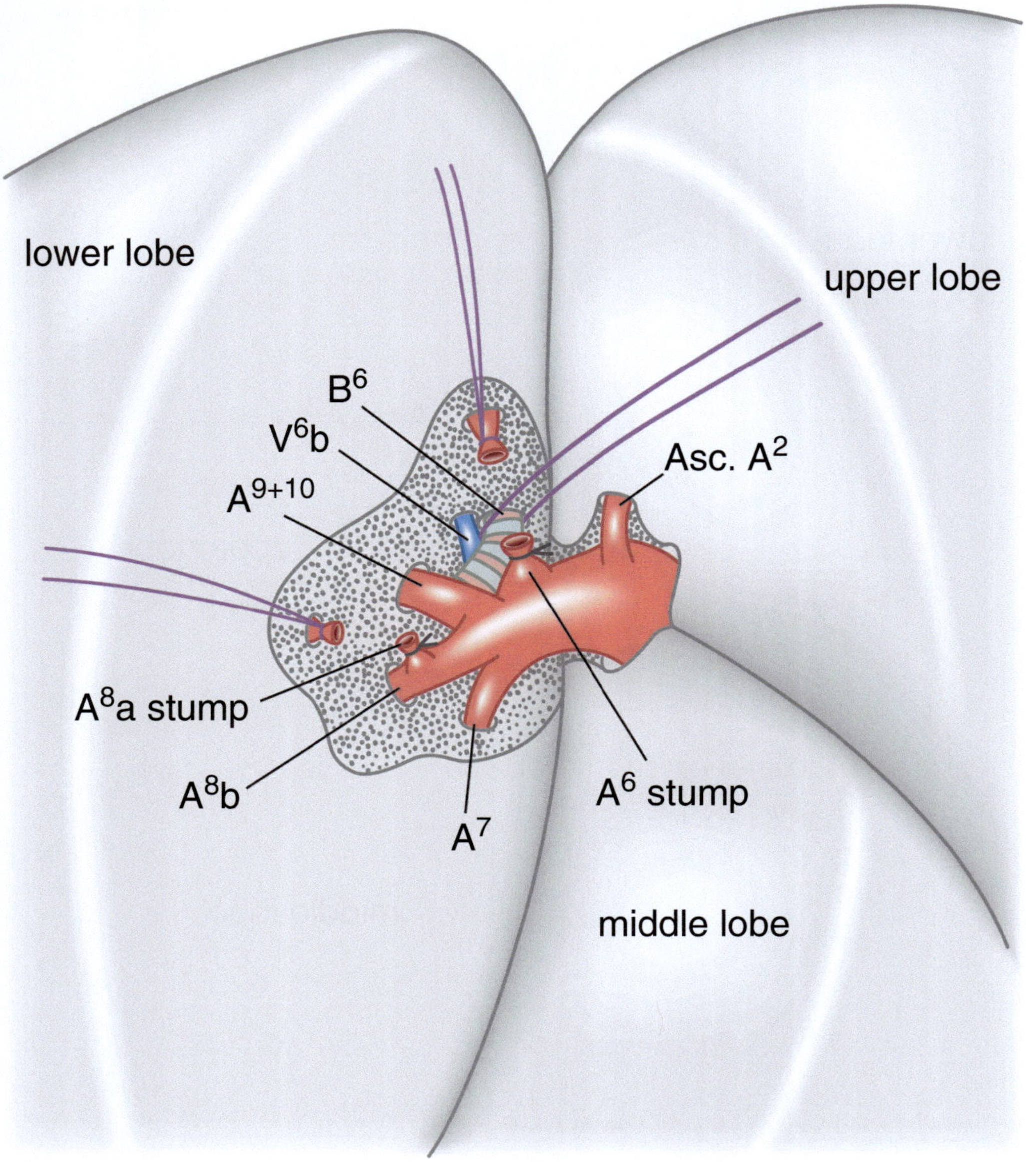

Fig. 4.6.4 A^6 is cut. The B^6, which runs in caudal and backside of A^6, is exposed. The B^6 is carefully encircled with thread to avoid damaging V^6b running at the back of it.

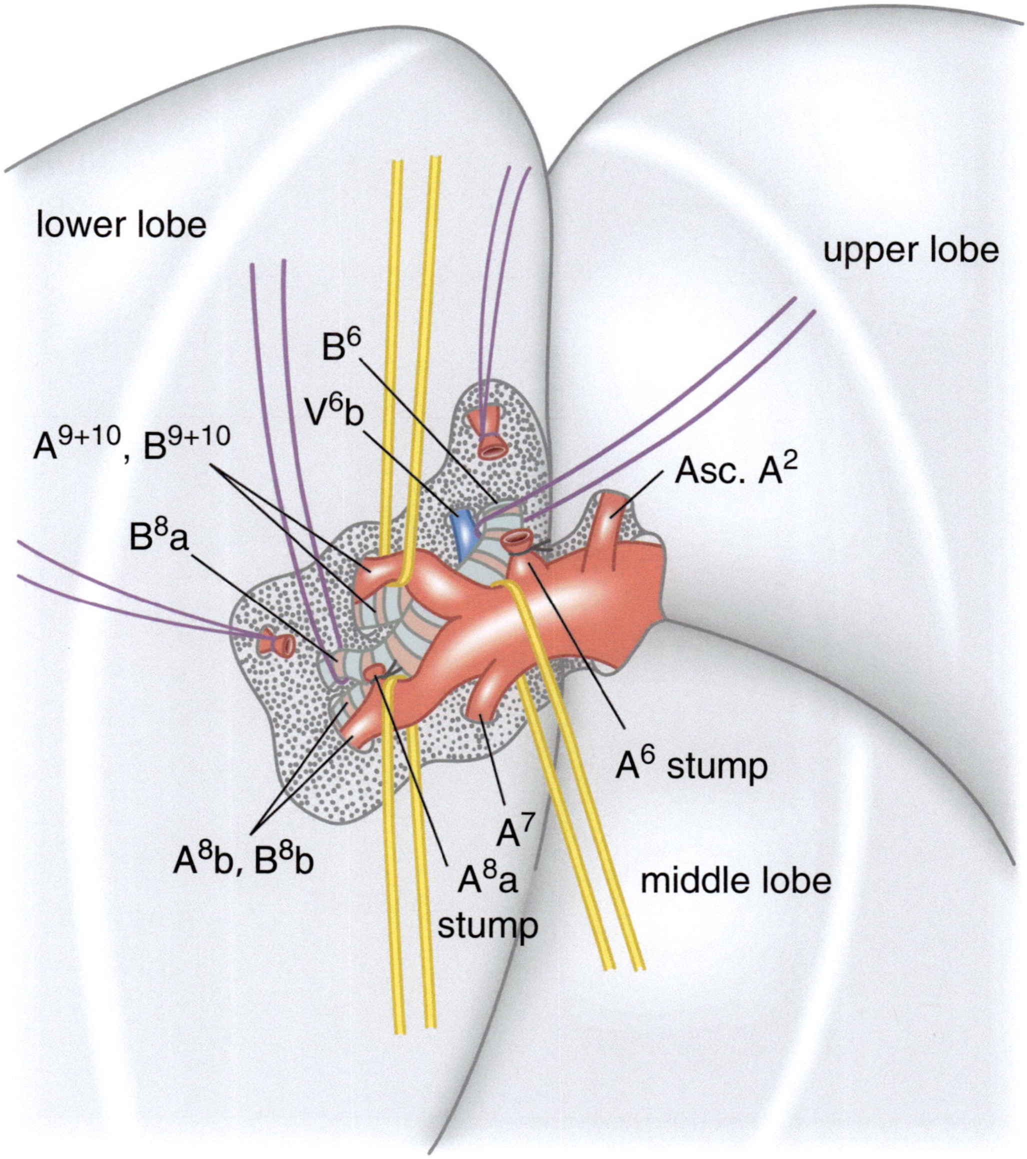

Fig. 4.6.5 A^8 is encircled with tape and exposed peripherally. Sometimes, A^8a branches from A^{9+10} and A^9a branches from A^8. Cutting A^8a reveals B^8a running behind.

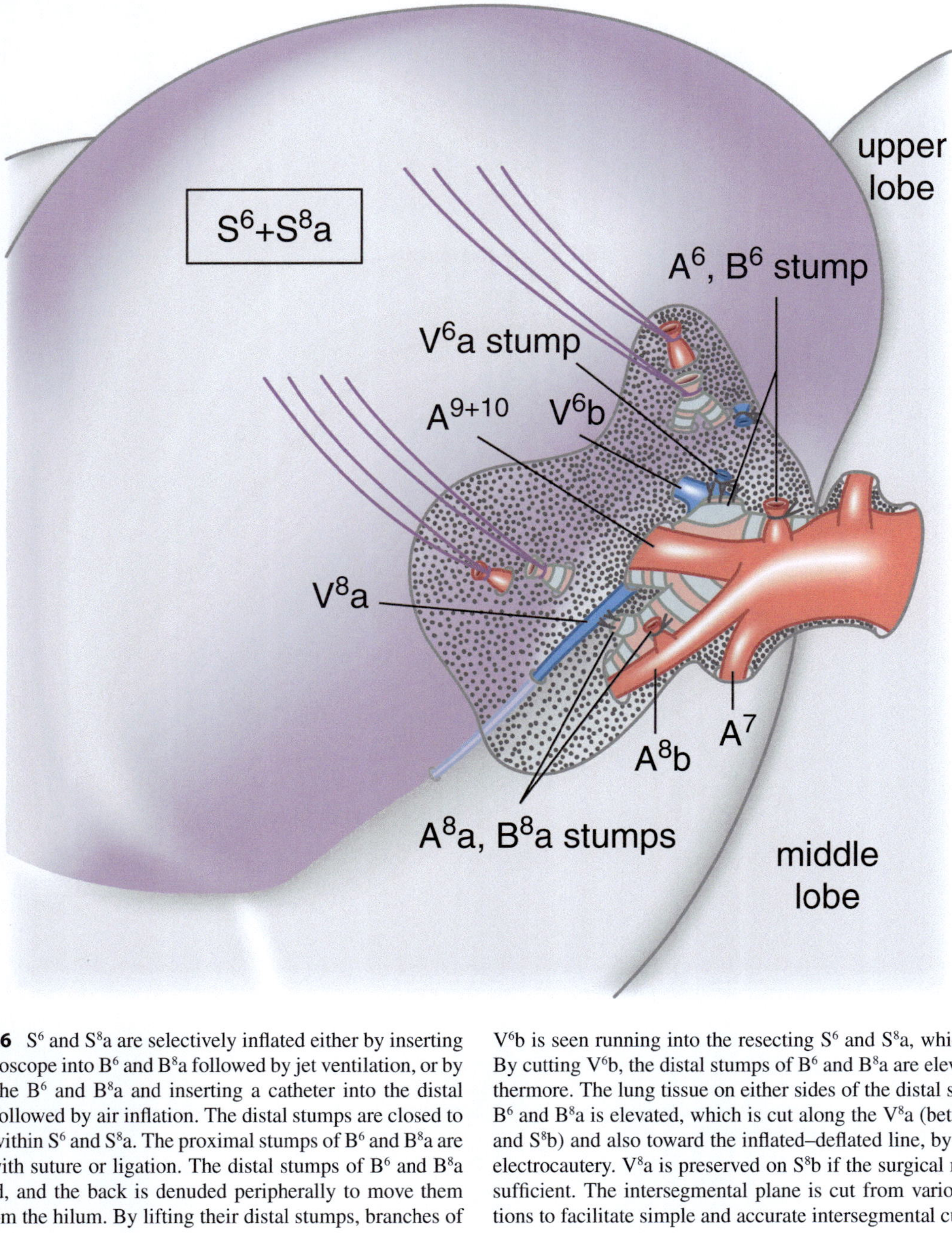

Fig. 4.6.6 S^6 and S^8a are selectively inflated either by inserting a bronchoscope into B^6 and B^8a followed by jet ventilation, or by cutting the B^6 and B^8a and inserting a catheter into the distal stumps followed by air inflation. The distal stumps are closed to trap air within S^6 and S^8a. The proximal stumps of B^6 and B^8a are closed with suture or ligation. The distal stumps of B^6 and B^8a are lifted, and the back is denuded peripherally to move them away from the hilum. By lifting their distal stumps, branches of V^6b is seen running into the resecting S^6 and S^8a, which is cut. By cutting V^6b, the distal stumps of B^6 and B^8a are elevated furthermore. The lung tissue on either sides of the distal stumps of B^6 and B^8a is elevated, which is cut along the V^8a (between S^8a and S^8b) and also toward the inflated–deflated line, by using an electrocautery. V^8a is preserved on S^8b if the surgical margin is sufficient. The intersegmental plane is cut from various directions to facilitate simple and accurate intersegmental cutting.

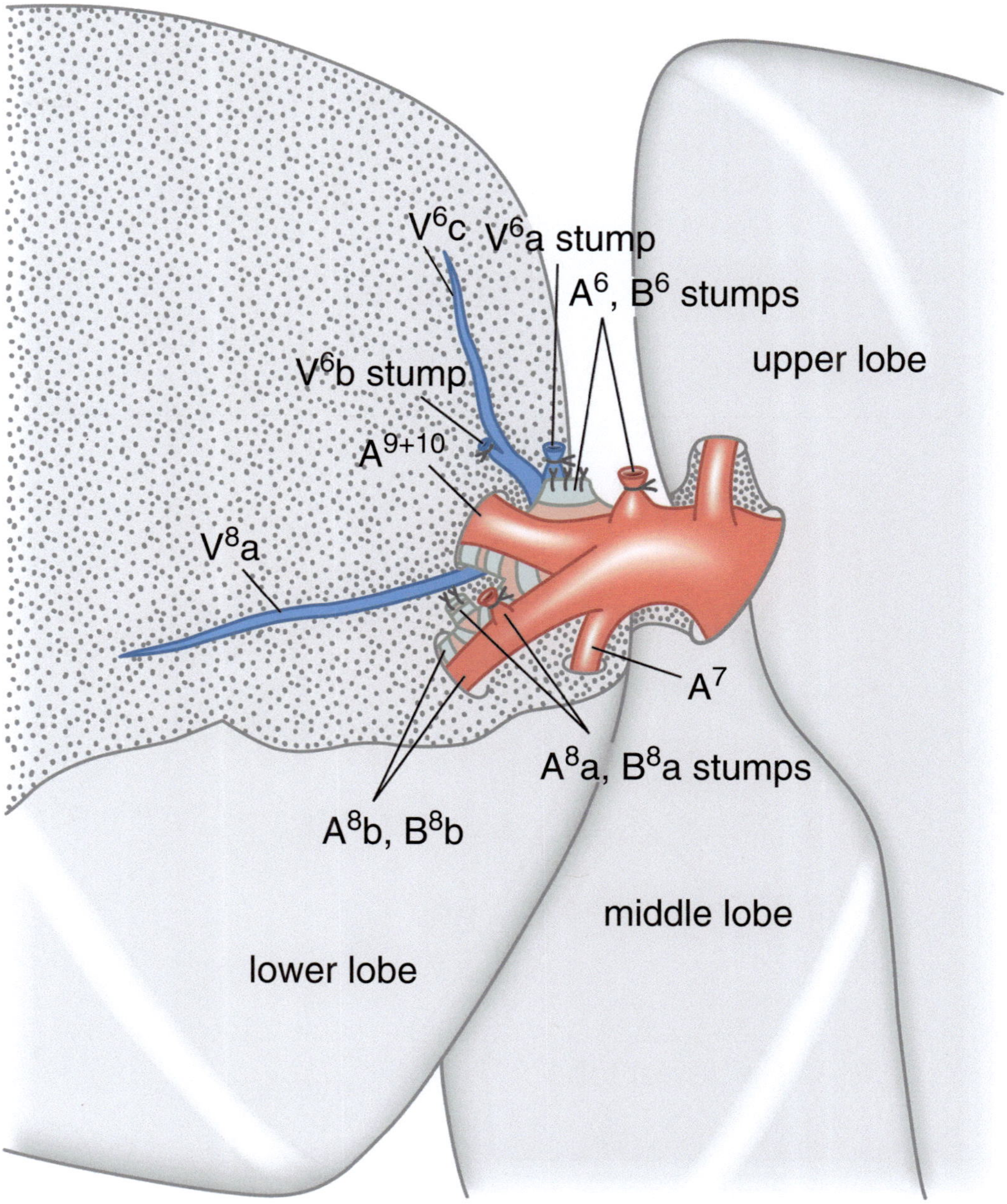

Fig. 4.6.7 The V^6c (between S^6c and $S^{10}a$) and V^8a (between S^8a and S^8b) are preserved on the segmental plane.

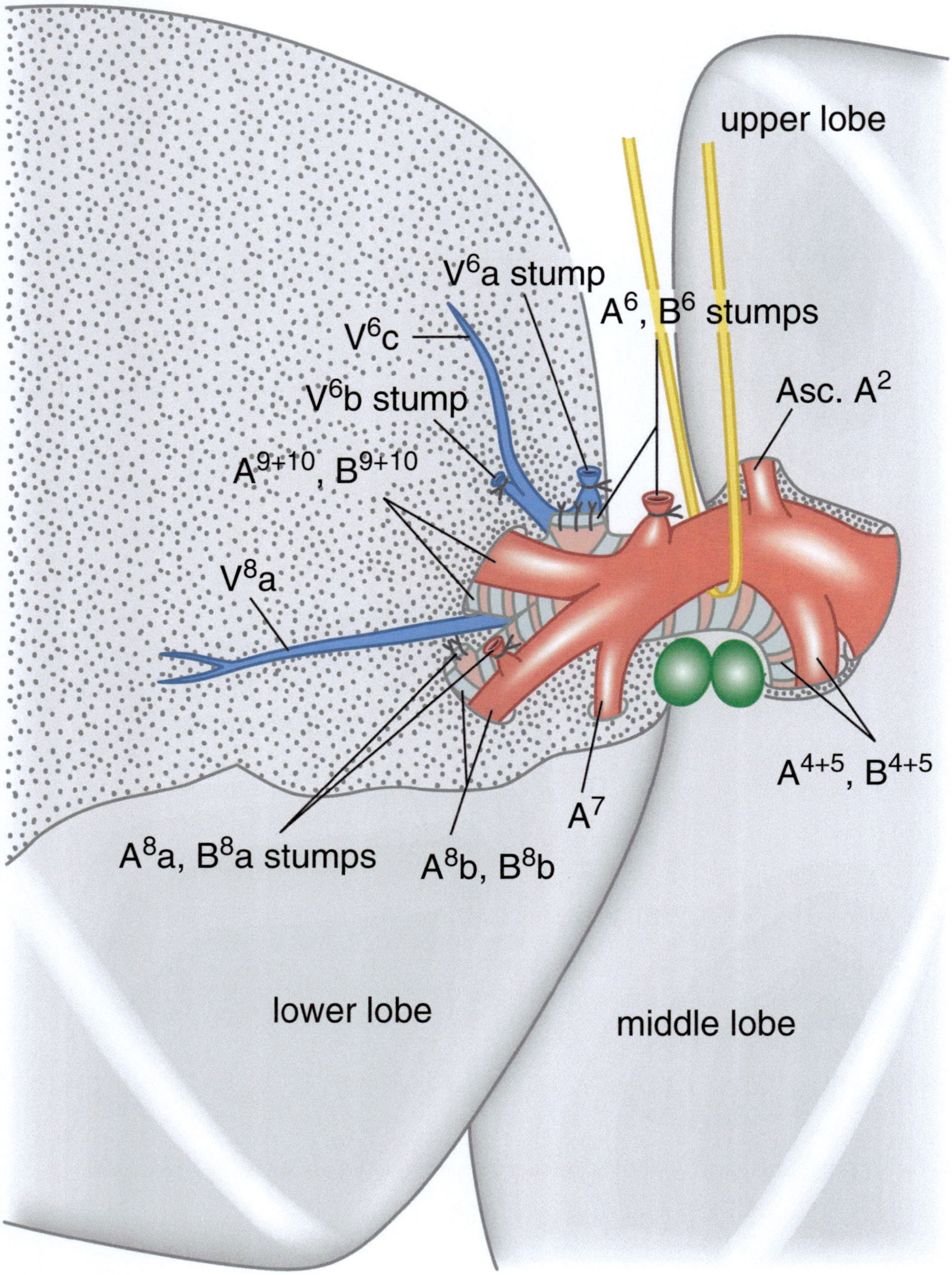

Fig. 4.6.8 A^{8-10} is encircled with tape followed by dissection of the #11i and anterior #12l lymph nodes.

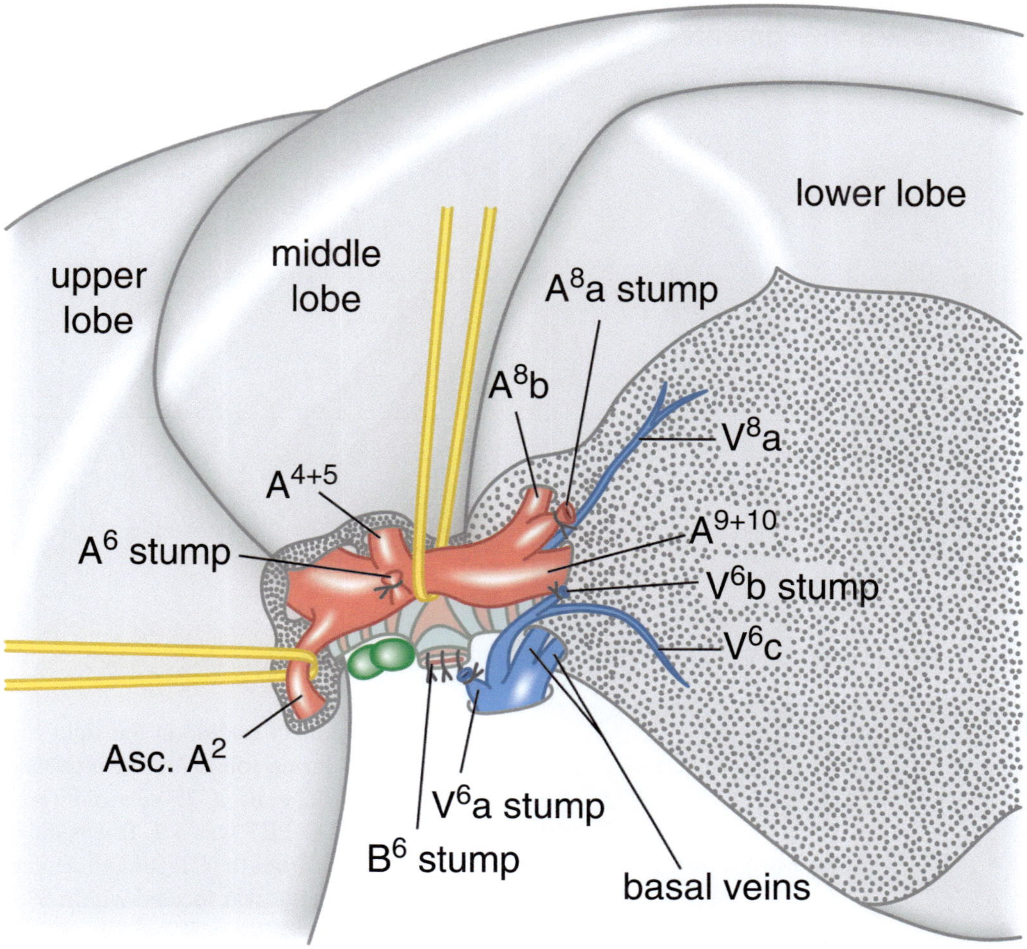

Fig. 4.6.9 The #11s lymph node is sampled with taping A^{8-10} and ascending A^2.

4.7 Right $S^6 + S^{10}a$ Segmentectomy

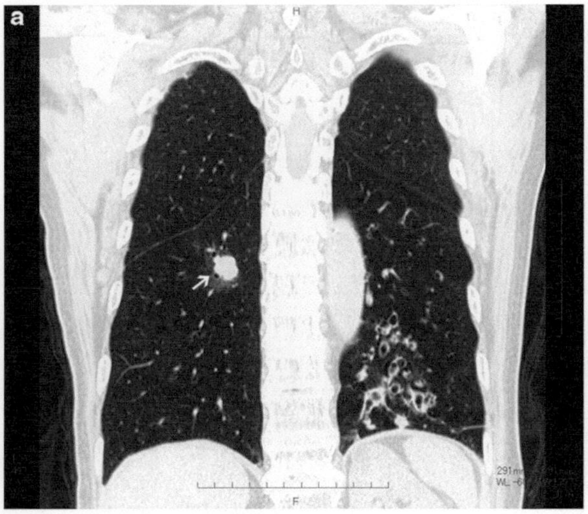

coronal view (CT scan)

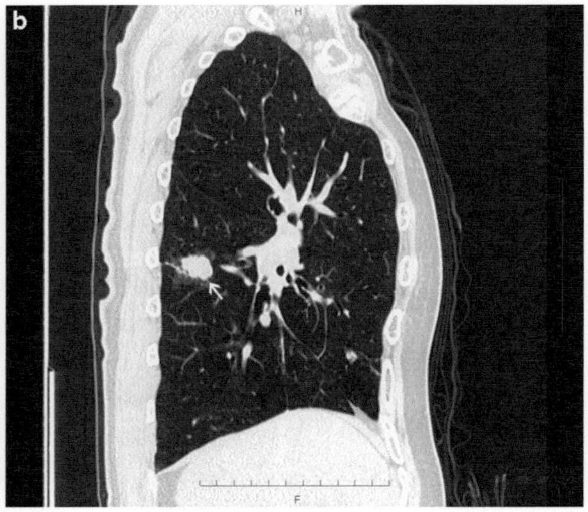

sagittal view (CT scan)

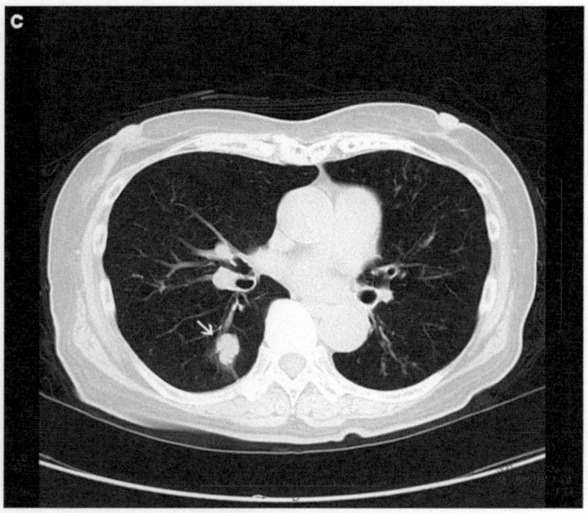

axial view (CT scan)

A 2.6-cm pulmonary nodule in the right S^6-segment was identified during follow-up for bronchiectasis in the left lower lobe of a 79-year-old female. The SUVmax on FDG-PET was 4.7. It was diagnosed as adenocarcinoma from a CT-guided needle biopsy specimen. The tumor was located within S^6 and close to V^6c, which runs between S^6 and $S^{10}a$. Therefore, the $S^6 + S^{10}a$-segmentectomy was proceeded, and the final pathological diagnosis was pT1bN0M0 papillary adenocarcinoma.

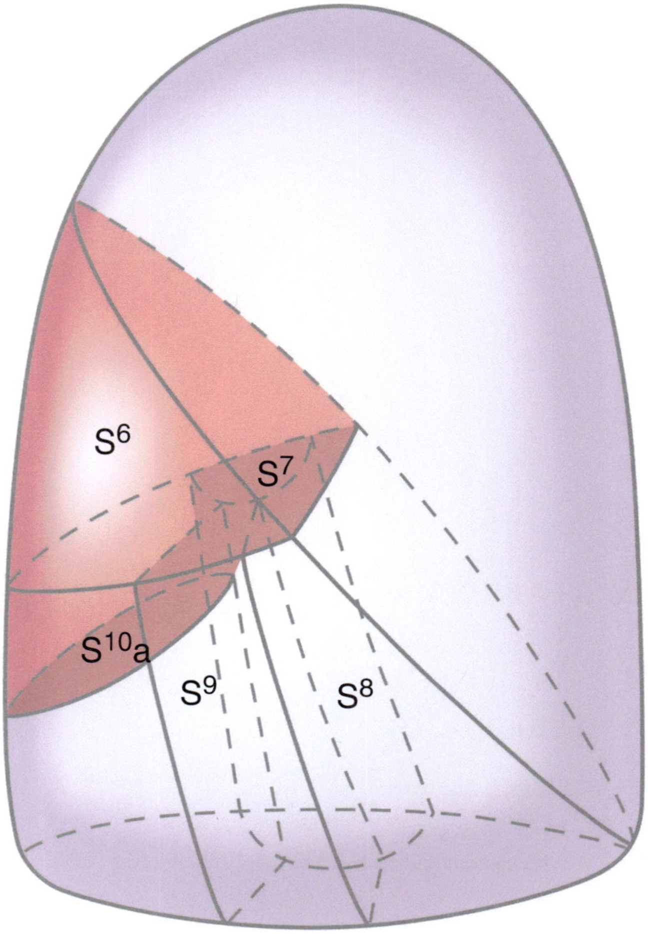

Fig. 4.7.1 This procedure is to resect a tumor in S^6c that is located near $S^{10}a$. When S^* is present, the procedure becomes S^6+S^* resection, of which technique is similar to that of $S^6+S^{10}a$-segmentectomy. The segmental arteries (A^{7-10}) and bronchi (B^{7-10}) are identified from axial, coronal, and sagittal views on HRCT. The branching pattern and size of B^7, B^8, B^9, and B^{10} are further examined by bronchoscopy after tracheal intubation. The branching pattern of $B^{10}a$, $B^{10}b$, and $B^{10}c$ is also further examined by bronchoscopy.

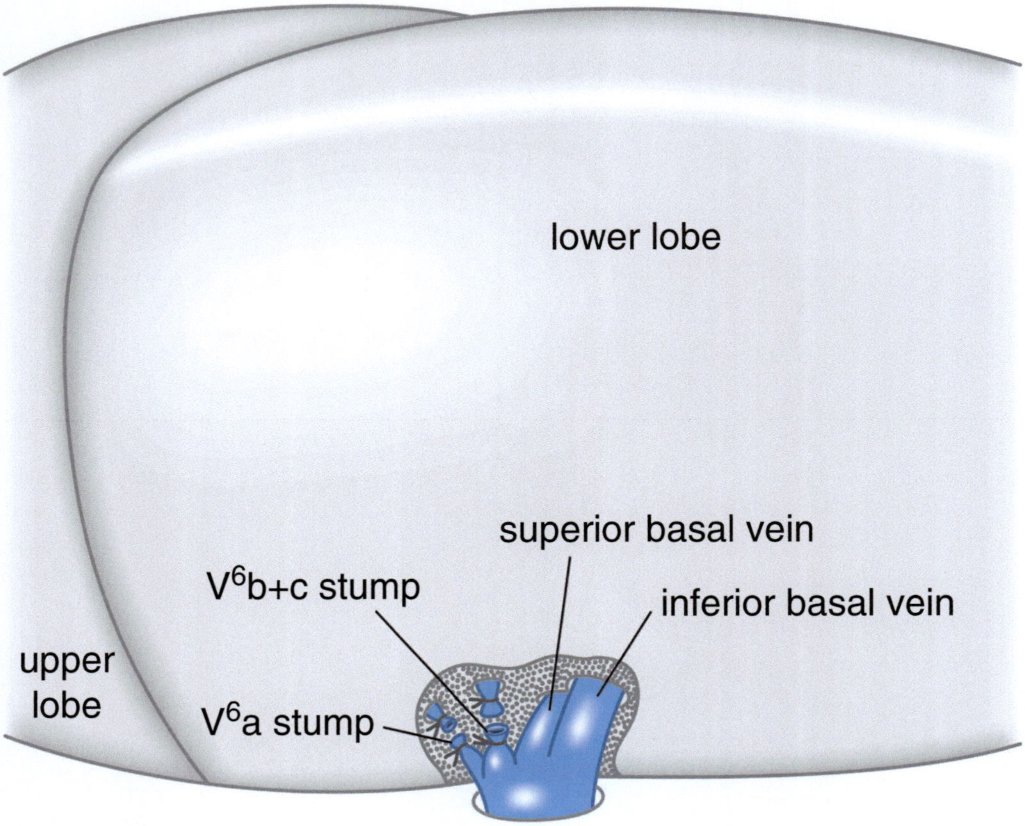

Fig. 4.7.2 The inferior pulmonary vein is exposed from behind. V^6 is cut.

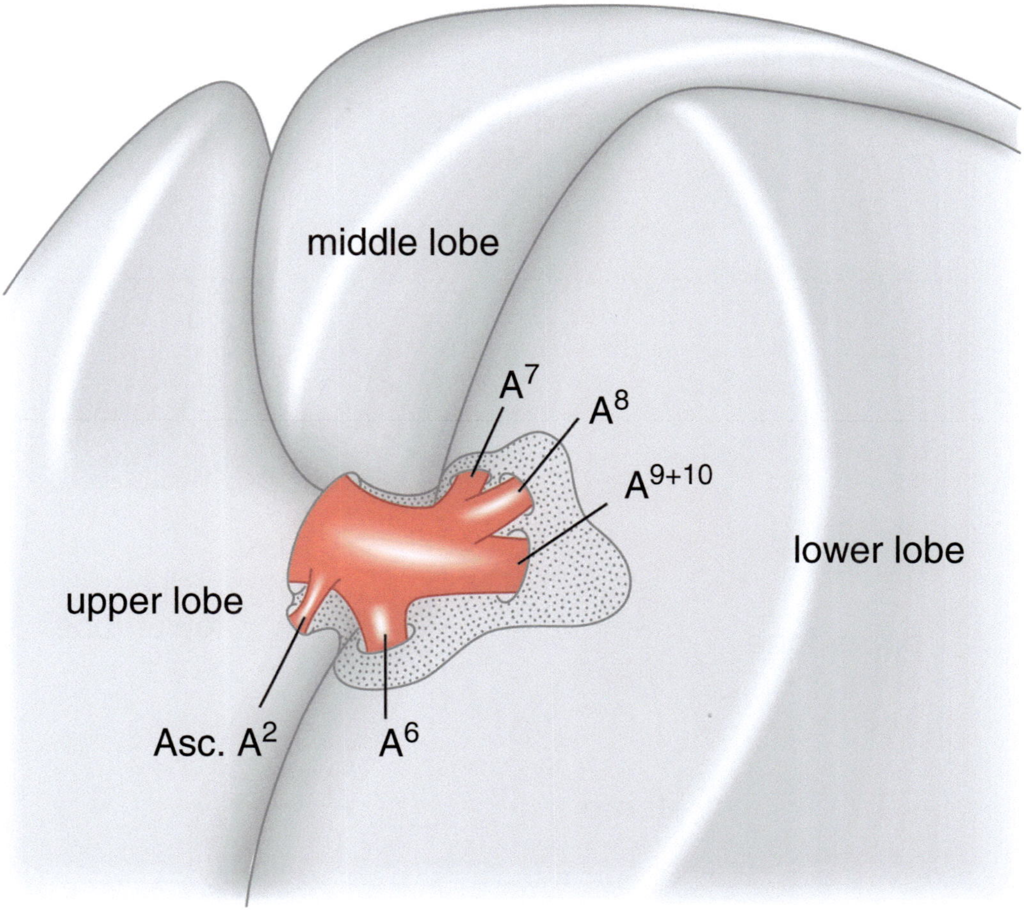

Fig. 4.7.3 The operator stands at the dorsal side in the figures of this session. The branches of A^6, A^7, A^8, and A^{9+10} are exposed. The branching patterns of A^6 are one branch in 78%, two branches in 20%, and three branches in 2%.

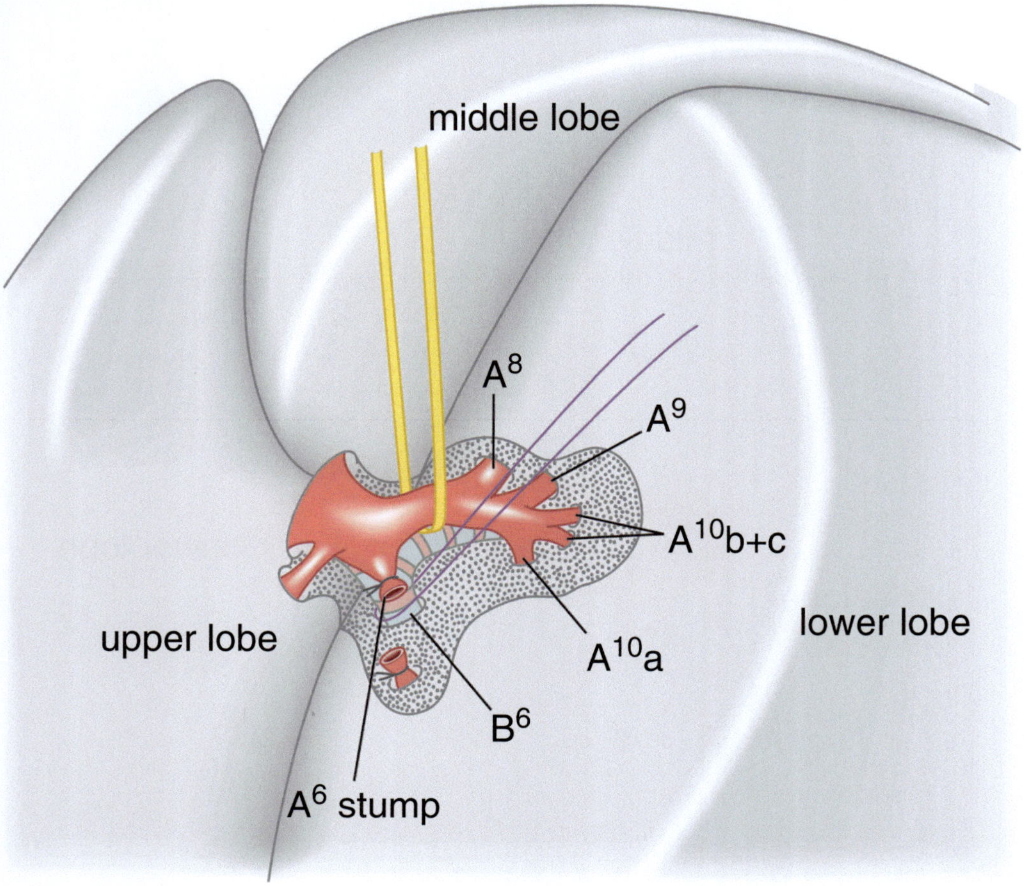

Fig. 4.7.4 A^6 is cut. B^6 is exposed, which runs caudally and behind A^6. The B^6 is encircled with thread taking care not to injure the V^6b running behind B^6.

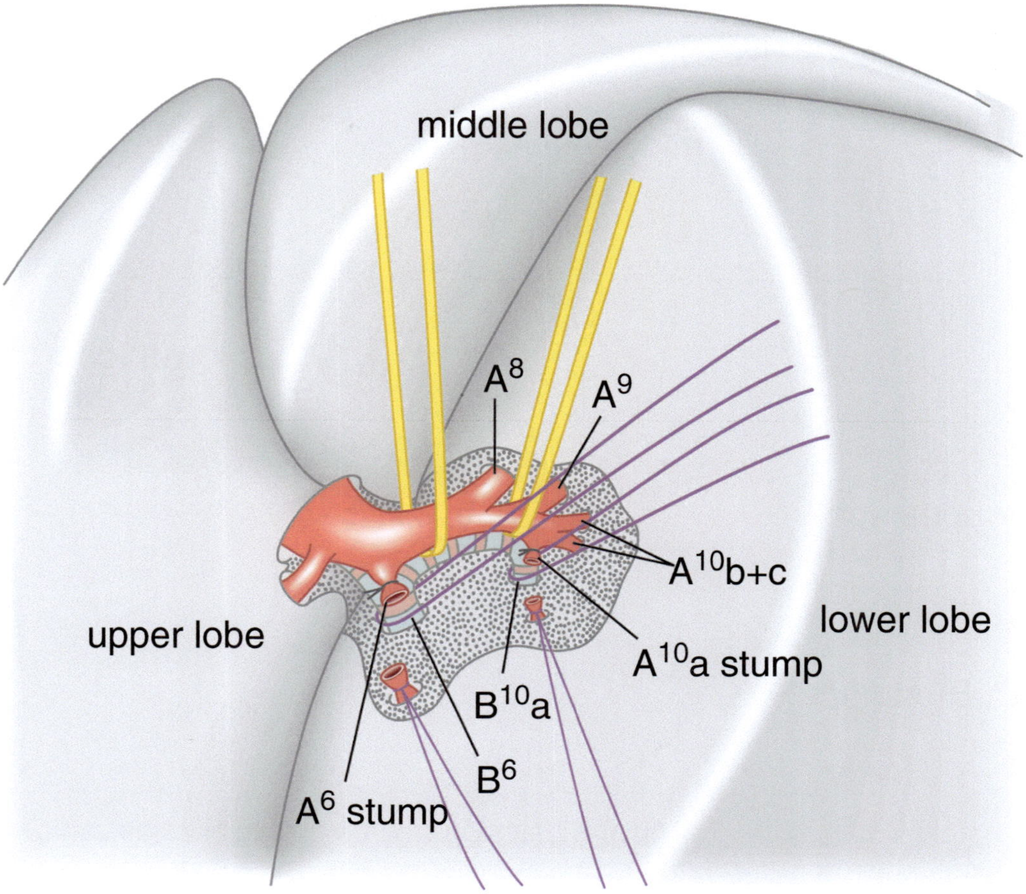

Fig. 4.7.5 A^{9+10} is exposed peripherally. $A^{10}a$ is identified. If the $A^{10}a$ is hard to be identified at this point, B^6 is cut first, which enables the $A^{10}a$ to be exposed without difficulty. $A^{10}a$ is cut. The $B^{10}a$ running behind $A^{10}a$ is encircled with thread.

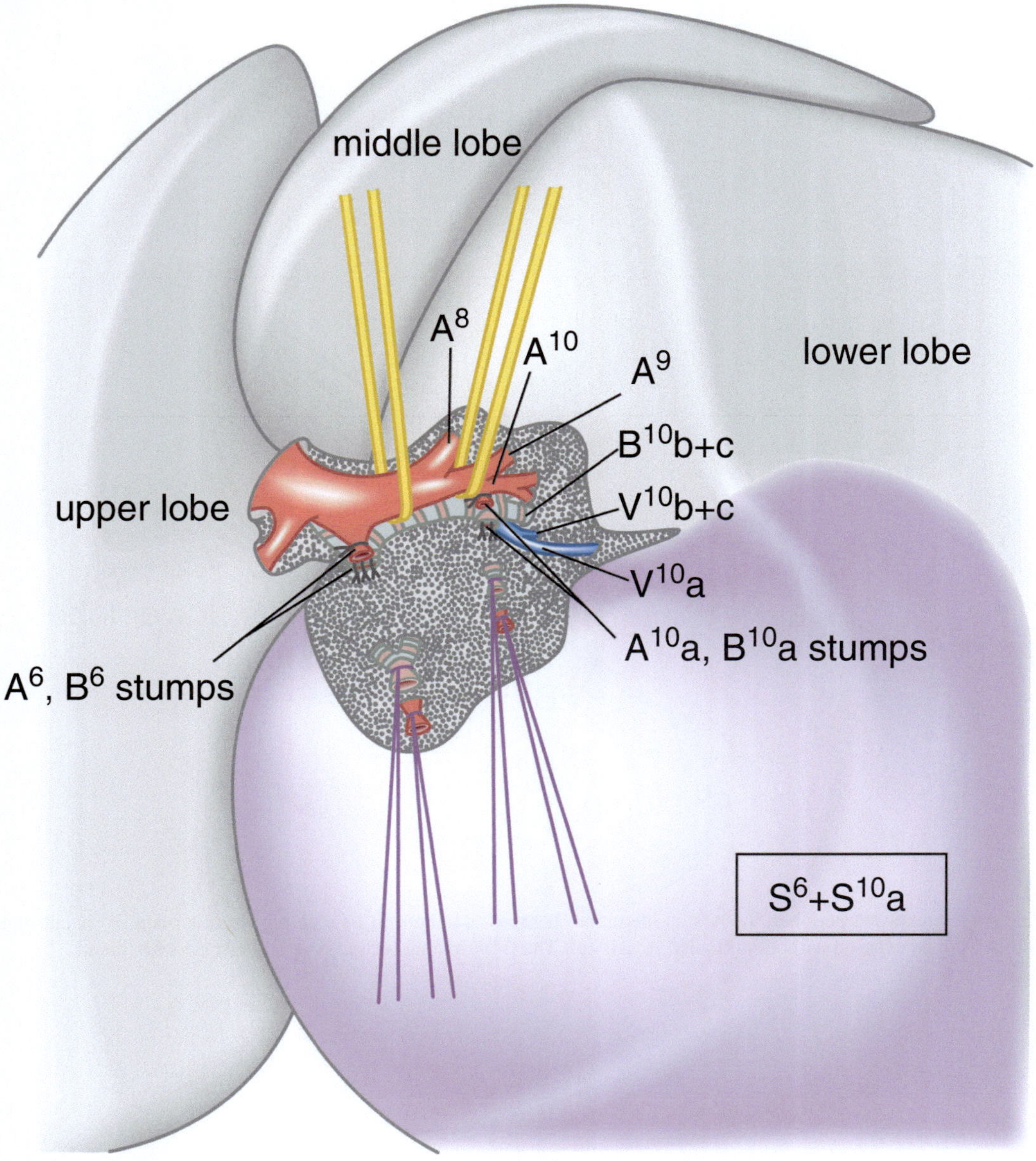

Fig. 4.7.6 S^6 and S^{10}a are selectively inflated either by inserting a bronchoscope into B^6 and B^{10}a followed by jet ventilation, or by cutting the B^6 and B^{10}a and inserting a catheter into the peripheral stumps followed by air inflation. The distal stumps are then closed to trap air within S^6 and S^{10}a. The proximal stumps of B^6 and B^{10}a are closed with suture or ligation. The distal stumps of B^6 and B^{10}a are lifted and denuded peripherally at the back to move them away from the hilum. By doing that, lung tissue on either side of these distal stumps is also elevated, which is cut along V^{10}a (between S^{10}a and S^{10}b+c) and also towards the inflation–deflation line by electrocautery. However, V^{10}a always cannot be found because of its wide variation. The intersegmental plane is cut from various directions to facilitate simple and accurate segmentectomy.

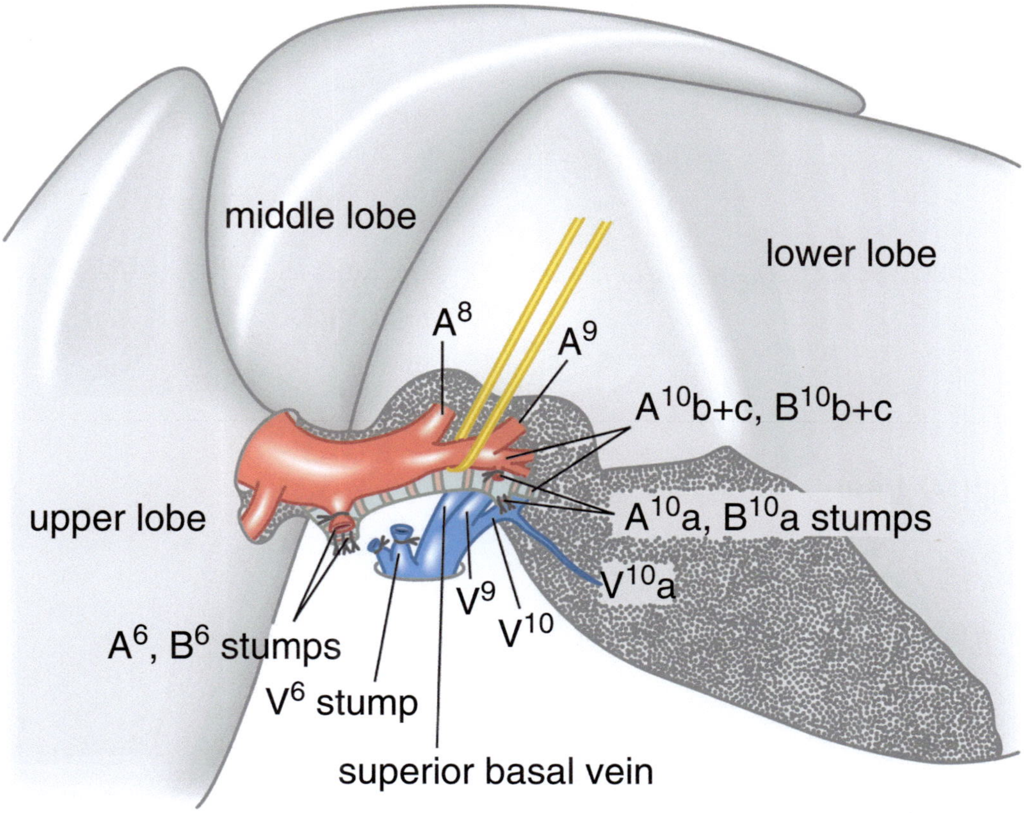

Fig. 4.7.7 After resecting S^6 and $S^{10}a$, $V^{10}a$ is preserved on $S^{10}b+c$.

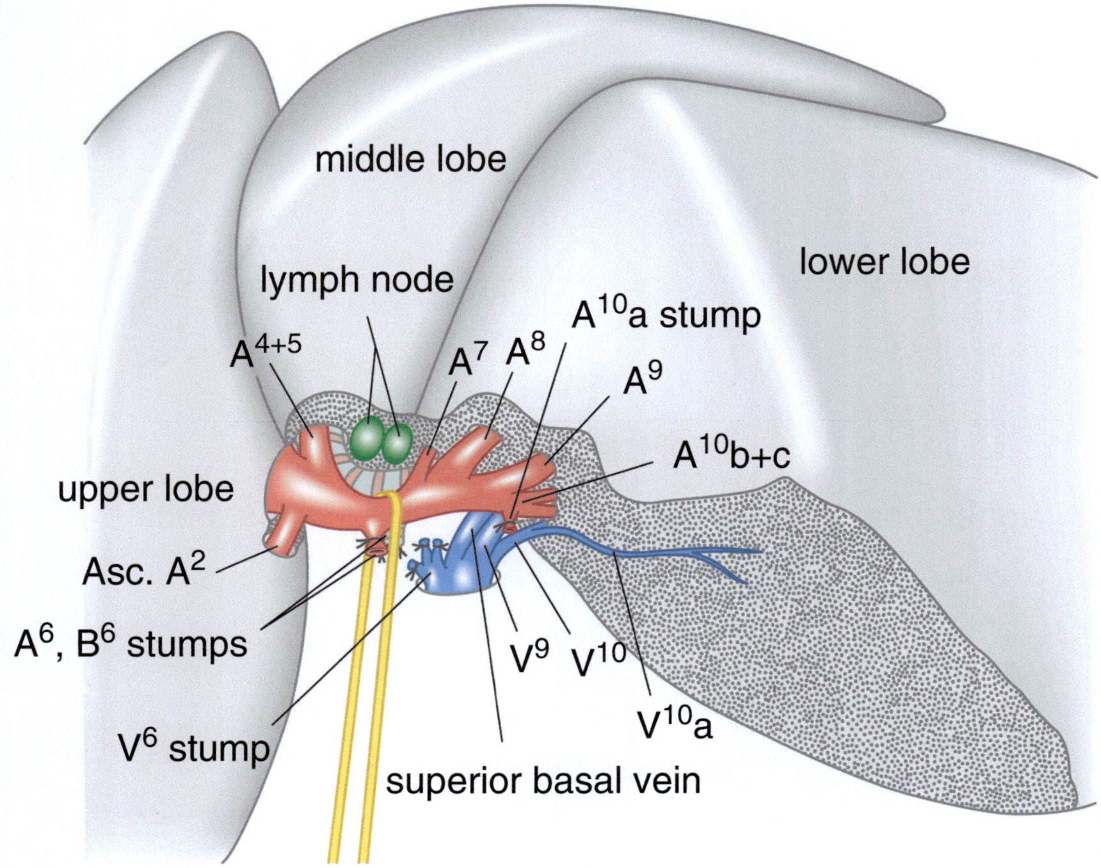

Fig. 4.7.8 A^{8-10} is encircled with tape and then the #11i and anterior #12l lymph nodes are dissected.

4.8 Right $S^6b + S^8a$ Segmentectomy

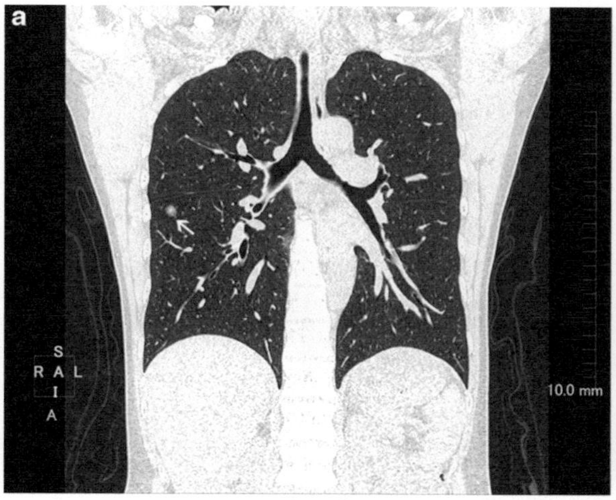

coronal view (CT scan)

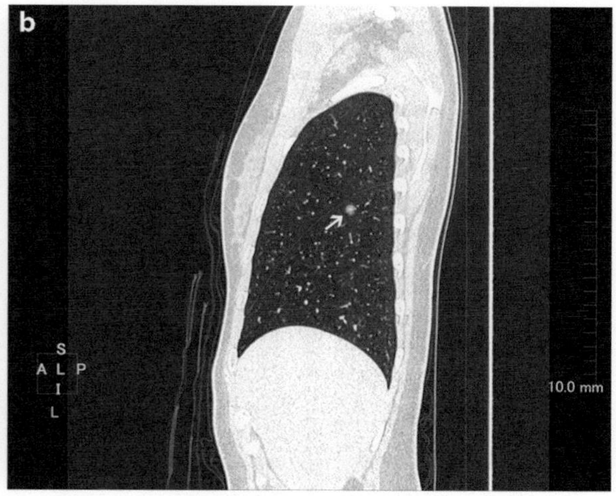

sagittal view (CT scan)

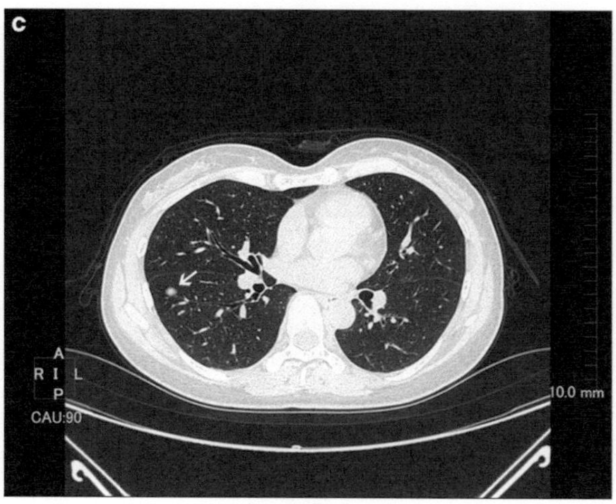

axial view (CT scan)

A CT scan revealed a 0.8-cm nodule in the right S^6b of a 46-year-old female. The nodule was located near V^6b, which runs between S^6b and S^8a. Although it was diagnosed as bronchioloalveolar carcinoma from a CT-guided needle biopsy specimen, a solid area on CT suggested the mixture of papillary adenocarcinoma. Therefore, $S^6b + S^8a$ segmentectomy was performed rather than wedge resection. The final pathological diagnosis was pT1aN0M0 bronchioloalveolar carcinoma.

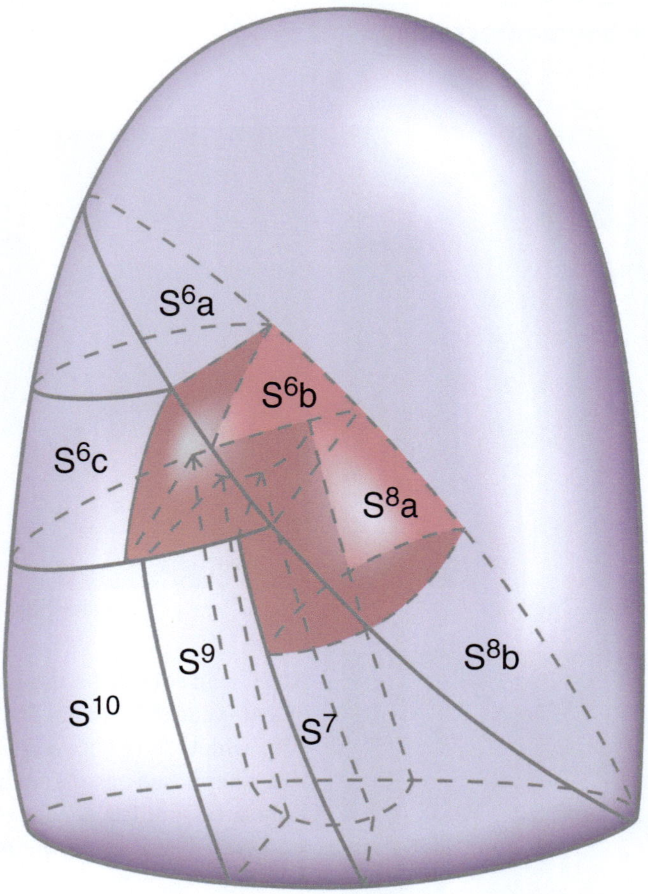

Fig. 4.8.1 Tumors such as bronchioloalveolar carcinoma nodules of <2 cm, which is deeply located between S^6b and S^8a, can be curatively resected using this procedure, whereas the resection of both S^6 and S^8 results in a major decrease in pulmonary function of lower lobe. The segmental arteries (A^{6-10}) and bronchi (B^{6-10}) are identified from axial, coronal, and sagittal views on HRCT. The size and branching of B^{6-10} and those of B^6b and B^8a are further determined by bronchoscopy after tracheal intubation. The patterns of B^6 branches are B^6a + c and B^6b (66% in frequency), B^6a + b and B^6c (28%), and B^6a, B^6b, and B^6c (6%).

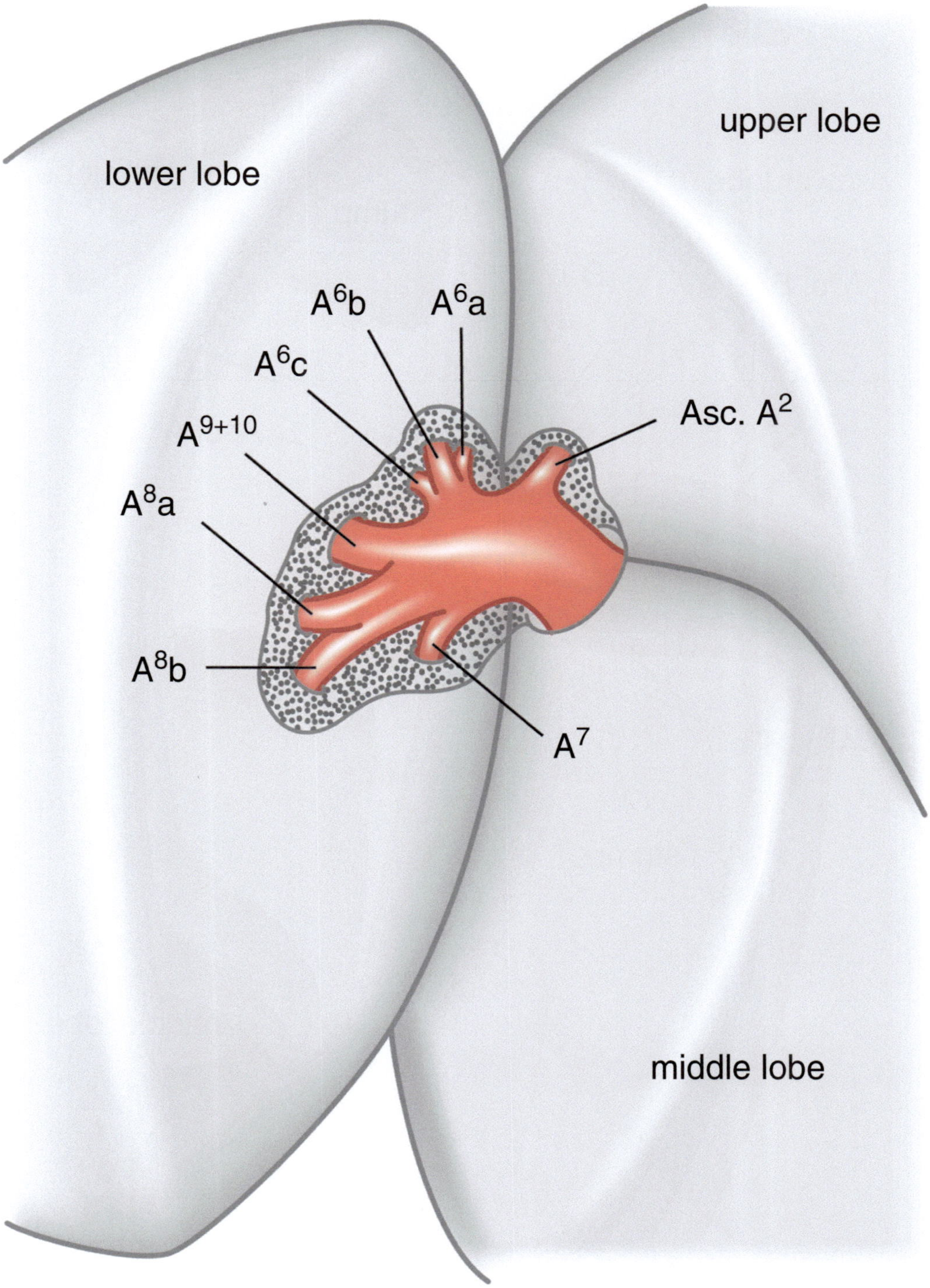

Fig. 4.8.2 The segmental bronchus and artery branch most frequently into B^8 and B^{9+10}, and A^8 and A^{9+10}. The figures of this session show that A^6 comprises one branch (78% in frequency) and B^6 branches into B^6a+c and B^6b (66% in frequency). The branches of A^6, A^7, A^8, and A^{9+10} are exposed sufficiently during this procedure, although exposing the inferior pulmonary vein is unnecessary. It should be taken into consideration that A^8a sometimes branches from A^{9+10}.

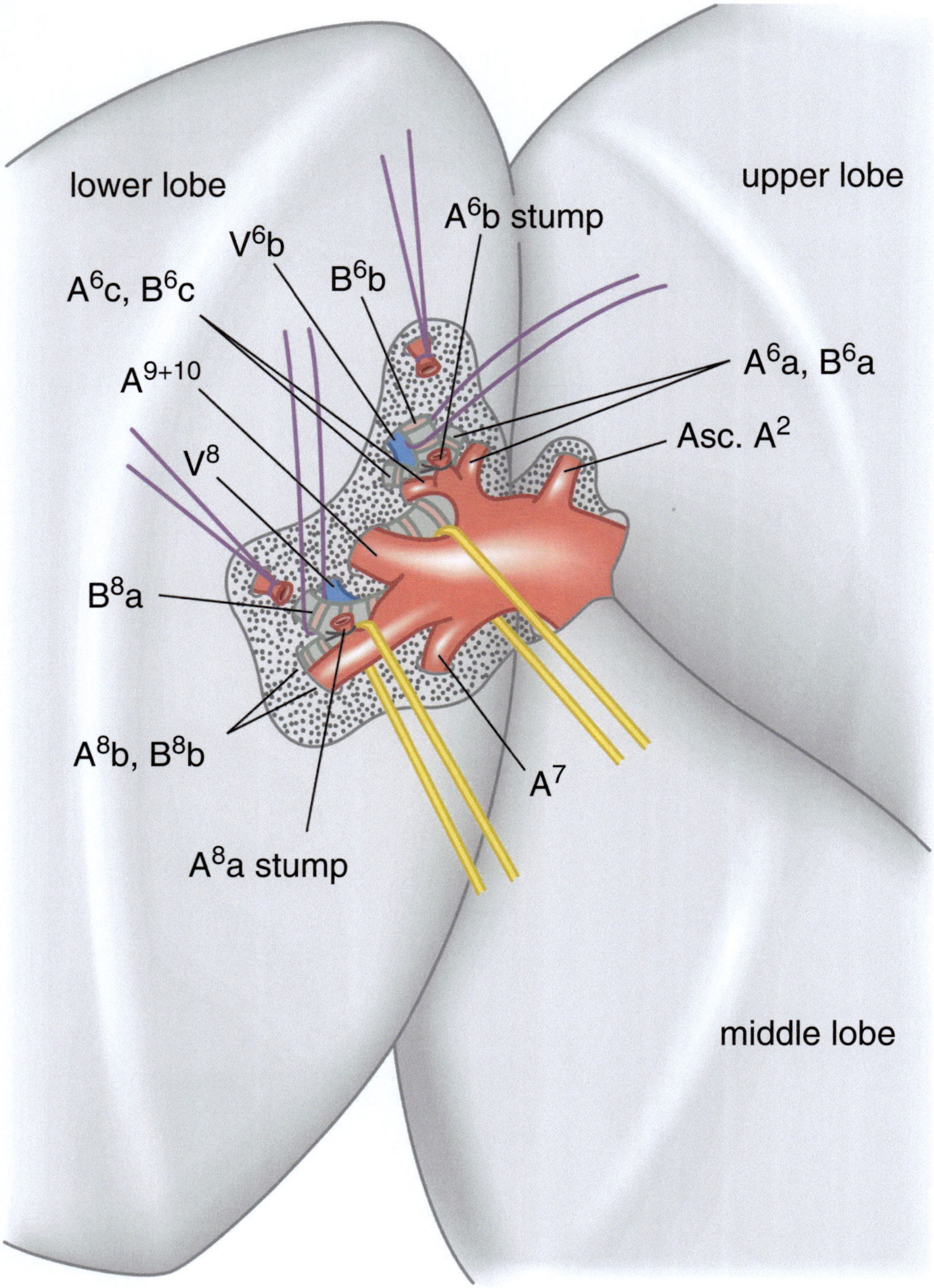

Fig. 4.8.3 A^6 is encircled with tape and exposed peripherally. A^6b runs most laterally when branching into A^6a+c and A^6b. The A^6b is cut, which reveals B^6b behind it. B^6b is encircled with thread. A^8a is cut, which reveals B^8a behind it. B^8a is encircled with thread.

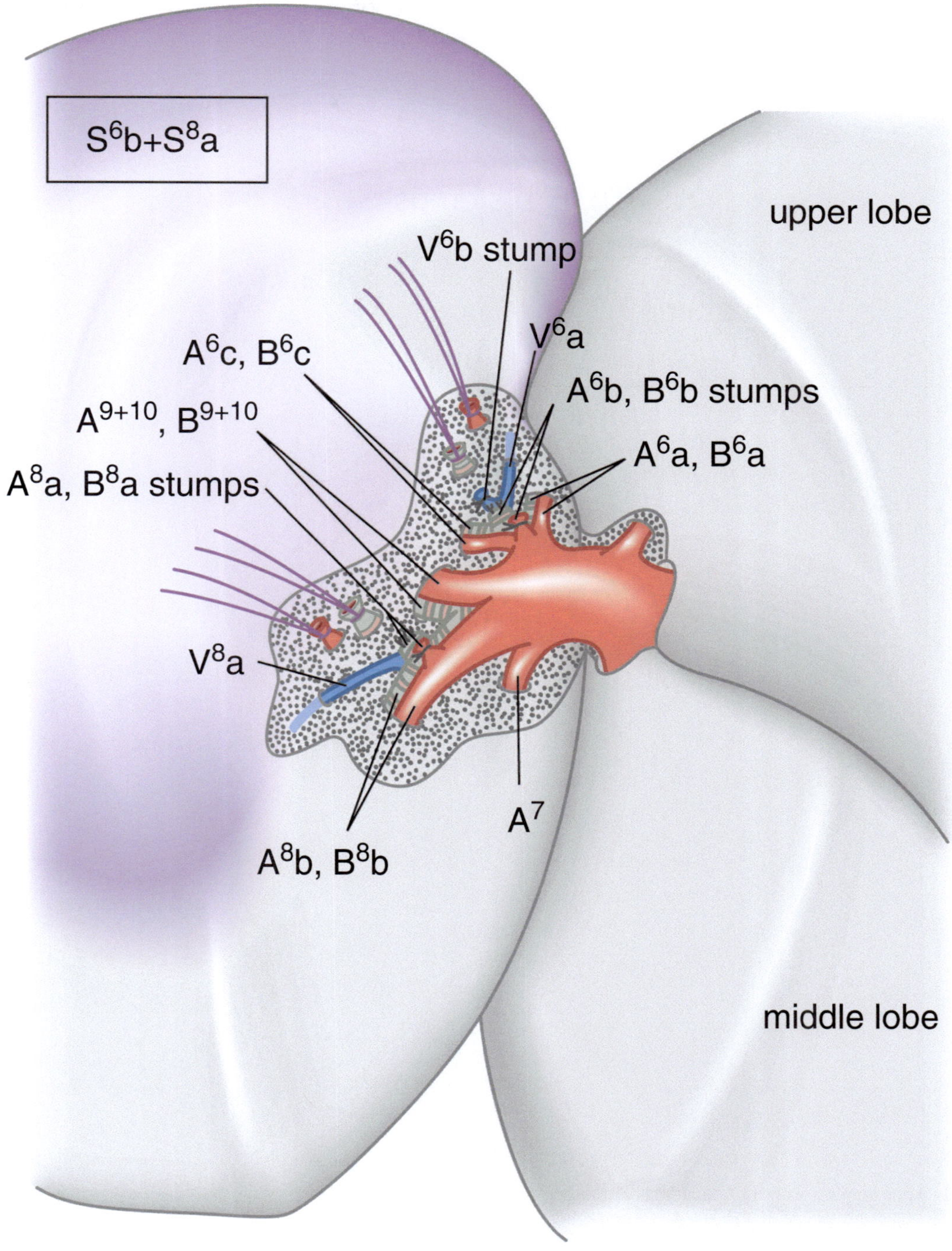

Fig. 4.8.4 S^6b and S^8a are inflated either by inserting a bronchoscope into B^6b and B^8a followed by jet ventilation, or by cutting the B^6b and B^8a and inserting a catheter into the distal stumps followed by air inflation. The distal stumps are closed to trap air within S^6b and S^8a. The proximal stumps of B^6b and B^8a are closed with suture or ligation. The distal stumps of B^6b and B^8a are lifted, and denuded peripherally at the back to move them away from the hilum. By lifting the distal stumps of B^6b and B^8a, V^6b is seen between S^6b and S^8a, which is cut. Lung tissue on both sides of the stumps is cut along V^6a (between S^6a and S^6b) and V^8a (between S^8a and S^8b) and also towards the inflation–deflation line using electrocautery. The intersegmental plane is cut from various directions to facilitate simple and accurate segmentectomy.

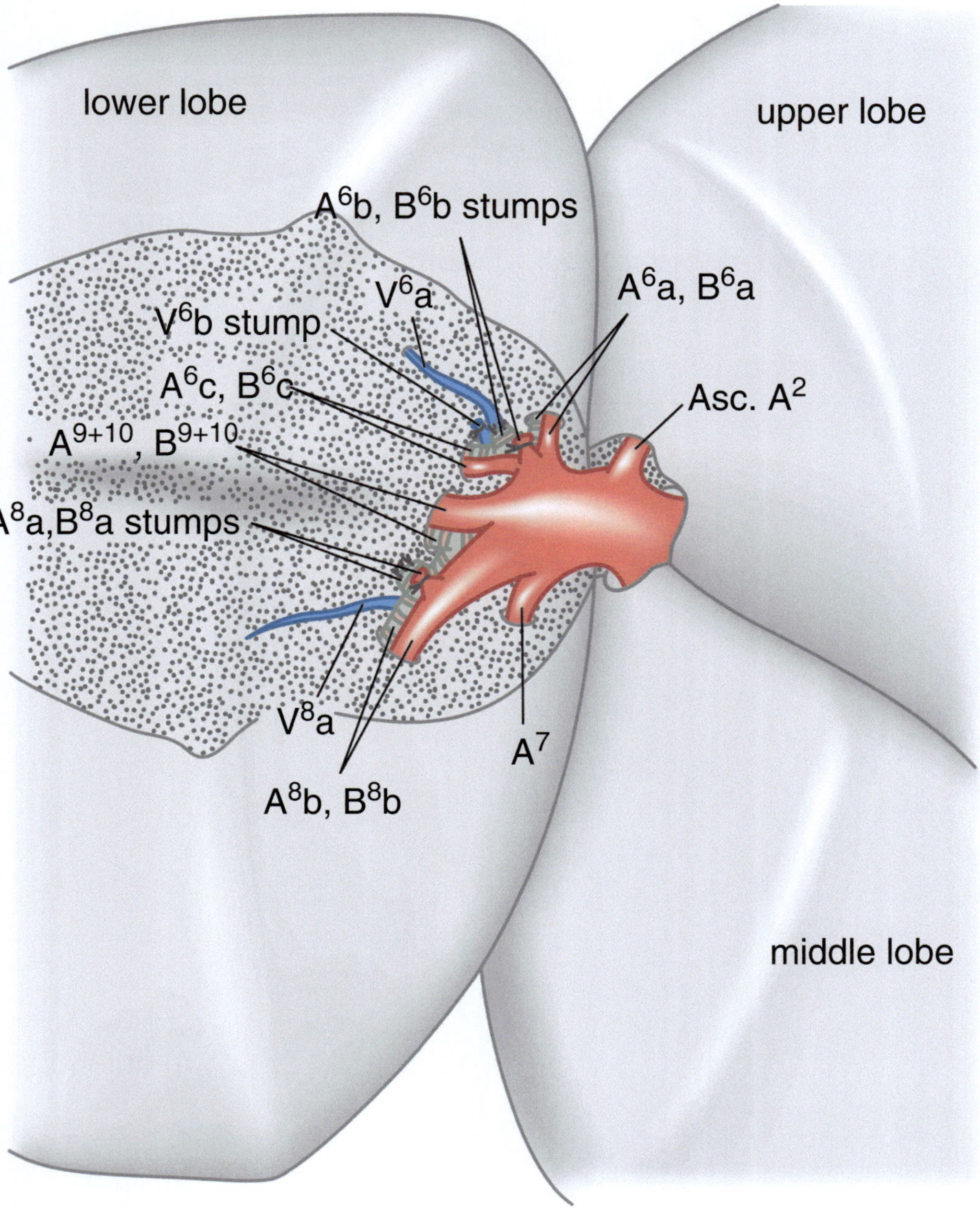

Fig. 4.8.5 After lung resection, V^6a and V^8a are preserved on S^6a and S^8b, respectively. A^6 is encircled with tape and hilar lymph nodes of #13 around B^6 and posterior #12l are dissected, which is important because these nodes lie along the route of lymphatic chain towards #7. A^{8-10} is also encircled with tape and then #11i and anterior #12l lymph nodes are dissected.

Segmentectomy of the Left Upper Lobe

5

The major branches of the right pulmonary artery are named herein as follows:
Truncus superior: first major branch to the left upper lobe
Truncus intermedius: pulmonary artery between the truncus superior artery and A^6
Interlobar artery: peripheral pulmonary artery after A^6 branches

Branching profile			Frequency (%)
Bronchus	B^{1-3}	B^{1+2} and B^3	46
		B^{1+2}, B^3a and B^3b + c	27
		B^{1+2}a + b, B^{1+2}c, and B^3	27
	B^{1+2}	B^{1+2}a + b and B^{1+2}c	65
		B^{1+2}a and B^{1+2}b + c	35
	B^3	B^3a and B^3b + c	90
	Other		10
Artery	A^{1+2}	A^{1+2}a + b and A^{1+2}c	31
		A^{1+2}a, A^{1+2}b, and A^{1+2}c	28
		A^{1+2}a and A^{1+2}b + c	26
		A^{1+2}a + b + c	15
	A^3	Mediastinal type: A^3 branches from main pulmonary artery mostly into A^3a and A^3b + c	90
		Mediastinal and interlobar type: A^3b + c branches from main pulmonary artery, and A^3a branches distal to A^{1+2}c and proximal to A^4a	10
	A^{4+5}	Interlobar type: A^4 and A^5 separately branch from interlobar artery	26
		Interlobar type: A^{4+5} branches from interlobar artery	44
		Mediastinal type: A^{4+5} branches from mediastinum (main pulmonary artery) and runs between V^{1+3} and B^3	18
		Mediastinal and interlobar type	12
Vein		Apical type: V^{1+2} and V^3 both branch from superior pulmonary vein	98
		Central type: entire V^{1+2} forms a common truncus with V^3, and runs into deep lung tissue	2

H. Nomori and M. Okada, *Illustrated Anatomical Segmentectomy for Lung Cancer*,
DOI 10.1007/978-4-431-54144-8_5, © Springer Japan 2012

5.1 Left $S^{1+2}+S^3$ (Upper Division) Segmentectomy

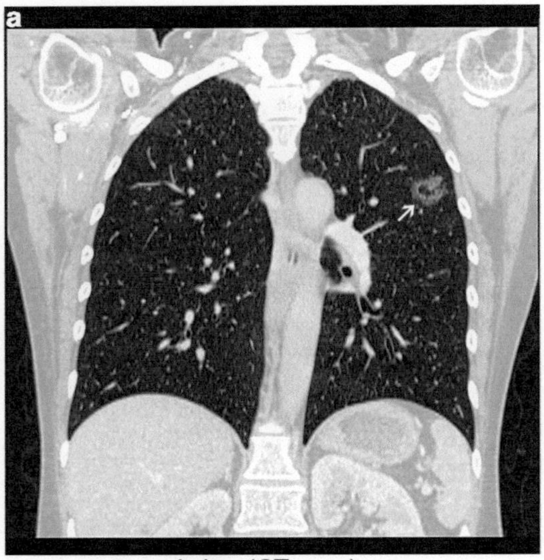

coronal view (CT scan)

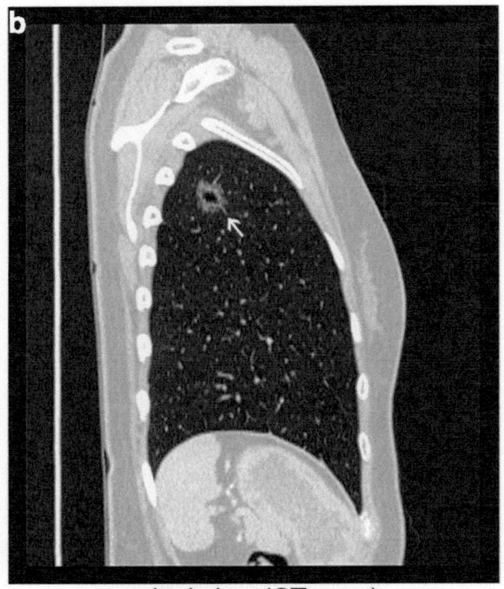

sagittal view (CT scan)

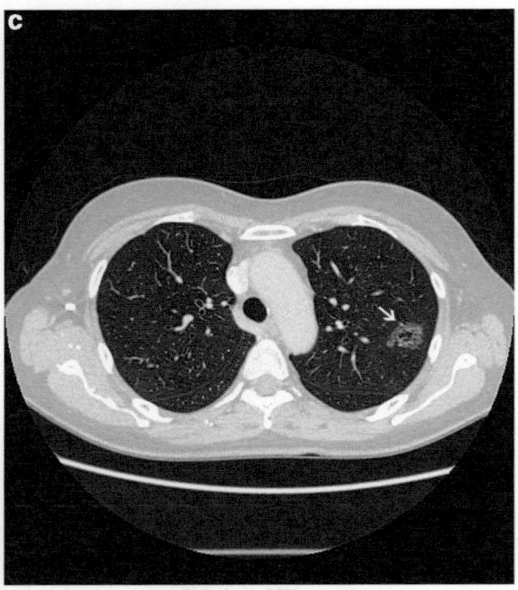

axial view (CT scan)

A CT scan of a 53-year-old female revealed a 2.3-cm GGO nodule with a central cavity in the left S^{1+2} that was diagnosed as adenocarcinoma from a CT-guided needle biopsy specimen. The tumor involved $V^{1+2}d$ (between $S^{1+2}c$ and S^3a). Therefore, upper division ($S^{1+2}+S^3$) segmentectomy was proceeded, and the final pathological diagnosis was pT1bN0M0 bronchioloalveolar carcinoma.

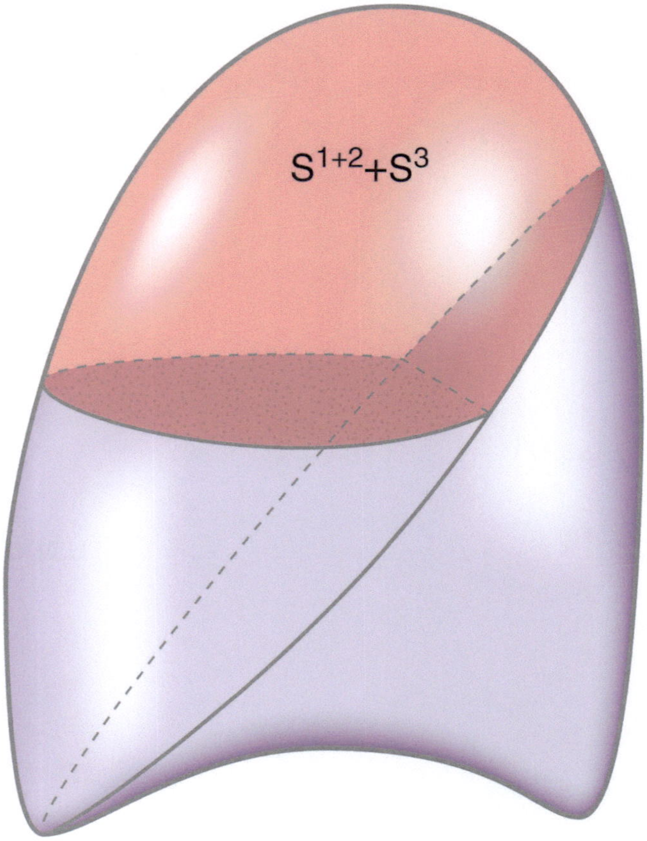

Fig. 5.1.1 Upper division segmentectomy and right upper lobectomy are quite similar. Therefore, describing the procedure as a segmentectomy has met with considerable resistance from the viewpoint of pulmonary function. Regardless, the most important aim is to preserve the pulmonary function of the small lingular division (S^4+S^5) as well as that of the right middle lobe. To achieve this, a stapler should not be used for dividing upper and lingular division, because it would impair expansion of the lingular division. Branching of the artery, vein, and bronchus is confirmed from axial, coronal, and sagittal views on HRCT. The branching and size of B^{1+2} and B^3 are further examined by bronchoscopy after tracheal intubation. The upper lobar bronchus usually branches into B^{1-3} and B^{4+5}, and occasionally into three branches with B^{1+2}, B^3, and B^{4+5}.

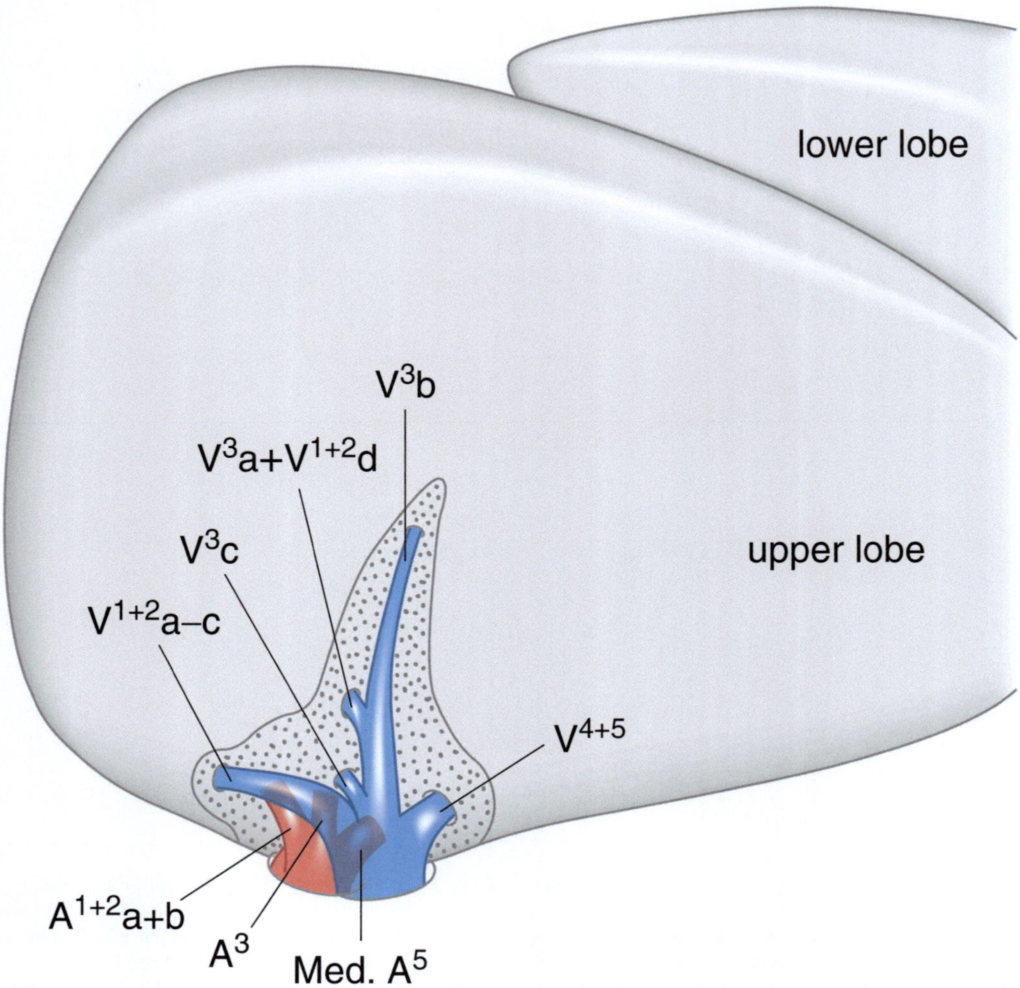

Fig. 5.1.2 The hilum of the left upper lobe is exposed from the ventral to the dorsal side to reveal the superior pulmonary vein, main pulmonary artery, truncus superior artery, truncus intermedius artery, and the proximal site of interlobar artery. The V^3b is identified, encircled with tape, and then exposed peripherally, which is the border of S^3b and S^4b. The V^3a and $V^{1+2}d$ usually form a common trunk branching from the rear of V^3b, which is barely visible at this point.

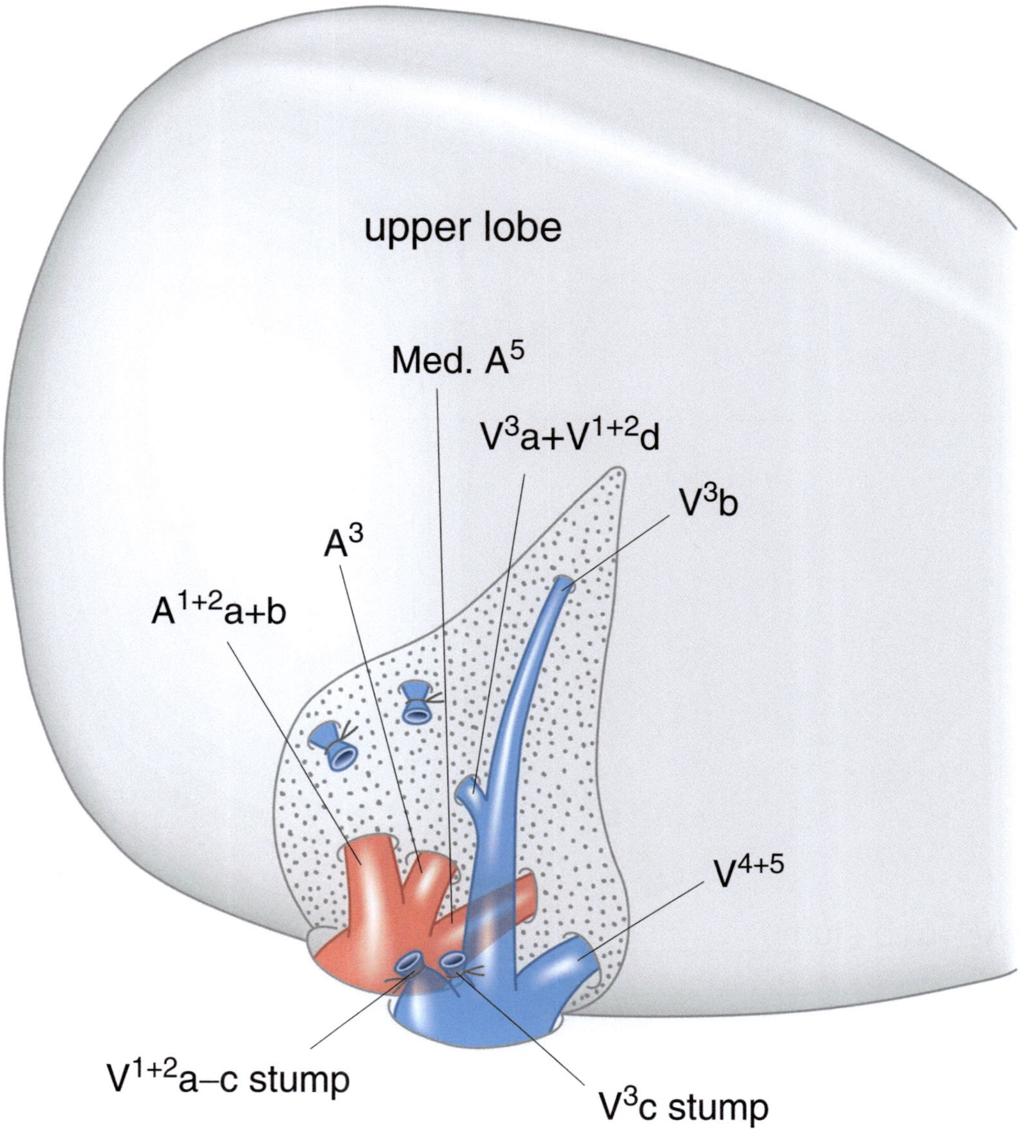

Fig. 5.1.3 The V^{1+2} and V^3c at the cranial side of V^3b are cut, which reveals the truncus superior artery. The presence of a mediastinal A^4 or A^5 running between V^3 and B^3 is verified, of which frequency is about 30 %. A mediastinal A^4 or A^5 is preserved if present. This figure shows a mediastinal A^5. The pulmonary artery is exposed from the dorsal side until A^6 branches, which exposes A^3, $A^{1+2}a+b$, and $A^{1+2}c$.

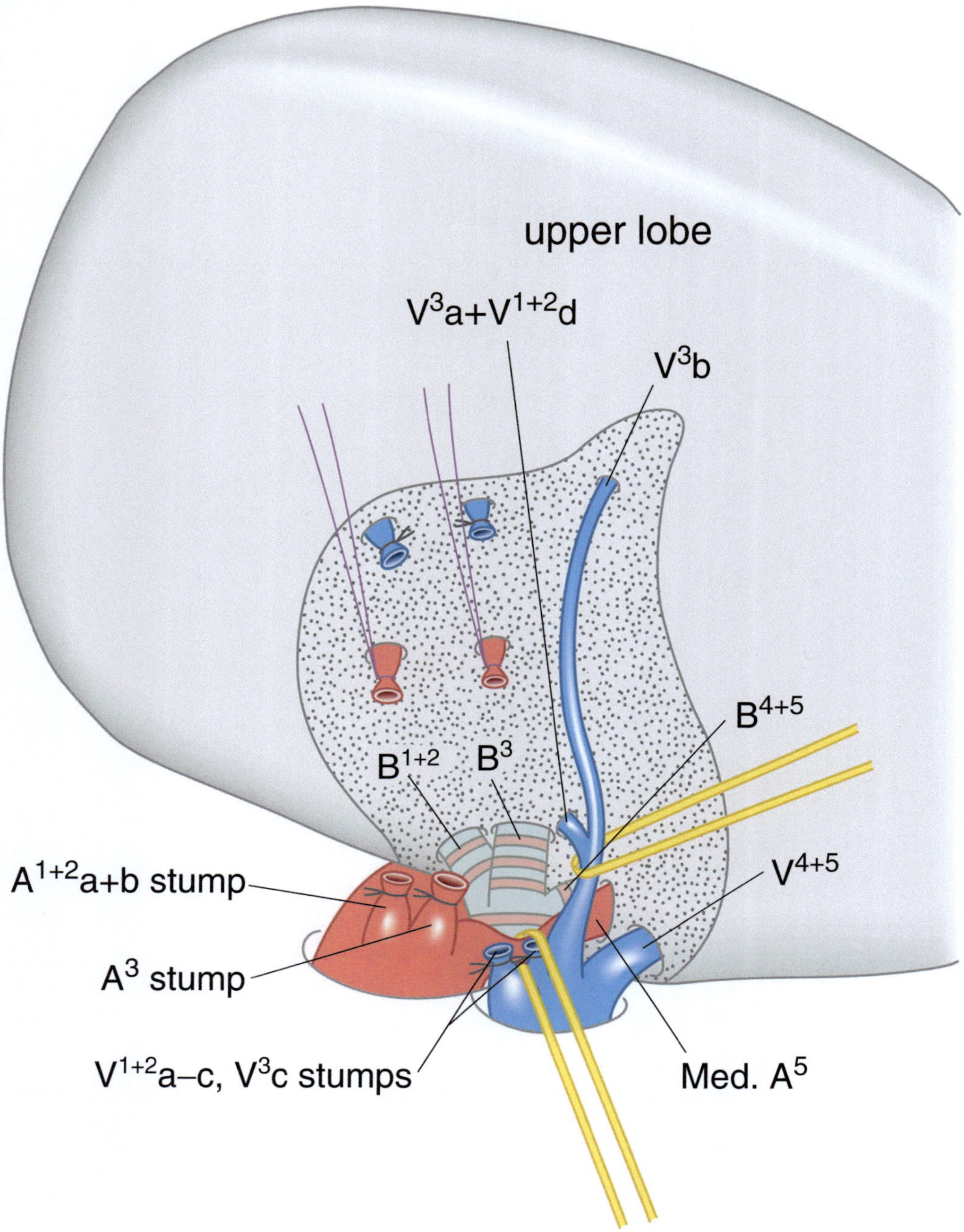

Fig. 5.1.4 A^3 and $A^{1+2}a+b$ are cut, which reveals the B^3 and B^{1+2} running behind them. The preoperative bronchoscopic findings can help to identify B^{1+2} and B^3 at this point based on their anatomical branching and size.

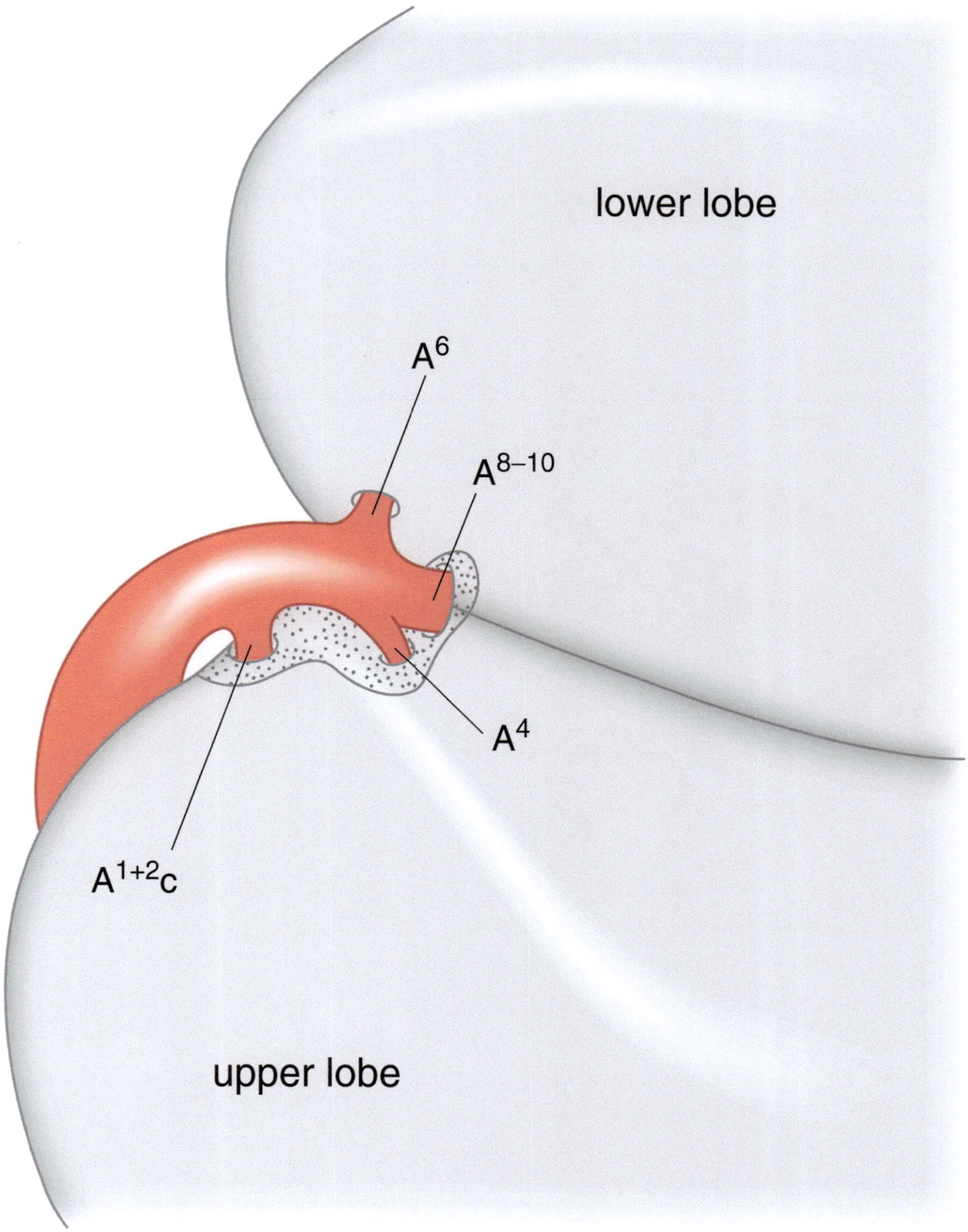

Fig. 5.1.5 The incomplete fissure between S^{1+2} and S^6 is divided using electrocautery but not using a stapler, because a staple line usually impairs identification of the intersegmental plane. The following procedure facilitates the fissure identification: a bronchoscope is inserted into B^{1+2} followed by jet ventilation, which forms an inflation-deflation line between the inflated S^{1+2} and deflated lower lobe. The fissure can be divided along the inflated-deflated line using electrocautery. $A^{1+2}c$ is identified. In principle, an artery branching at the proximal side of A^6 would be $A^{1+2}c$, but it is sometimes difficult to differentiate from A^4a, especially when it branches near the level of A^6. Therefore, an arterial branch near A^6 is preserved at this point, because it might be A^4a. It can be identified after cutting B^{1-3} or creating an inflation–deflation line later.

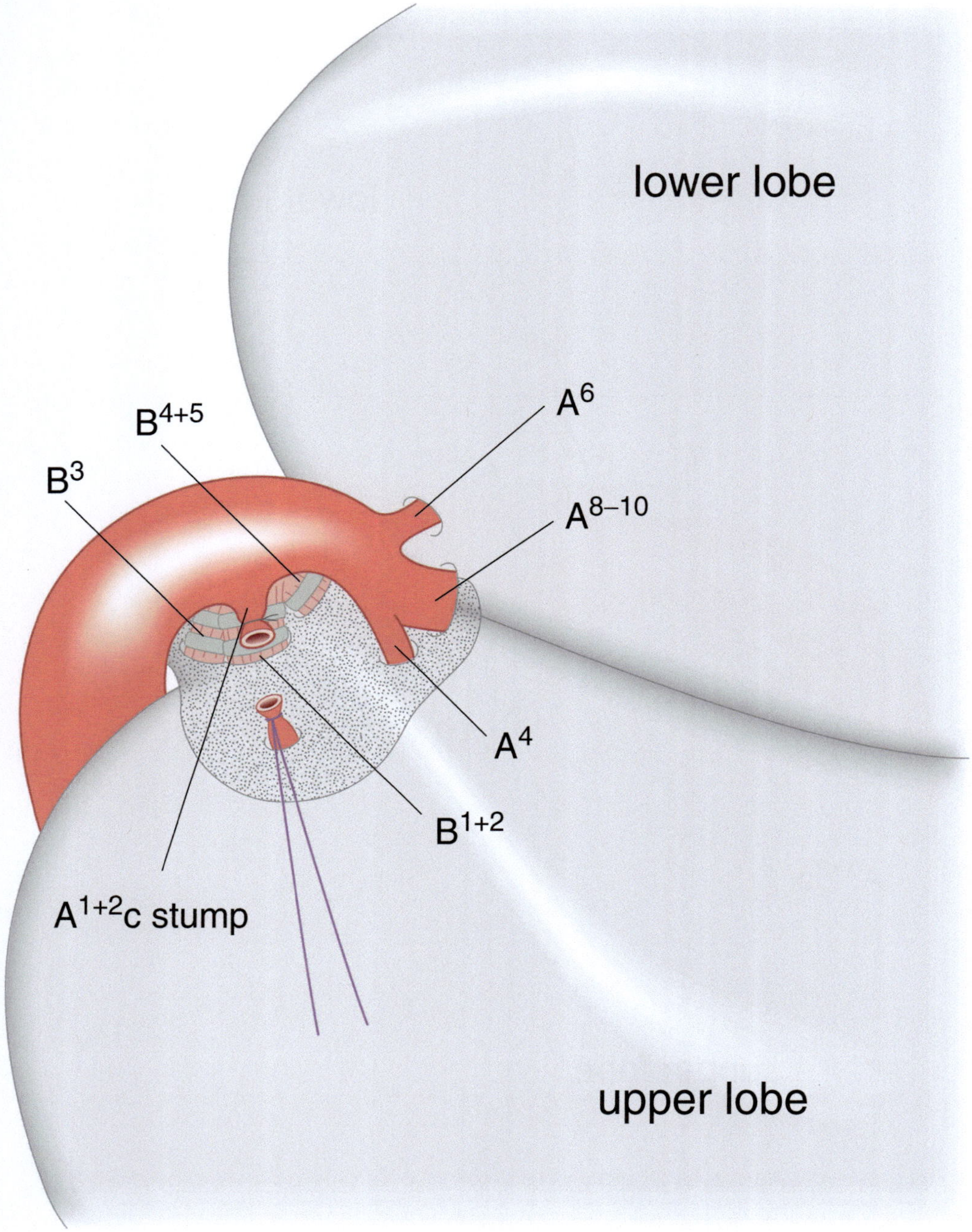

Fig. 5.1.6 Cutting $A^{1+2}c$ can expose B^{1+2} and B^3, which can also be confirmed from the illumination of bronchoscope inserted into B^{1-3} and B^{4+5}.

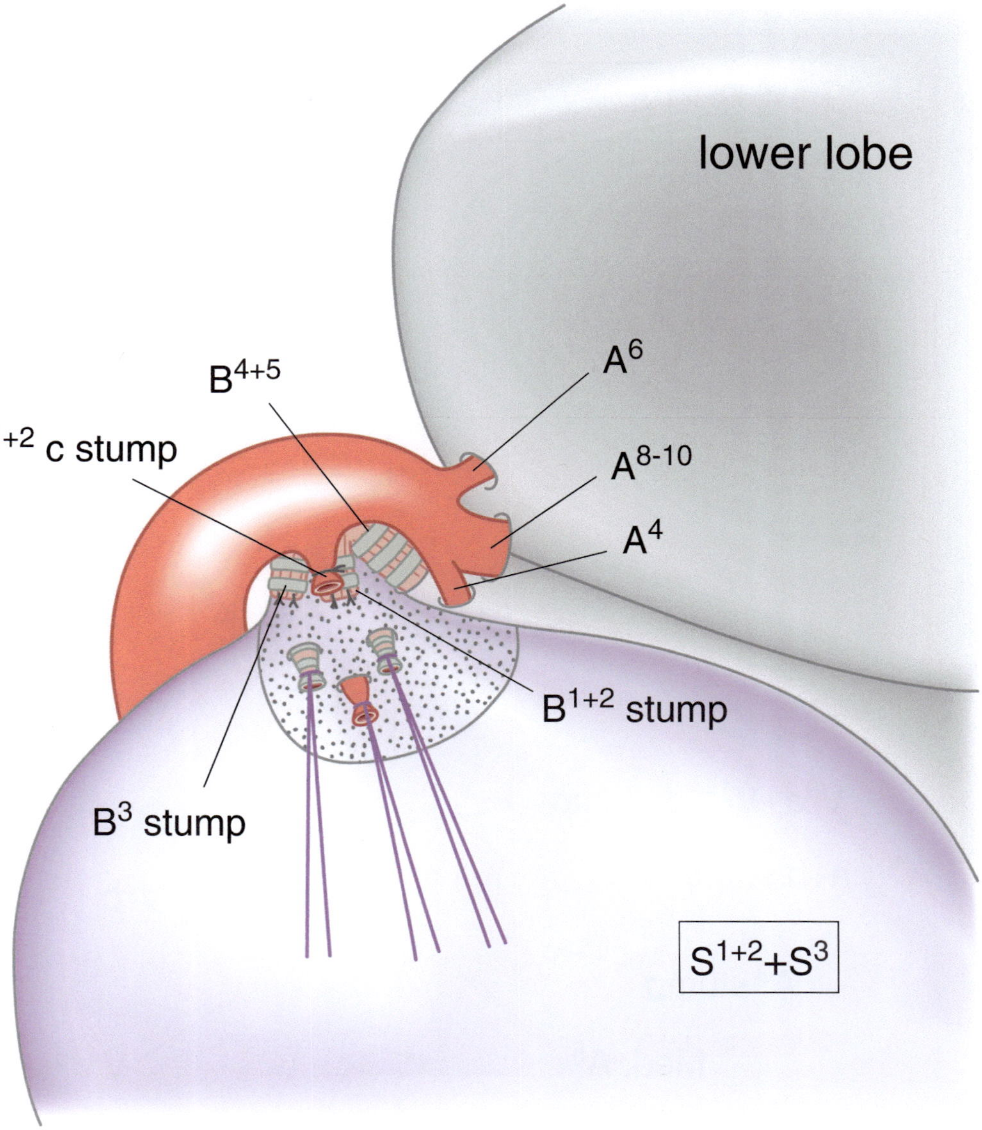

Fig. 5.1.7 $S^{1+2}+S^3$ is selectively inflated either by inserting a bronchoscope into B^{1-3} followed by jet ventilation, or by cutting the B^{1-3} and inserting a catheter into the peripheral stump followed by air inflation. The distal stump is closed to trap air within $S^{1+2}+S^3$. The proximal stump of B^{1-3} is closed with suture. When using jet ventilation via bronchoscope to inflate $S^{1+2}+S^3$, B^{1-3} can be cut using a stapler. The distal stump of B^{1-3} is lifted and denuded peripherally at the back to move the stump away from the hilum. Lifting the distal B^{1-3} stump also elevates lung tissue on both sides of the stump, and this lung tissue is cut towards the inflation–deflation line using electrocautery. Cutting the lung tissue reveals $V^{1+2}d$ (between $S^{1+2}c$ and S^3a), V^3a (between S^3a and S^3b), and V^3b (between S^3b and S^4b). While $V^{1+2}d$ and V^3a are cut, V^3b is preserved to preserve the lingular division (S^4+S^5) sufficiently if the surgical margin is enough.

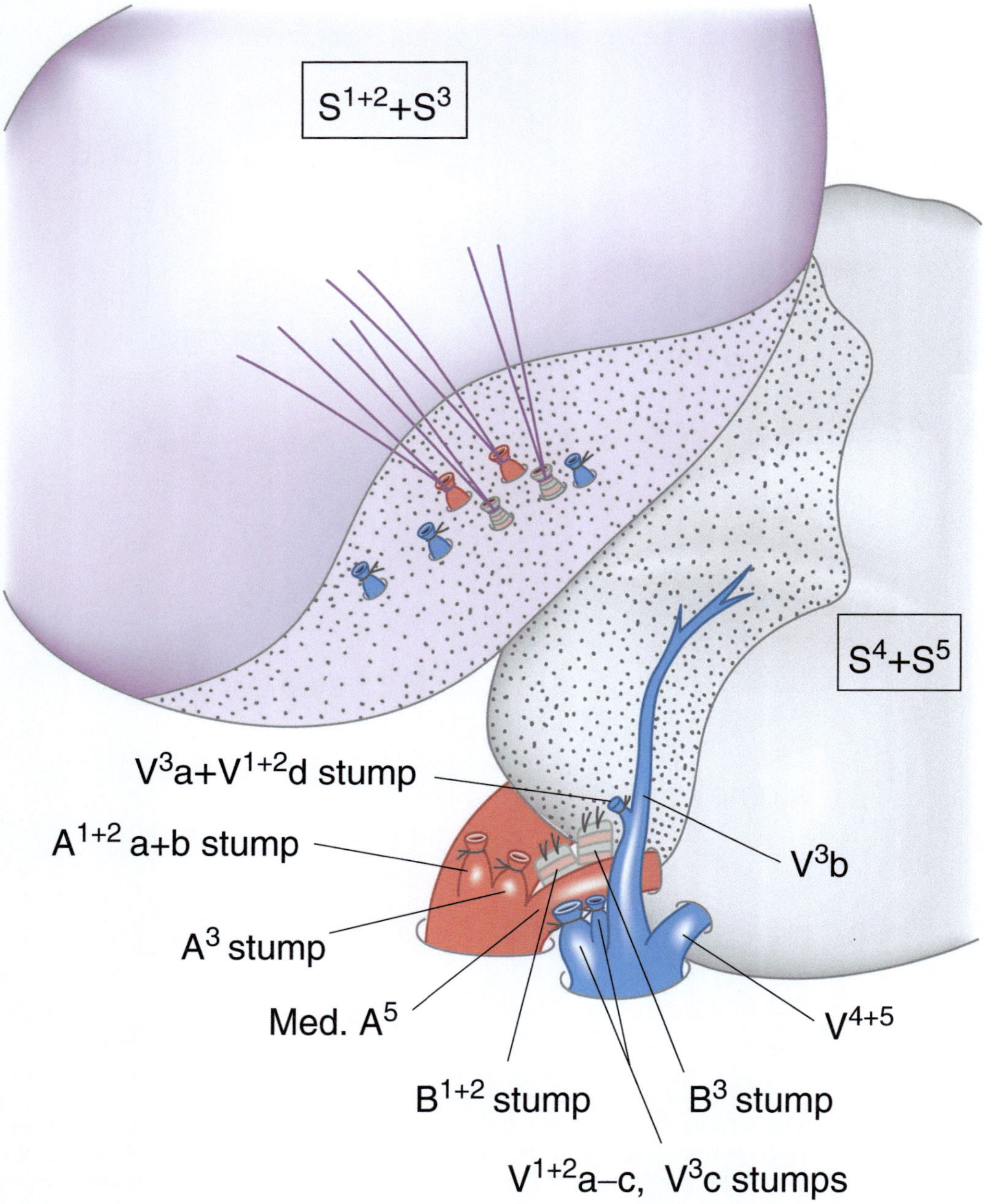

Fig. 5.1.8 Lung tissue is not cut with a stapler especially in upper division segmentectomy, as the lingular division (S^4+S^5) shrinks when whole lung tissue including the visceral pleura is cut by a stapler. A stapler can be used only for deep lung tissue after cutting shallow lung tissue using electrocautery. However, the intersegmental plane between $S^{1+2}+S^3$ and S^4+S^5 can usually be easily identified during cutting by electrocautery. The #11 lymph nodes are dissected after taping both B^{4+5} and A^4 or A^{4+5}.

5.2 Left S^{1+2} Segmentectomy

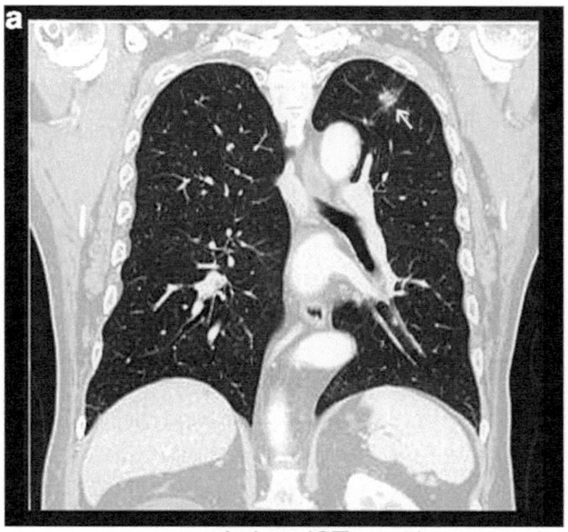

coronal view (CT scan)

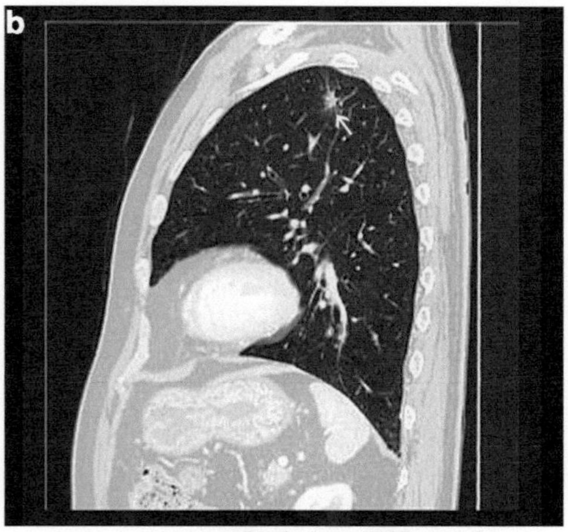

sagittal view (CT scan)

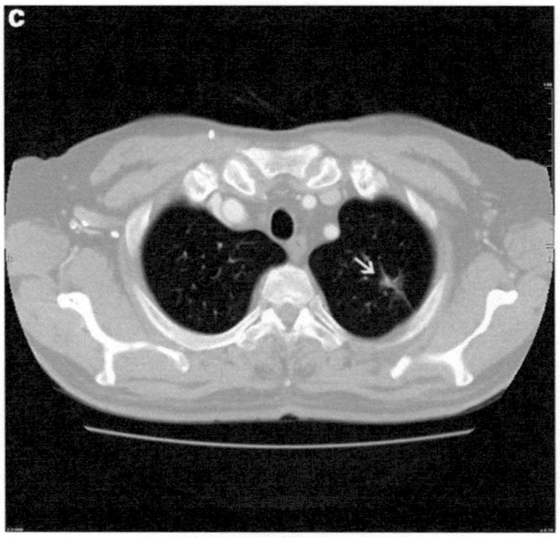

axial view (CT scan)

A GGO lesion was discovered in a 74-year-old male 2 years previously. A follow-up CT showed that the lesion had increased and had a solid region. A CT scan showed a 1.6-cm nodule with spicular formation and pleural indentation. The nodule was diagnosed as adenocarcinoma from the CT-guided needle biopsy specimen. The tumor was located within S^{1+2}. The S^{1+2}-segmentectomy was proceeded, and the final pathological diagnosis was pT1aN0M0 papillary adenocarcinoma.

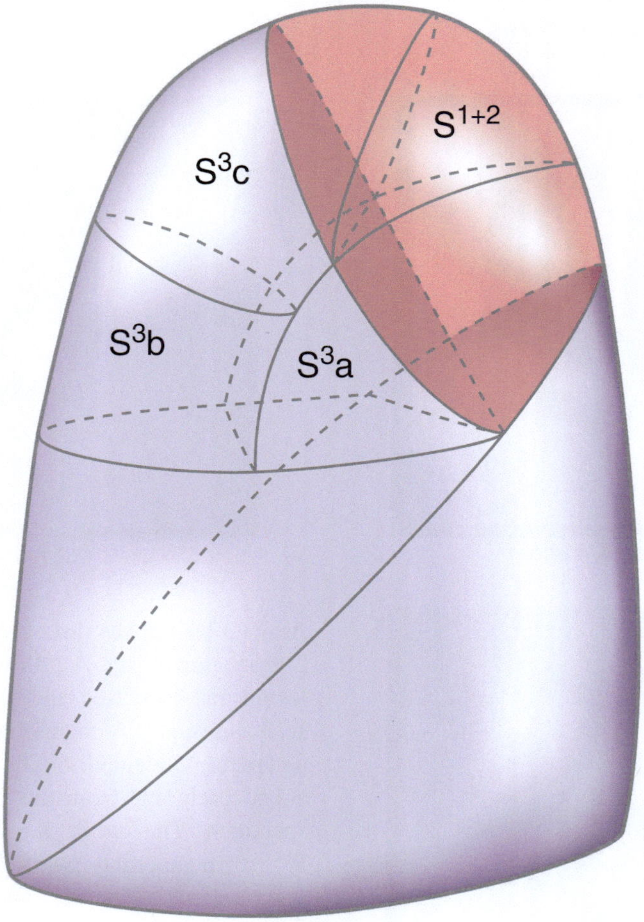

Fig. 5.2.1 Artery, vein, and bronchus branching is confirmed from axial, coronal, and sagittal views on HRCT, and the branching and size of B^{1+2} and B^3 are further examined by bronchoscope after tracheal intubation. The bronchus most frequently branches into B^{1-3} and B^{4+5}, and sometimes into B^{1+2}, B^3, and B^{4+5}. The anatomical branching configuration in the figures of this session is that the B^{1-3} is branched into B^{1+2} and B^3 (46% in frequency), A^{1+2} is branched into A^{1+2}a+b and A^{1+2}c (31%), and A^5 is the mediastinal type (12%).

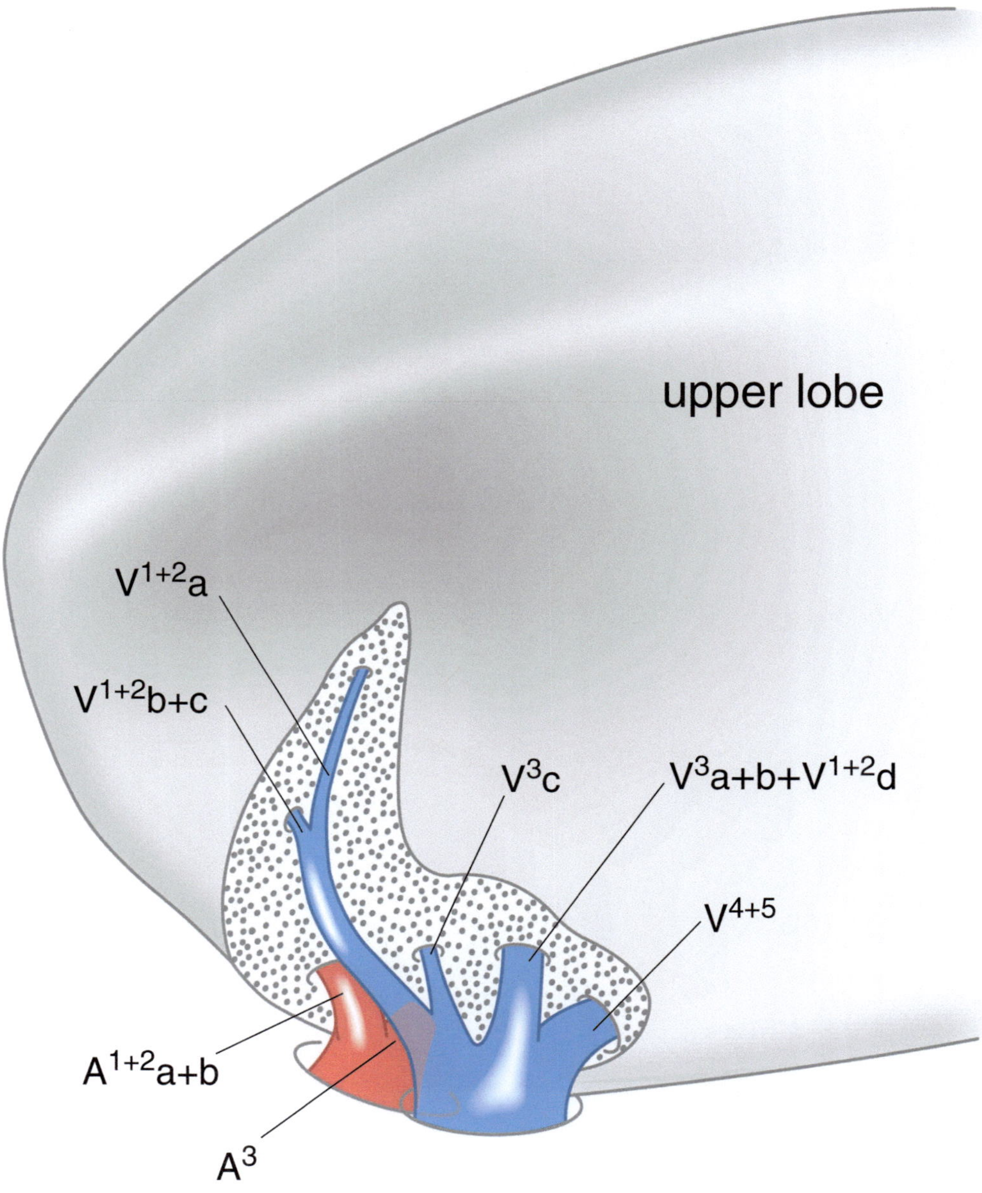

Fig. 5.2.2 The hilum of the left upper lobe is exposed from the ventral to the dorsal side to reveal the superior pulmonary vein and pulmonary arteries. The V^{1+2} is encircled with tape and exposed peripherally to identify $V^{1+2}a$. The $V^{1+2}a$ runs near the surface layer and towards the apex between S^{1+2} and S^3. At this point, $V^{1+2}b+c$ is not usually visible. A thin V^{1+2} superior sometimes branches from the proximal site of V^{1+2}, which runs dorsally and crosses A^{1+2}. The V^{1+2} superior is cut. The $V^{1+2}a$ is exposed peripherally which identifies the border between S^{1+2} and S^3. Exposing the $V^{1+2}a$ can identify A^{1+2} and A^3 which, respectively, run dorsally and ventrally to $V^{1+2}a$.

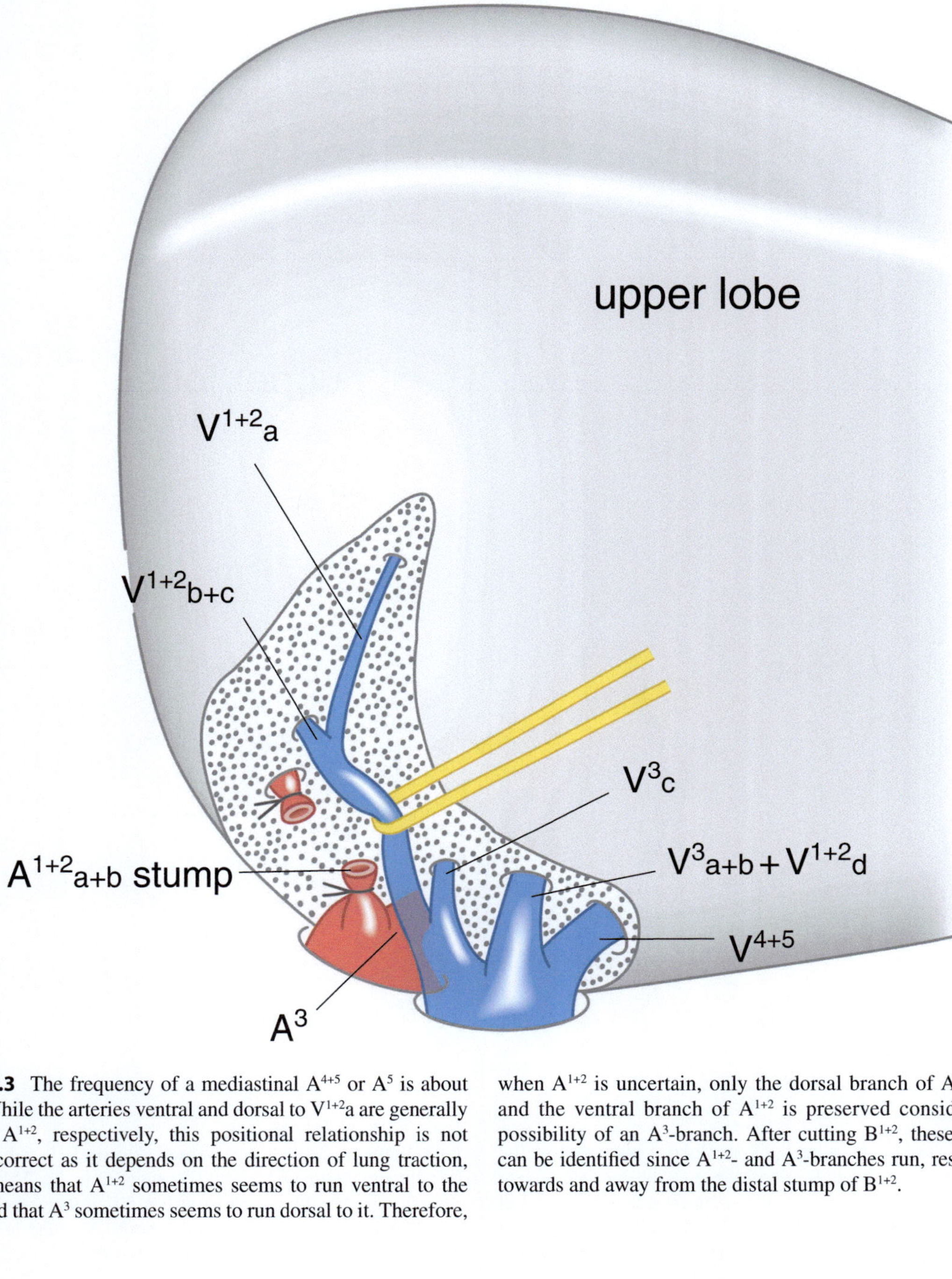

Fig. 5.2.3 The frequency of a mediastinal A^{4+5} or A^5 is about 30 %. While the arteries ventral and dorsal to V^{1+2}a are generally A^3 and A^{1+2}, respectively, this positional relationship is not always correct as it depends on the direction of lung traction, which means that A^{1+2} sometimes seems to run ventral to the V^{1+2}a and that A^3 sometimes seems to run dorsal to it. Therefore, when A^{1+2} is uncertain, only the dorsal branch of A^{1+2} is cut, and the ventral branch of A^{1+2} is preserved considering the possibility of an A^3-branch. After cutting B^{1+2}, these branches can be identified since A^{1+2}- and A^3-branches run, respectively, towards and away from the distal stump of B^{1+2}.

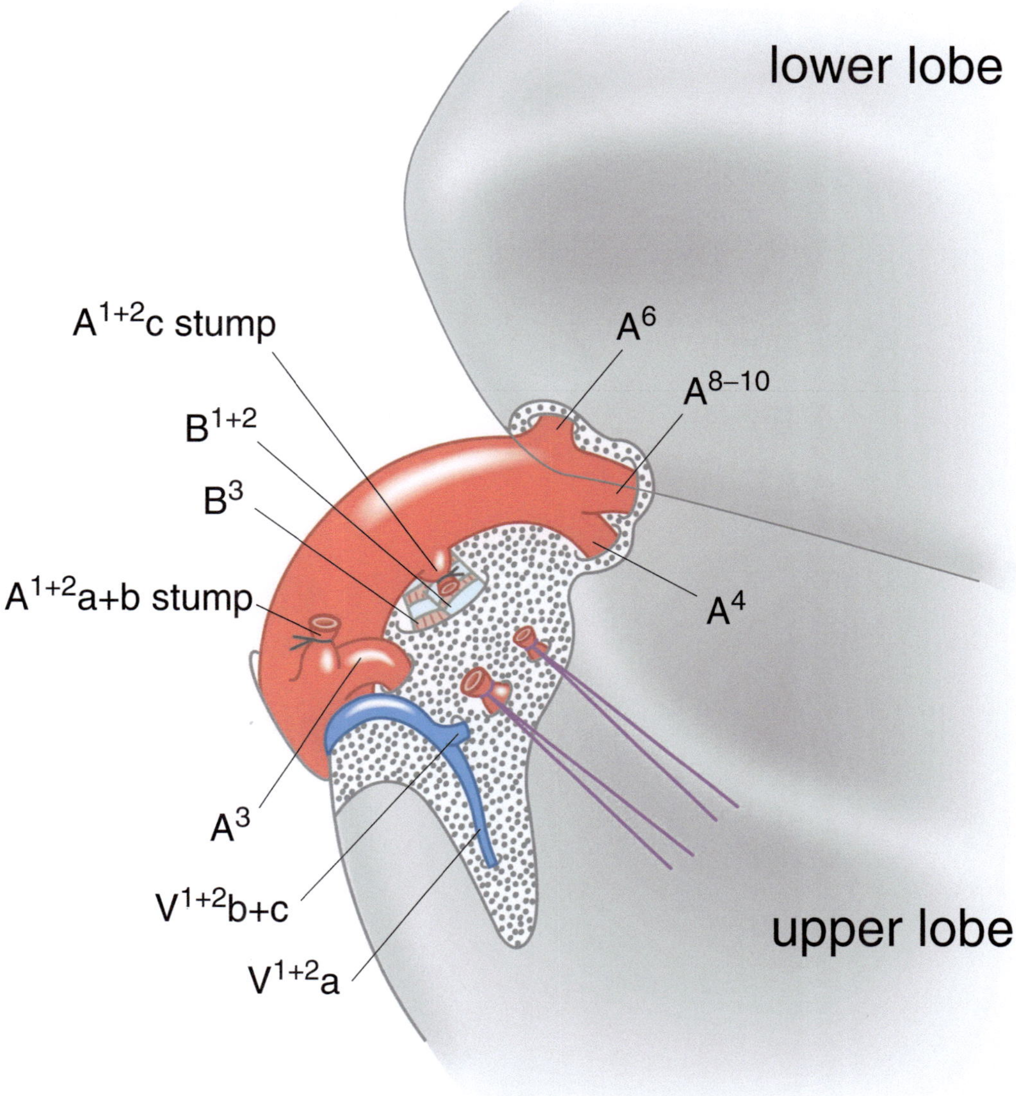

Fig. 5.2.4 The incomplete fissure between S^{1+2} and S^{6} is divided using electrocautery but not a stapler, because a staple line usually impairs identification of the intersegmental plane. The following procedure facilitates the fissure identification: a bronchoscope is inserted into B^{1+2} followed by jet ventilation, which forms an inflation-deflation line between the inflated S^{1+2} and deflated lower lobe. The fissure can be divided along the inflated-deflated line using electrocautery. A^{1+2}c branching from the truncus intermedius artery is identified. While an artery branching at proximal side of A^{6} is usually A^{1+2}c, it is sometimes difficult to differentiate from A^{4}a, especially when it branches near the level of A^{6}. Therefore, an arterial branch near A^{6} is preserved at this point, because it might be A^{4}a. It can be identified later after cutting the B^{1+2}. Cutting A^{1+2}a+b and A^{1+2}c exposes lymph nodes around B^{1+2}. Dissecting these lymph nodes reveals B^{1+2}, which is encircled with thread. A precaution at this point is that the bronchus visible here is not usually B^{1+2}, which might be B$^{1-3}$ or B^{1+2}c. The following point is important to identify B^{1+2} correctly: preoperative bronchoscopic findings of the anatomical branching and size of B^{1+2}; the B^{1+2} and B^{3} run, respectively, towards the dorsal and ventral side of A^{3}; and intraoperative bronchoscopic identification by illuminating the B^{1+2} and B^{3}.

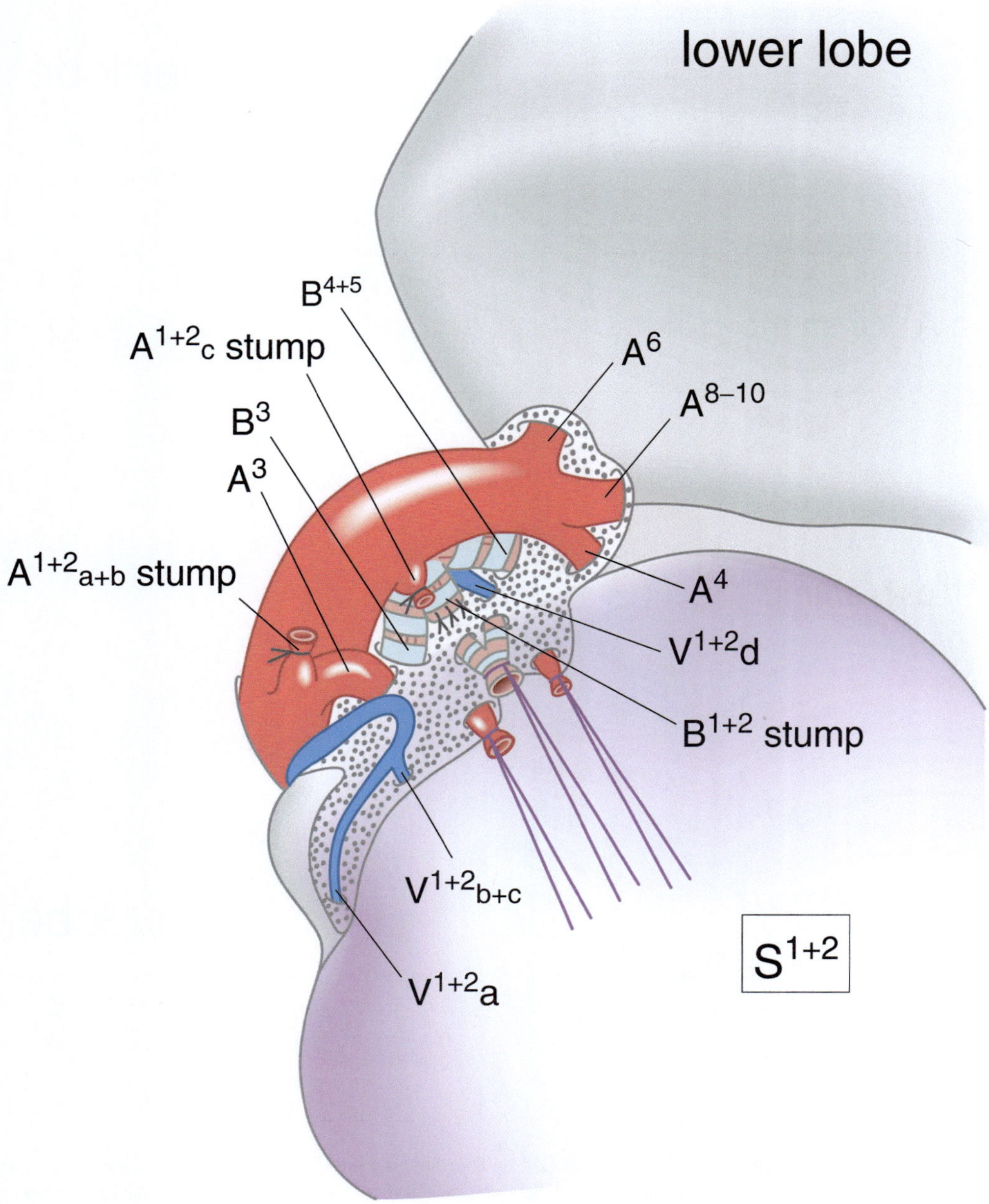

Fig. 5.2.5 S^{1+2} is selectively inflated either by inserting a bronchoscope into B^{1+2} followed by jet ventilation, or by cutting the B^{1+2} and inserting a catheter into the distal stump followed by air inflation. The distal stump is closed to trap air within S^{1+2}. The proximal stump of B^{1+2} is closed with suture or ligation. When using S^{1+2} is inflated by jet ventilation via bronchoscope, B^{1+2} can be cut using a stapler. The distal stump of B^{1+2} is lifted and is denuded peripherally at the back to move the stump away from the hilum. Lifting the distal B^{1+2} stump also elevates lung tissue at both sides of the stump, which is cut toward the inflation–deflation line using electrocautery.

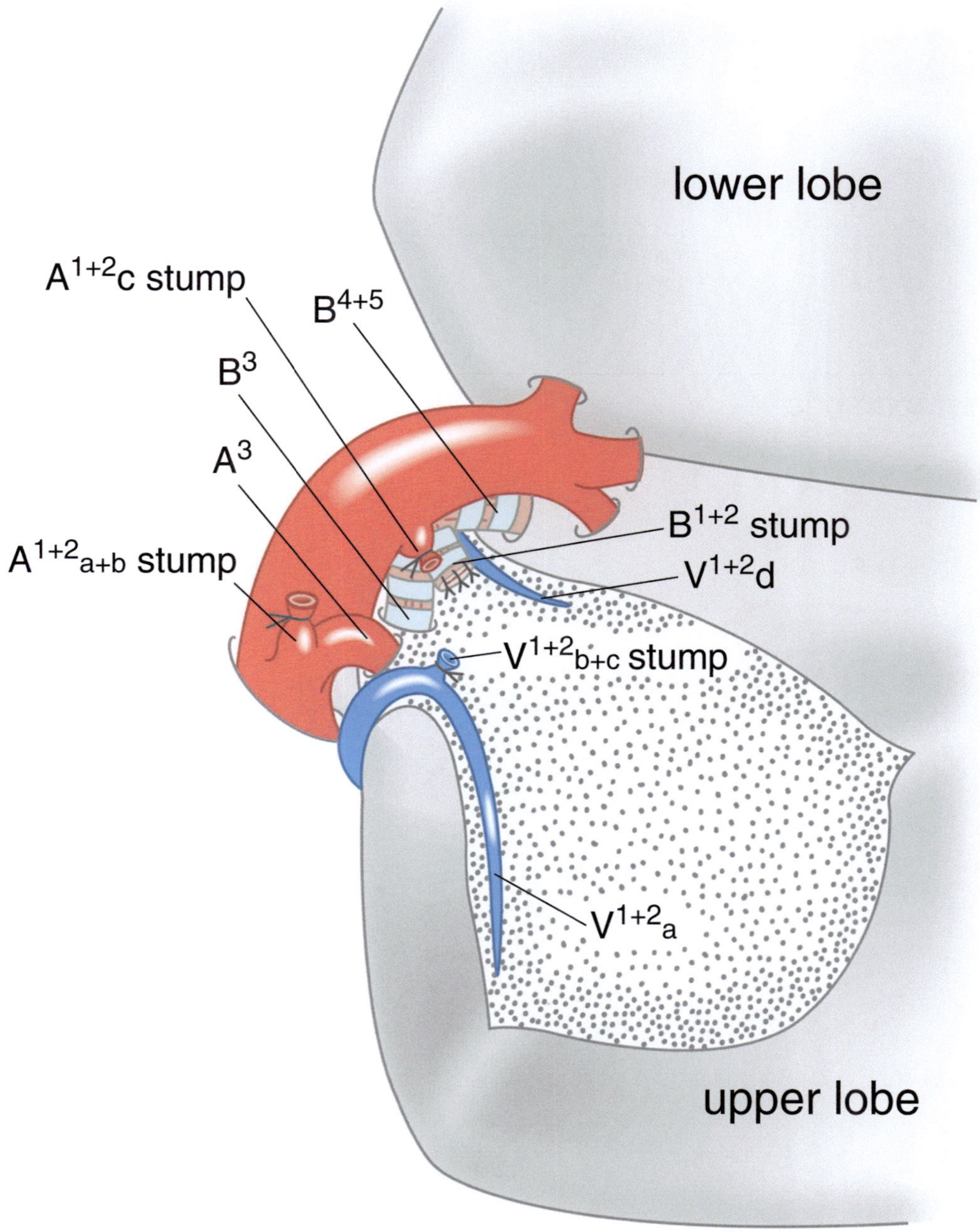

Fig. 5.2.6 Lung tissue is cut along the inflation–deflation line. While cutting the lung tissue, $V^{1+2}b$ and $V^{1+2}c$ running into the S^{1+2} are cut. $V^{1+2}d$ (between $S^{1+2}c$ and $S^{3}a$), which runs from the ventral side, is preserved on S^{3}. The intersegmental plane is cut from various directions to facilitate simple and accurate intersegmental cutting.

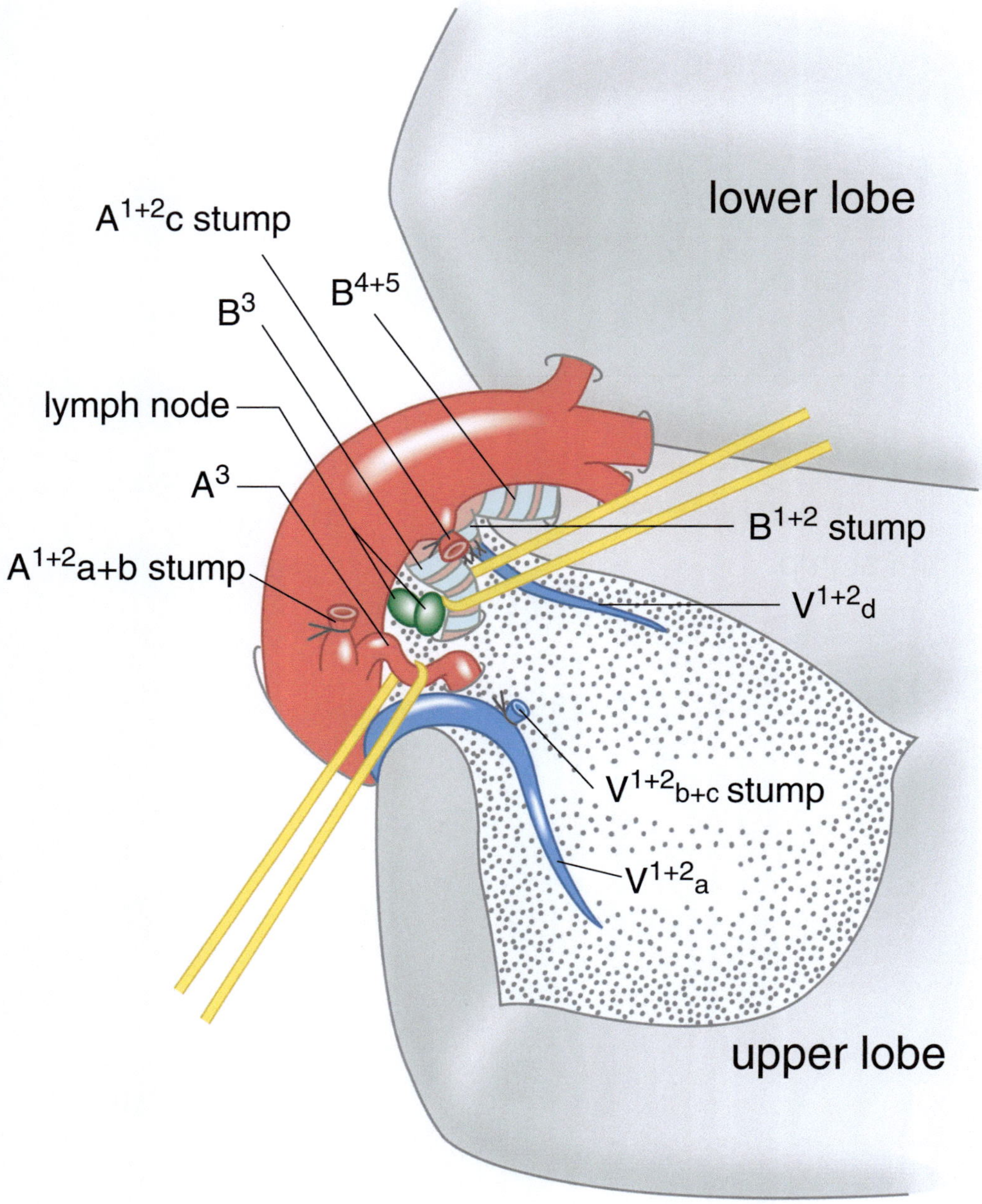

Fig. 5.2.7 The branches of B^3, A^3, and V^{1+2} are encircled with tape to show the #12u and #13 lymph nodes for dissection. One dissection technique is to peel the lymph nodes from both the B^3 and A^3 from the dorsal side first and then pass them through A^3 towards the ventral side. This enables dissection of #12u and #13 lymph nodes altogether from the ventral side. The #13 node between the B^{1-3} and B^{4+5} is then dissected. The A^4 or A^{4+5} are encircled with tape and the interlobar fissure is opened to the ventral side to expose the #11 node for sampling.

5.3 Left S³ Segmentectomy

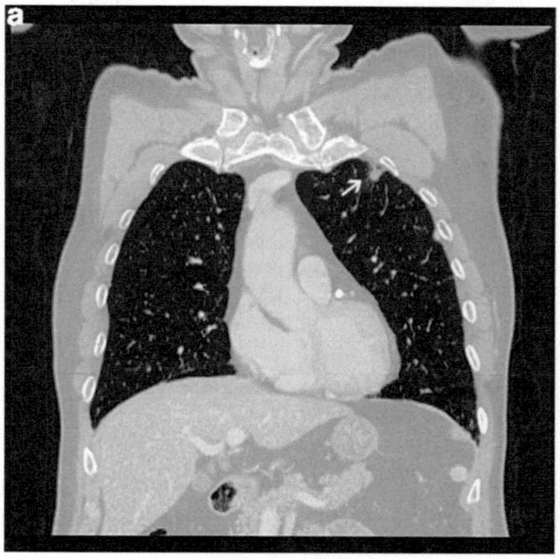

coronal view (CT scan)

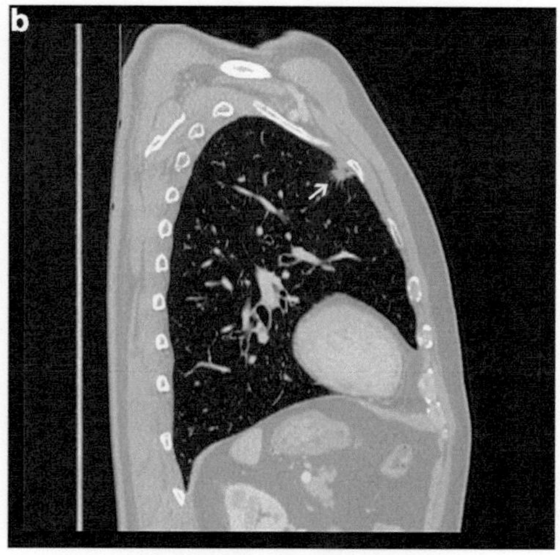

sagittal view (CT scan)

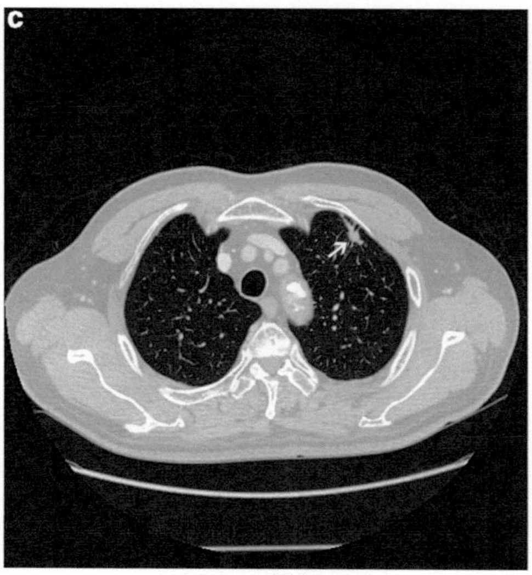

axial view (CT scan)

A follow-up CT scan of a 71-year-old male with angina revealed a 1.6-cm nodule in the left S^3b that was diagnosed as adenocarcinoma from a CT-guided needle biopsy specimen. The final diagnosis after left S^3-segmentectomy was pT1aN0M0 papillary adenocarcinoma.

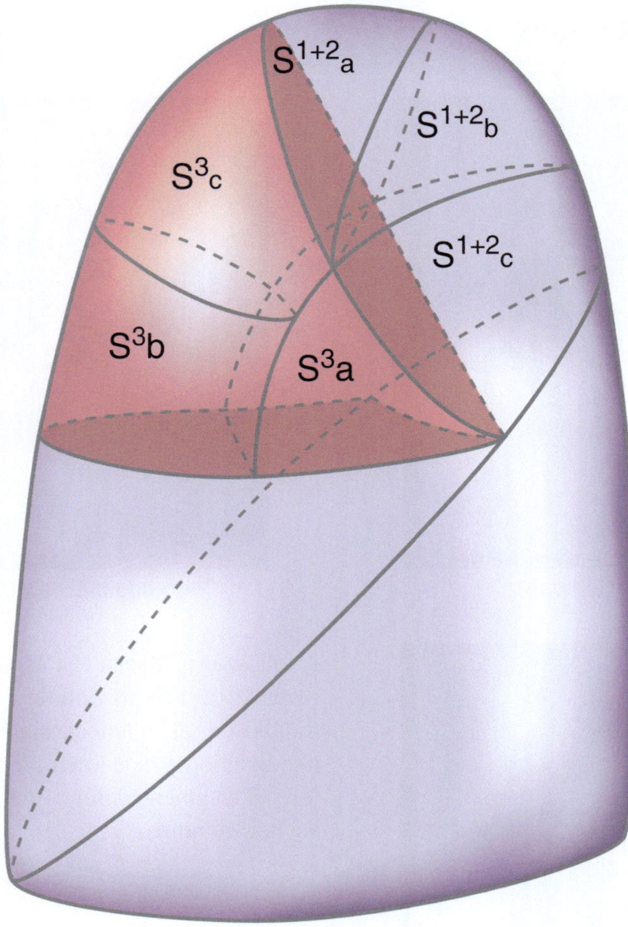

Fig. 5.3.1 Anatomical branching of artery, vein, and bronchus is confirmed from axial, coronal, and sagittal views on HRCT. The branches and sizes of B^{1+2} and B^3 are further examined using bronchoscope after tracheal intubation. One of the most important points of S^3-segmentecotmy is to preserve sufficient pulmonary function of the neighboring lingular division (S^4+S^5), which has a small volume as well as the right middle lobe. The following points are important to achieve this. Lung tissue between S^3 and the lingular division is not cut using a stapler, which would impair sufficient expansion of the lingular division. V^3b is preserved on lingular division, because it can help the sufficient preservation of lingular division.

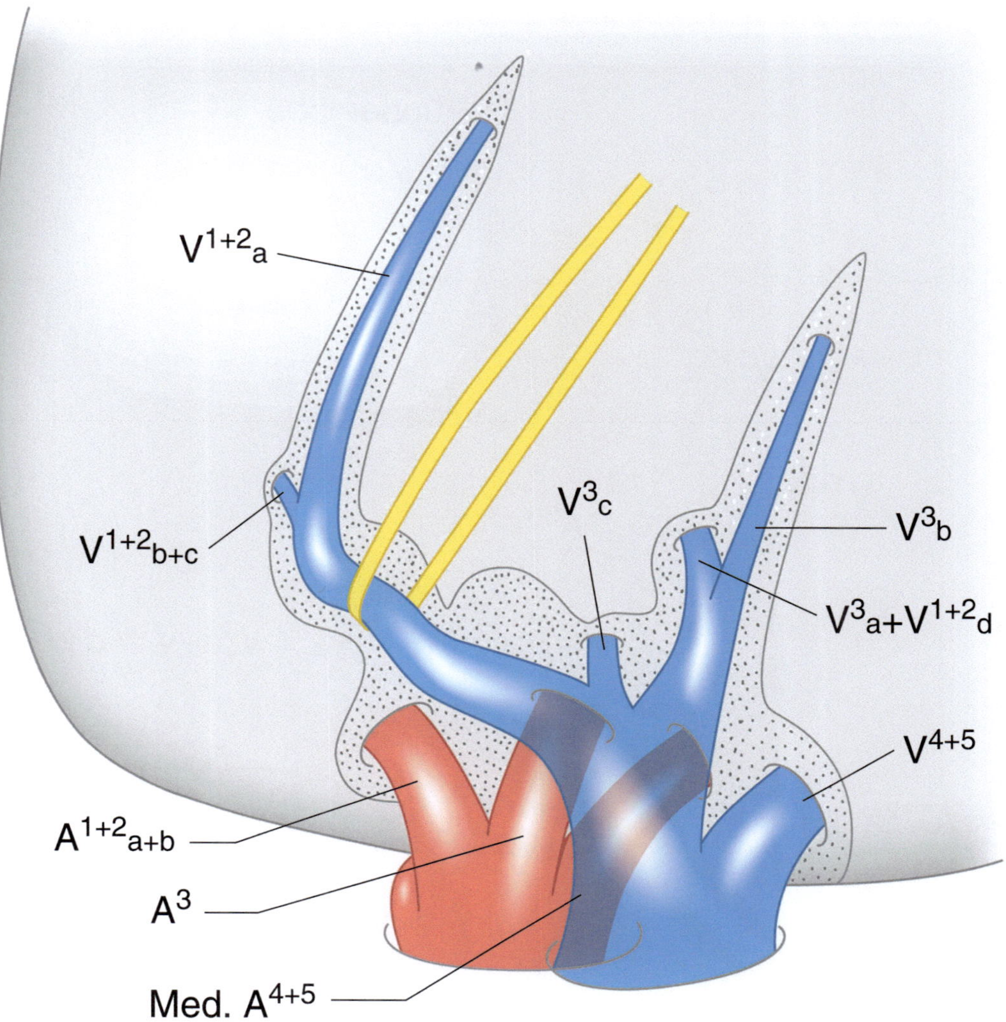

Fig. 5.3.2 The segmental bronchus in the figures of this session branches with B^{1+2} and B^3 (46 % frequency). It is known that A^3 almost always forms one or two branches from the main pulmonary artery (90 % in frequency). The hilum of the left upper lobe is exposed from the ventral to the dorsal side to reveal the superior pulmonary vein, and the main pulmonary artery, truncus superior artery, truncus intermedius artery, and proximal site of the interlobar artery. V^{1+2} is encircled with tape and exposed peripherally to identify $V^{1+2}a$. The $V^{1+2}a$ is exposed peripherally to identify the border between S^{1+2} and S^3. The $V^{1+2}a$ runs towards the apex and near the surface layer. Exposing $V^{1+2}a$ can identify A^{1+2} and A^3 running at the dorsal and ventral side of $V^{1+2}a$, respectively. Next, V^3b running ventrally near the surface of lung between S^3 and S^4 is exposed peripherally to reveal the border between S^3 and S^4. The V^3a and $V^{1+2}d$, usually forming a common trunk, branches from the back of V^3b.

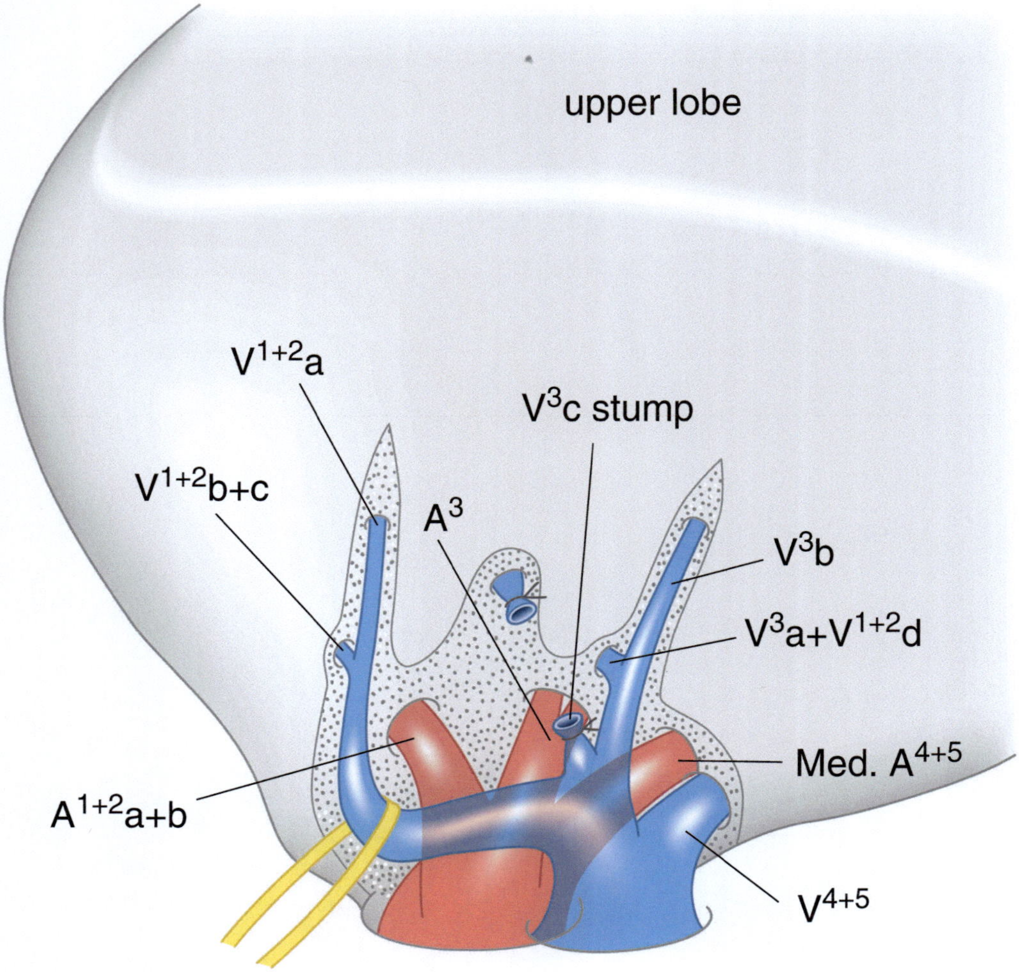

Fig. 5.3.3 V^3c running between S^3b and S^3c is cut, which visualizes the course of A^3. Mediastinal A^{4+5} or A^5 runs between V^3 and B^3. The A^3 is cut after confirming the presence or absence of a mediastinal A^{4+5}. Depending on the direction of traction of the lung, a branch of A^{1+2} sometimes seems to run at the ventral side of $V^{1+2}a$. Therefore, a dorsal branch of A^3 that might be A^{1+2}-branch is preserved at this point. Its identification can be easily confirmed later by cutting B^3, because the A^{1+2}-branch runs away from the distal stump of B^3, whereas the A^3-branch runs toward it.

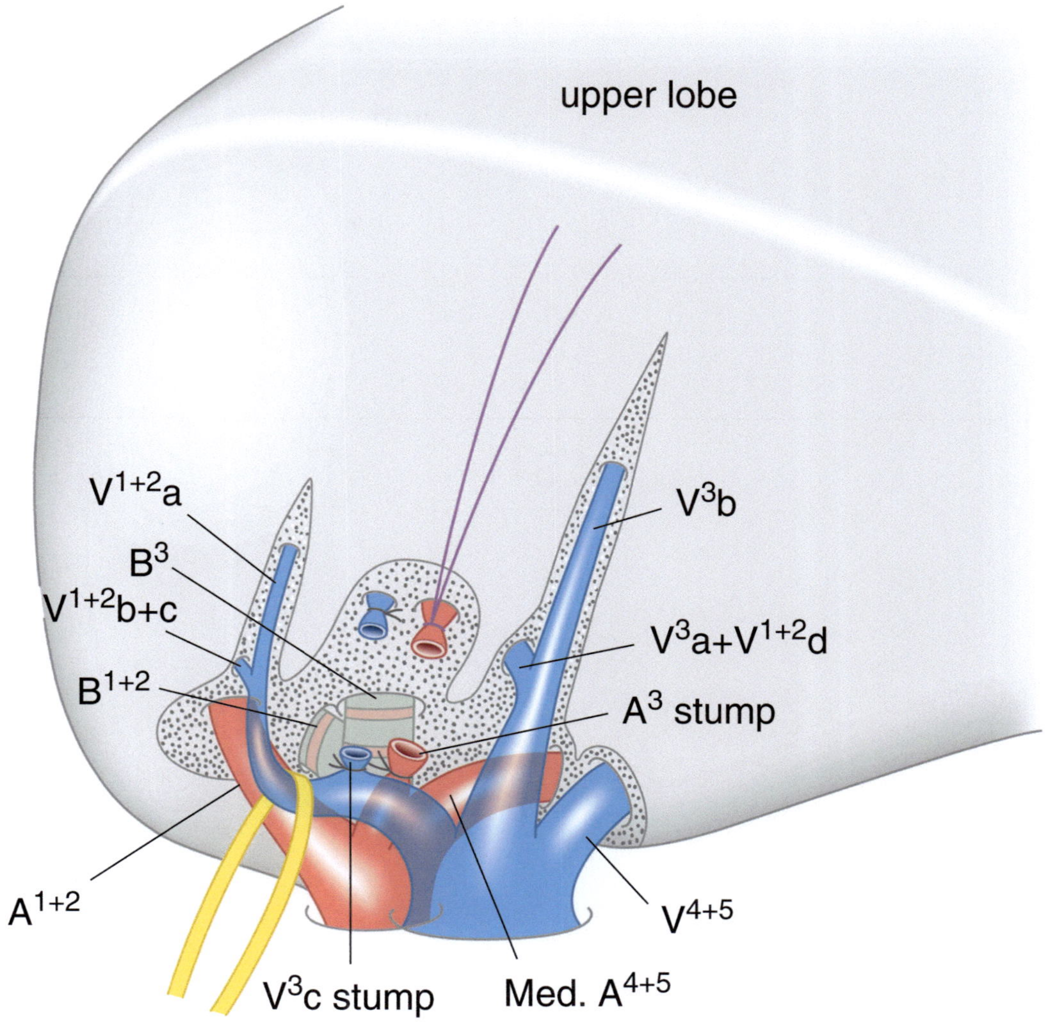

Fig. 5.3.4 After cutting A^3, B^3 can be seen at its backside. The lymph nodes are visible in front of B^3, which are dissected. B^3 is encircled with thread. However, B^3a which branches from the backside of B^3 would be missed when B^3a and B^3b+c branches at the root of B^3. Preoperative bronchoscopic findings could help to identify B^3a and B^3b+c, and illumination from a bronchoscope inserted into B^3 can also provide a confirmation.

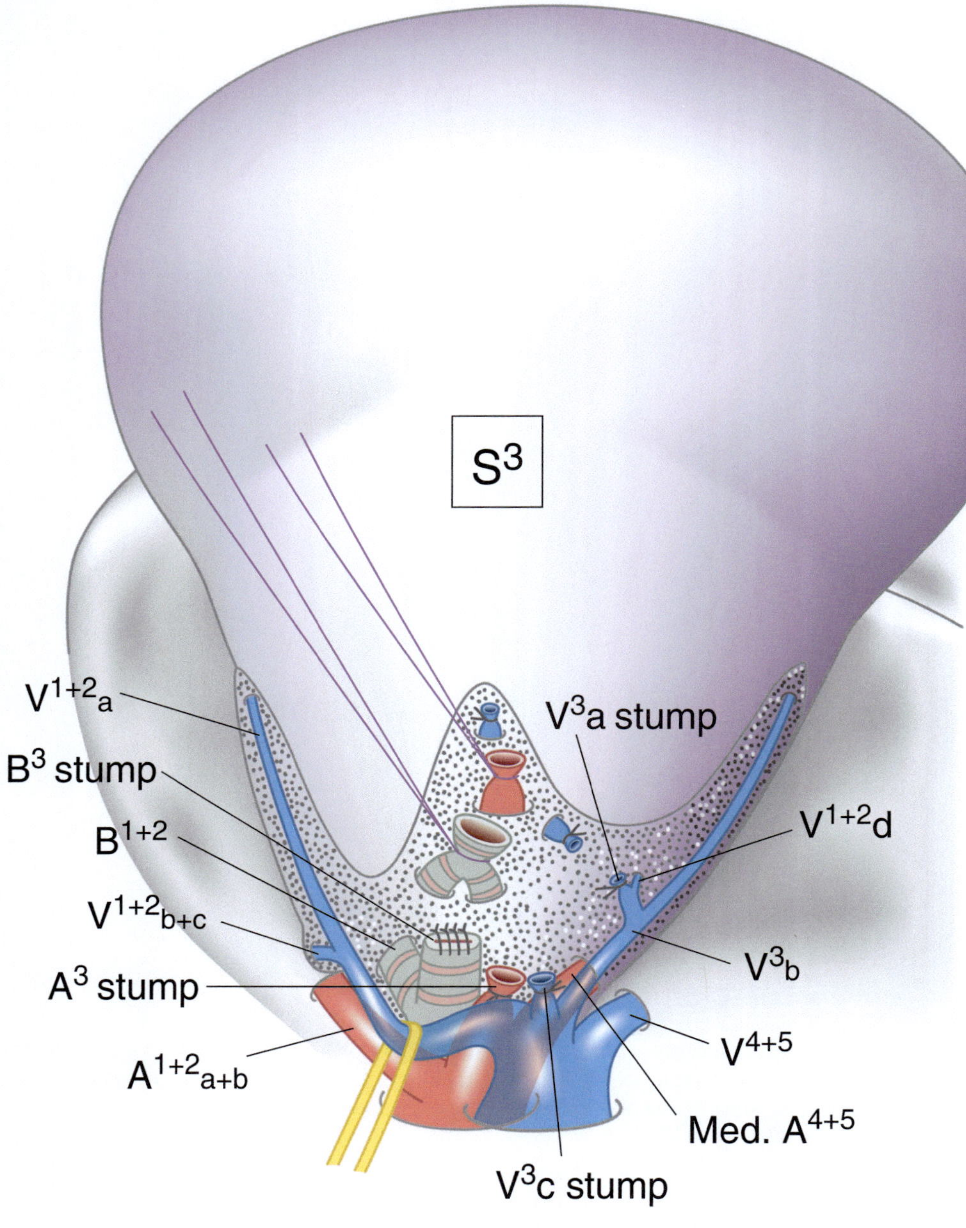

Fig. 5.3.5 S^3 is selectively inflated either by inserting a bronchoscope into B^3 followed by jet ventilation, or by cutting the B^3 and inserting a catheter into the distal stump followed by air inflation. The distal stump is closed to trap air within S^3. The proximal stump of B^3 is closed with suture or ligation. The distal stump of B^3 is lifted and denuded peripherally at the back which moves the stump away from the hilum. Lifting the stump also elevates lung tissue at both sides of the stump, which is cut towards the inflation–deflation line using electrocautery and also along V^3b and V^{1+2}a. The V^3b is preserved on the lingular division ($S^4 + S^5$), which help to identify the segmental plane and also to preserve the lingular division sufficiently. Cutting the lung tissue reveals V^3a (between S^3a and S^3b) and V^{1+2}d (between S^3a and S^{1+2}c) branching from the back of V^3b. The V^3a is cut, whereas V^{1+2}d is preserved for not only the guide of intersegmental plane but also preservation of venous return from S^{1+2}c. The intersegmental plane is cut from various directions to facilitate simple and accurate segmentectomy.

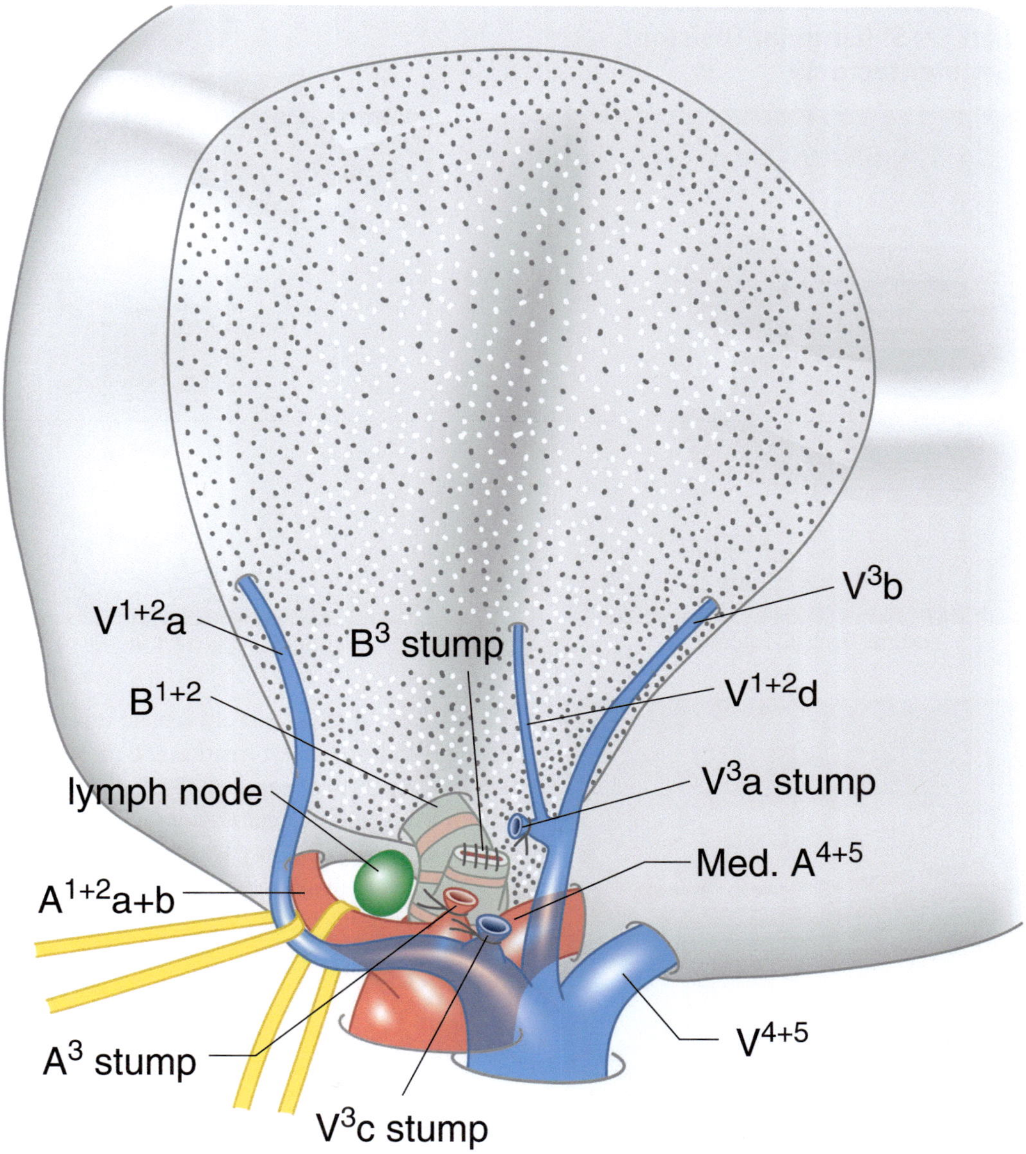

Fig. 5.3.6 Hilar lymph node dissection differs somewhat between S^3- and S^{1+2}-segmentectomy. Because $A^{1+2}c$ is not cut in S^3-segmentectomy, the lymph node dissection from the dorsal side is a little difficult. The $A^{1+2}a+b$ and B^{1+2} are encircled with tape. The #12u and #13 lymph nodes are then peeled away from the artery and bronchus from the dorsal side, passed through the artery and bronchus, and then dissected from the ventral side, which enables dissecting these nodes together.

5.4 Left S^4+S^5 (Lingular Division) Segmentectomy

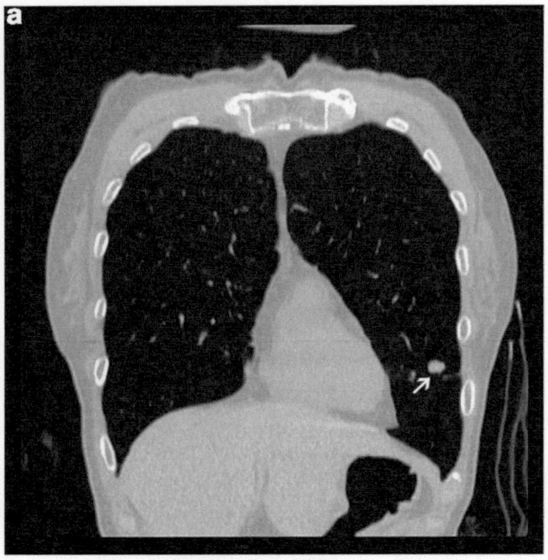

coronal view (CT scan)

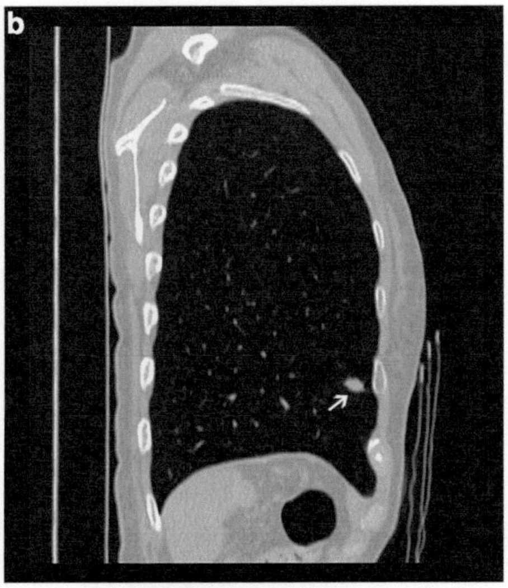

sagittal view (CT scan)

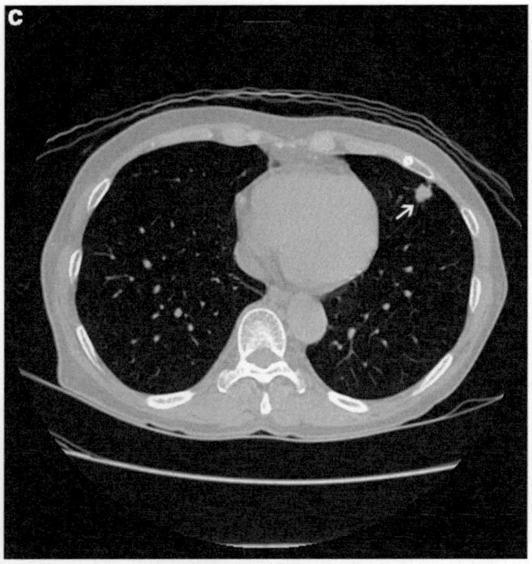

axial view (CT scan)

A CT scan of a 73-year-old female revealed a 1.2-cm nodule with spicular formation and pleural indentation in the left S^5 that was diagnosed as adenocarcinoma from a CT-guided needle biopsy specimen. Lingular division segmentectomy was proceeded, and the final pathological diagnosis was pT1aN0M0 papillary adenocarcinoma.

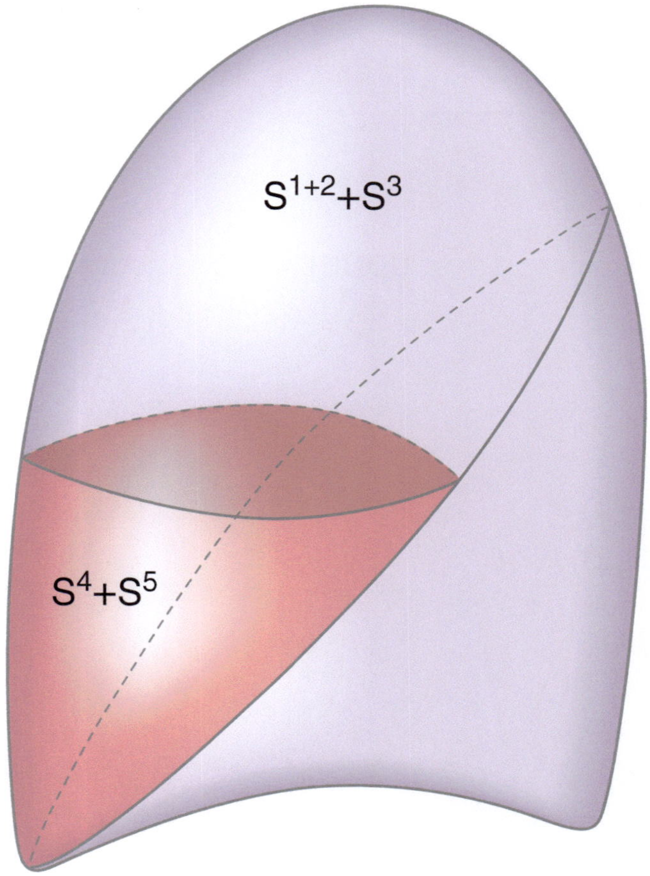

Fig. 5.4.1 The branching patterns of artery, vein, and bronchus are confirmed from axial, coronal, and sagittal views on HRCT. The branching profiles and size of B^{1-3} and B^{4+5} are further examined by bronchoscopy after tracheal intubation. Although the branching pattern with B^{1-3} and B^{4+5} is the most frequent, the pattern of three branches with B^{1+2}, B^3, and B^{4+5} or independent B^4a branching is occasionally encountered.

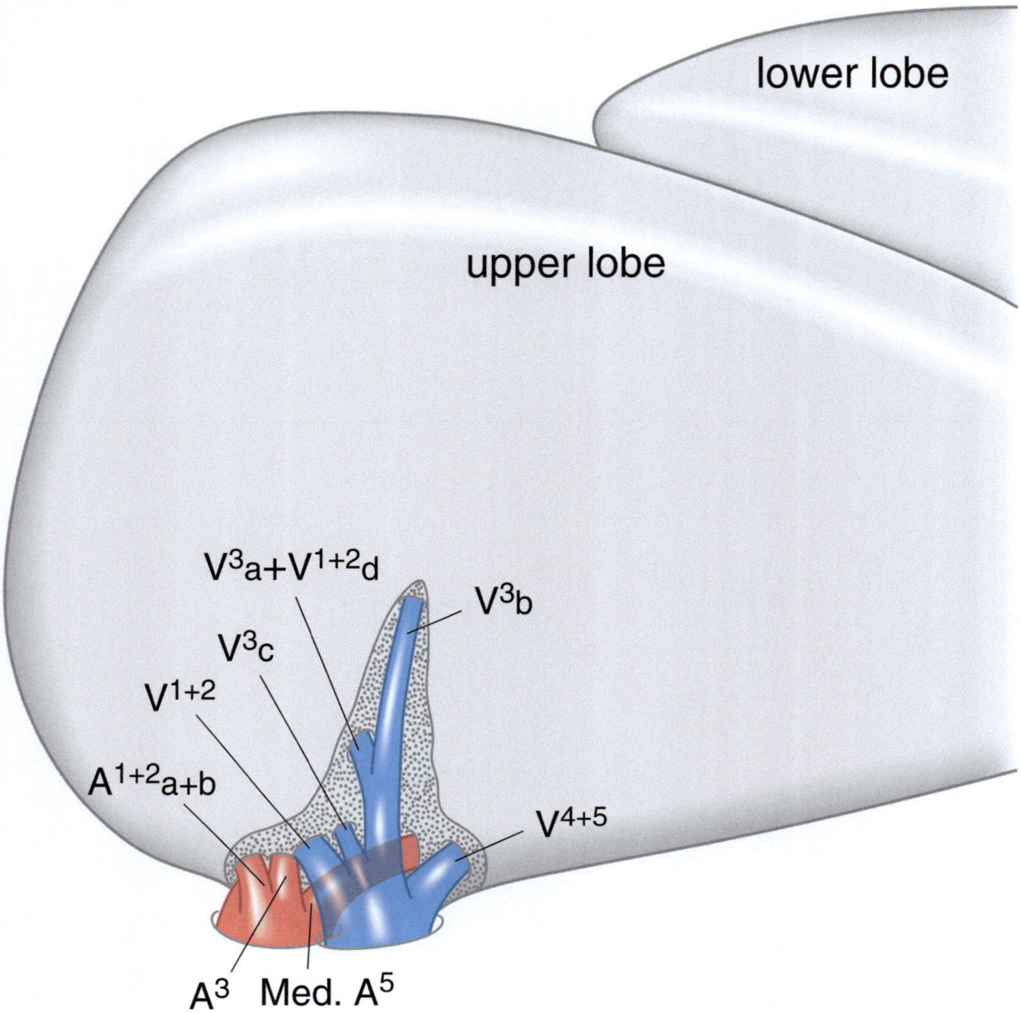

Fig. 5.4.2 The hilum of the left upper lobe is exposed from the ventral to the dorsal side to expose the superior pulmonary vein and the arteries from the left main to the proximal site of the interlobar artery. The frequency of having a mediastinal A^{4+5} or A^5 is about 30%. The figures in this session show a mediastinal A^5. The V^3b, which runs at the ventral side in the superficial layer, is identified, encircled with tape, and exposed peripherally to reveal the border between S^3 and S^4.

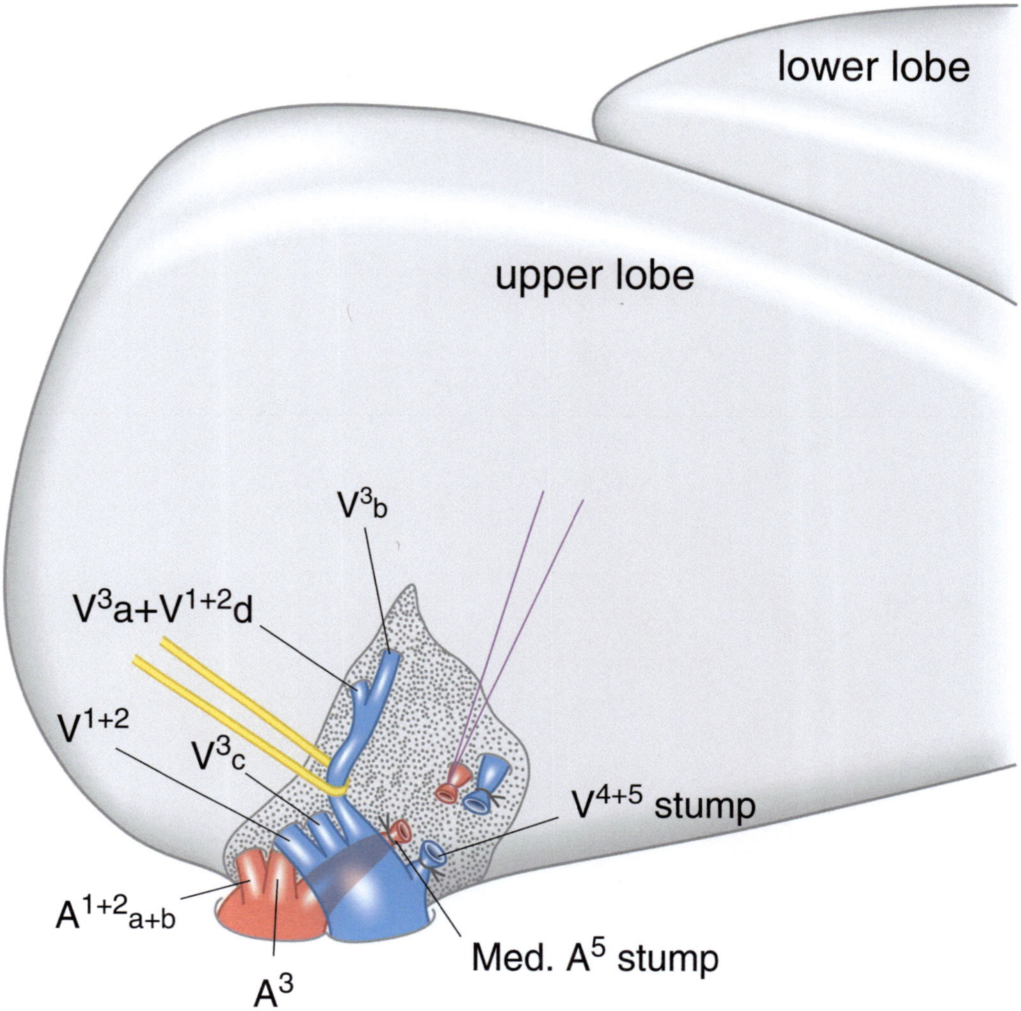

Fig. 5.4.3 V^{4+5} is cut. The V^{1+2}, V^3, and V^{4+5} sometimes branch independently each other, and if so, they should be carefully identified. In rare cases, V^{4+5} branches from the inferior pulmonary vein. Mediastinal A^5 running between V^3 and B^3 is cut.

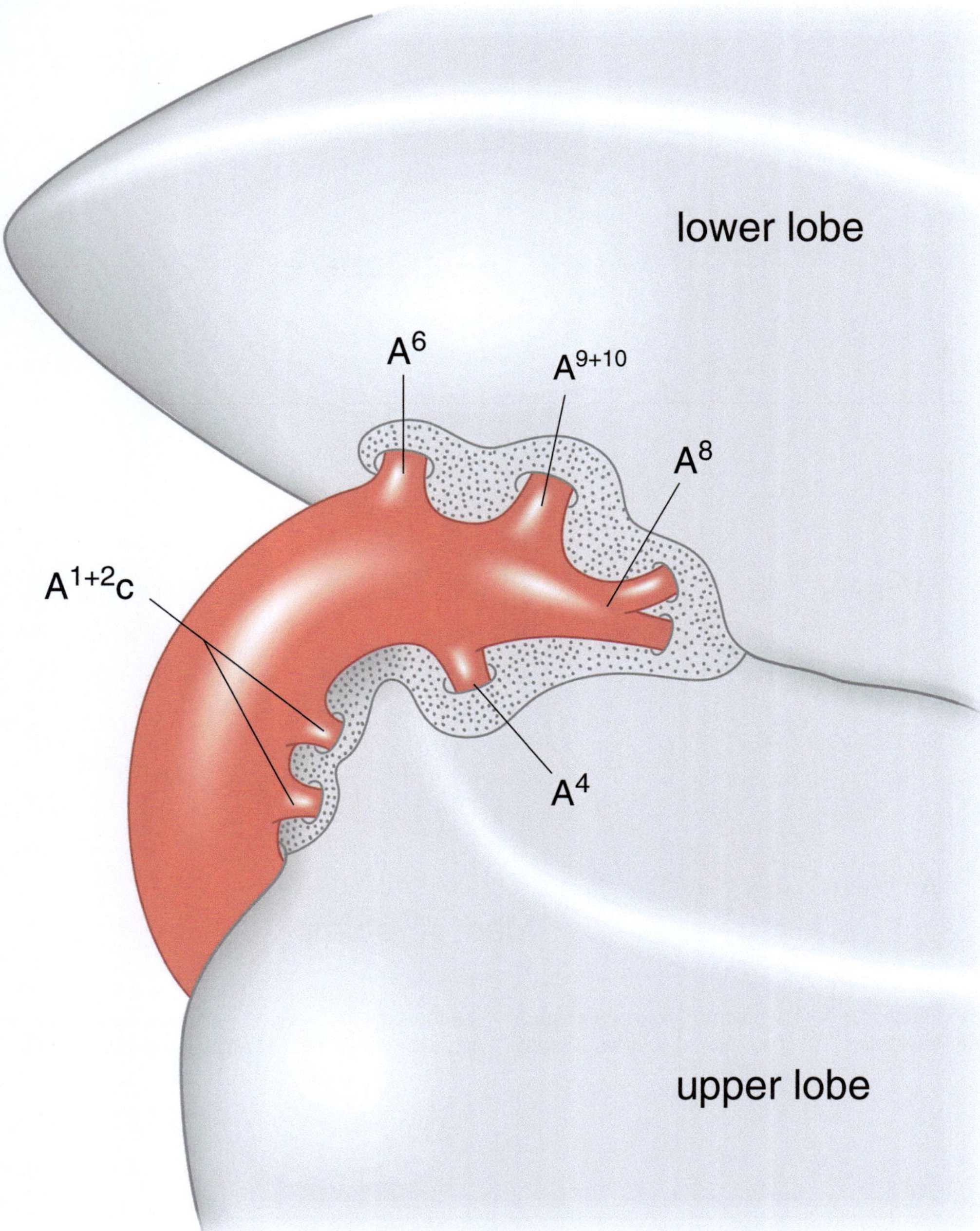

Fig. 5.4.4 A^4 branching from the interlobar pulmonary artery is cut. The interlobar fissure is cut using electrocautery but not a stapler, because a staple line would impair later identification of the inflation–deflation line.

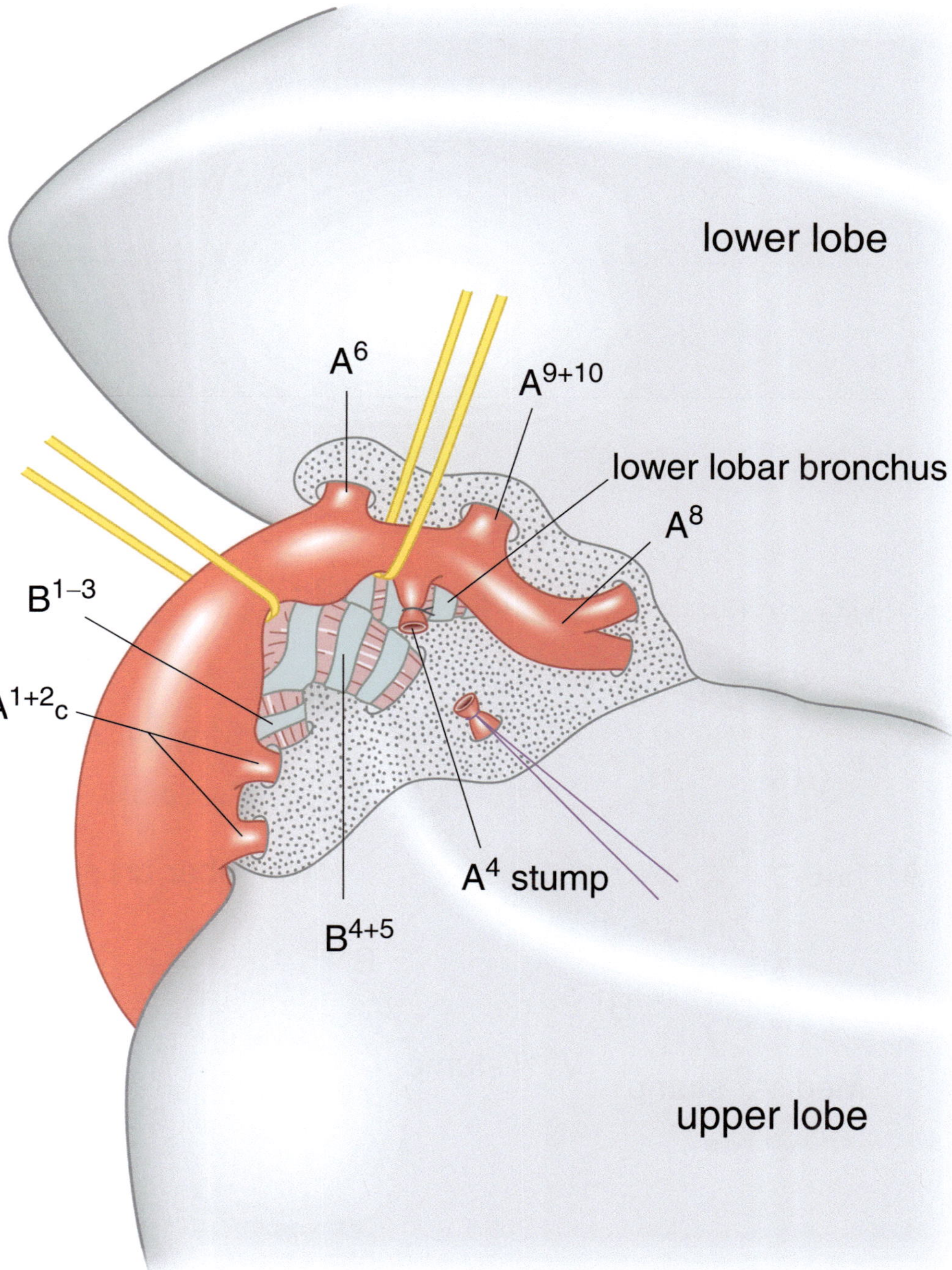

Fig. 5.4.5 B^{4+5} can be visualized behind A^4. To confirm the identification of B^{4+5}, illumination from bronchoscope inserted into B^{1-3} or B^{4+5} can guide it.

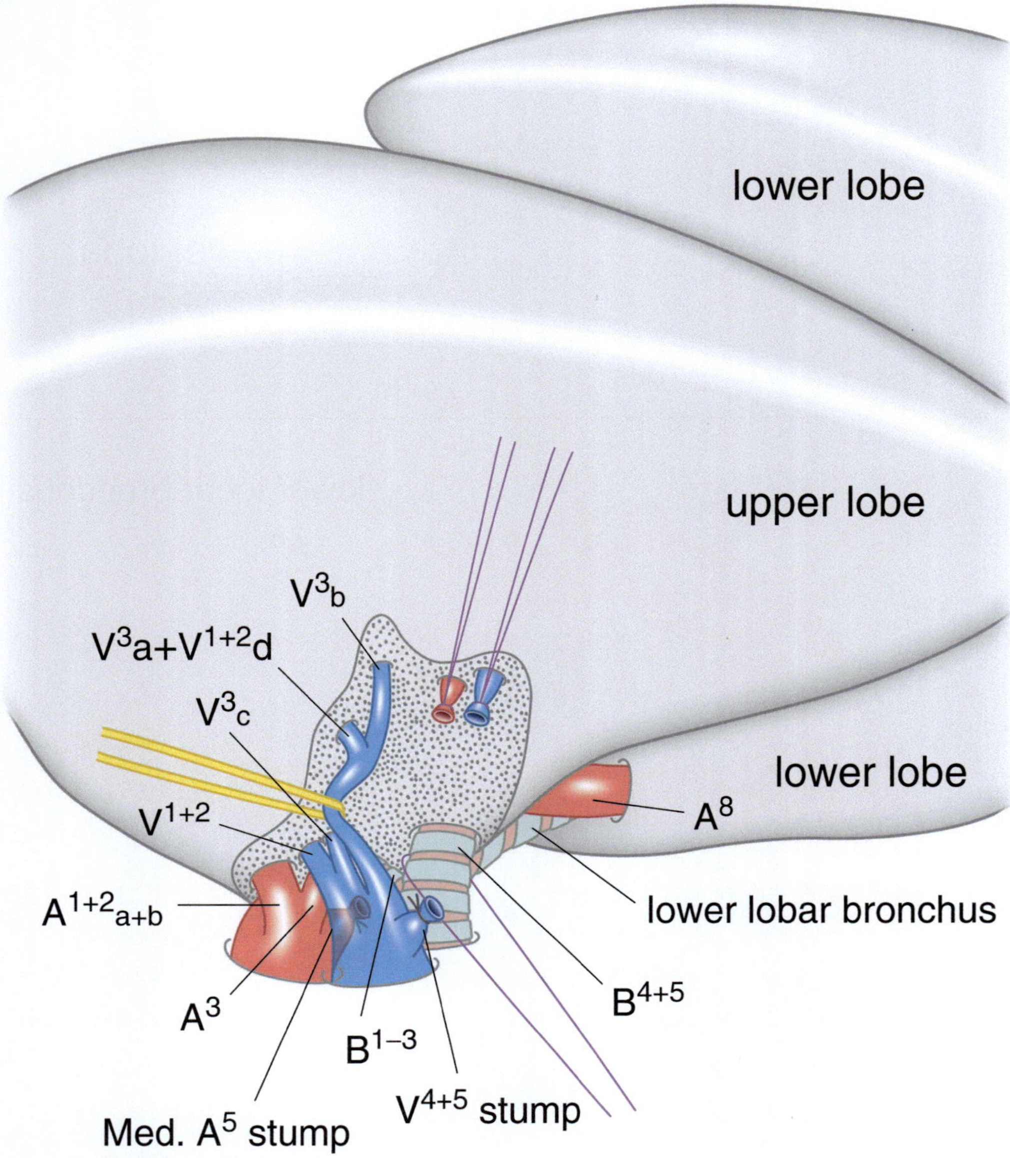

Fig. 5.4.6 B^{4+5} is encircled with thread.

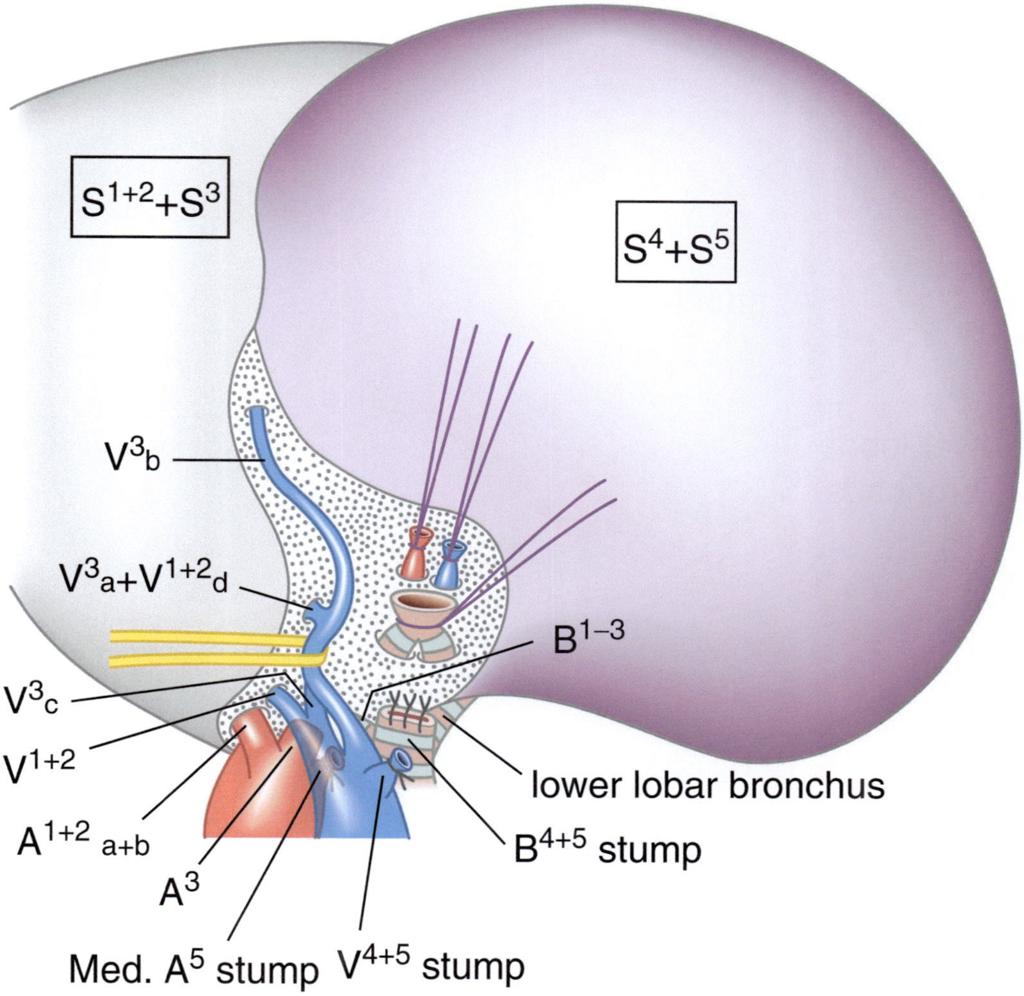

Fig. 5.4.7 S^4+S^5 is selectively inflated either by inserting a bronchoscope into B^{4+5} followed by jet ventilation, or by cutting the B^{4+5} and inserting a catheter into the distal stump followed by air inflation. The distal stump is closed to trap air within S^4+S^5. The proximal stump of B^{4+5} is closed with suture or ligation. When S^4+S^5 is inflated using jet ventilation via bronchoscope, B^{4+5} can be cut using a stapler. The distal stump of B^{4+5} is lifted and denuded peripherally at the back which moves the stump away from the hilum. Lifting the distal B^{4+5} stump also elevates lung tissue at the lateral side of the stump, which is cut towards the inflation–deflation line using electrocautery. V^3b is preserved on S^3, which is useful to identify the segmental plane. Cutting the lung tissue reveals V^3a (between S^3a and S^3b) and V^{1+2}d (between S^3a and S^{1+2}c) branching from the backside of V^3b, both of which are preserved.

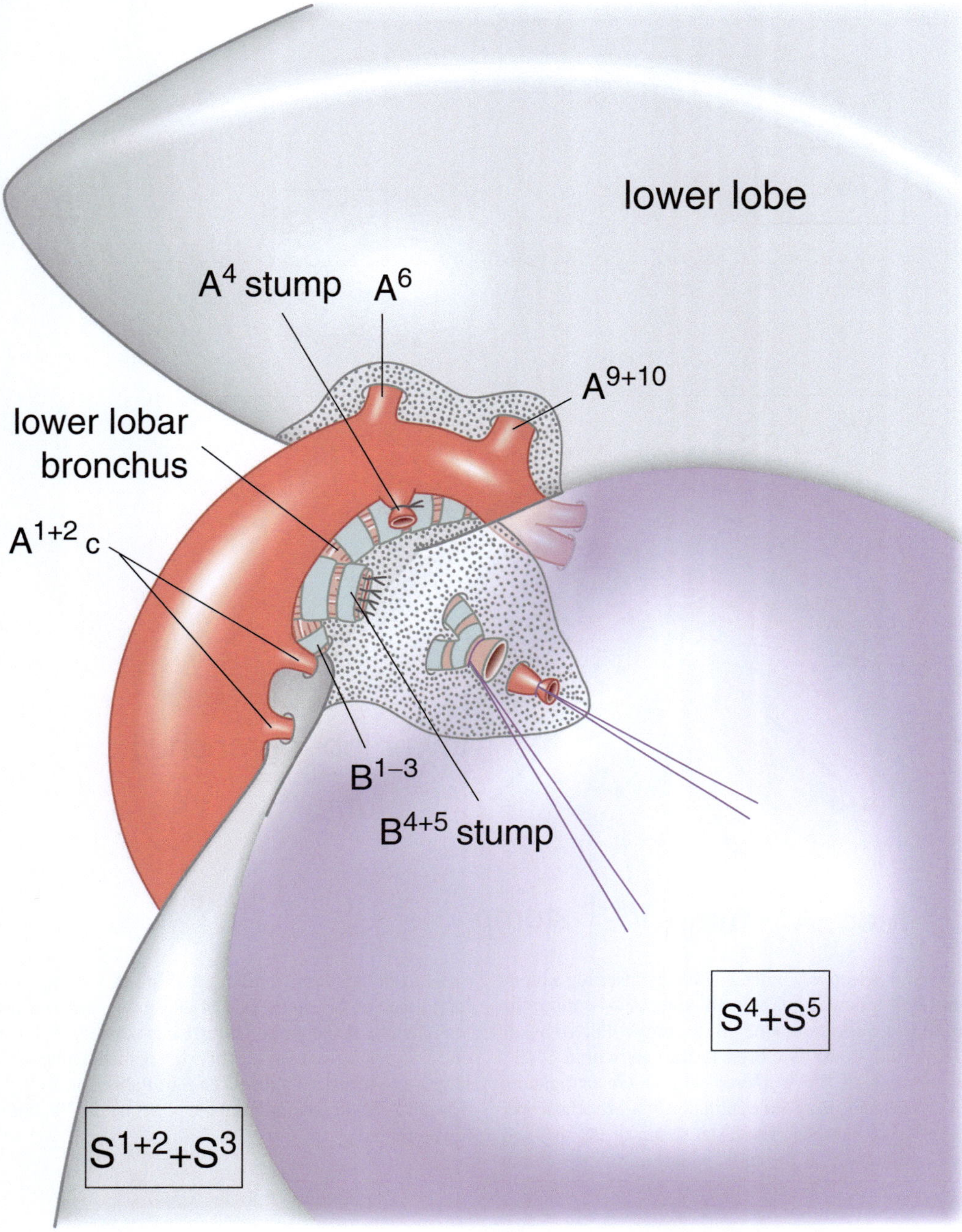

Fig. 5.4.8 The lung is cut along the inflation–deflation line. The intersegmental plane is cut from various directions to facilitate simple and accurate intersegmental cutting.

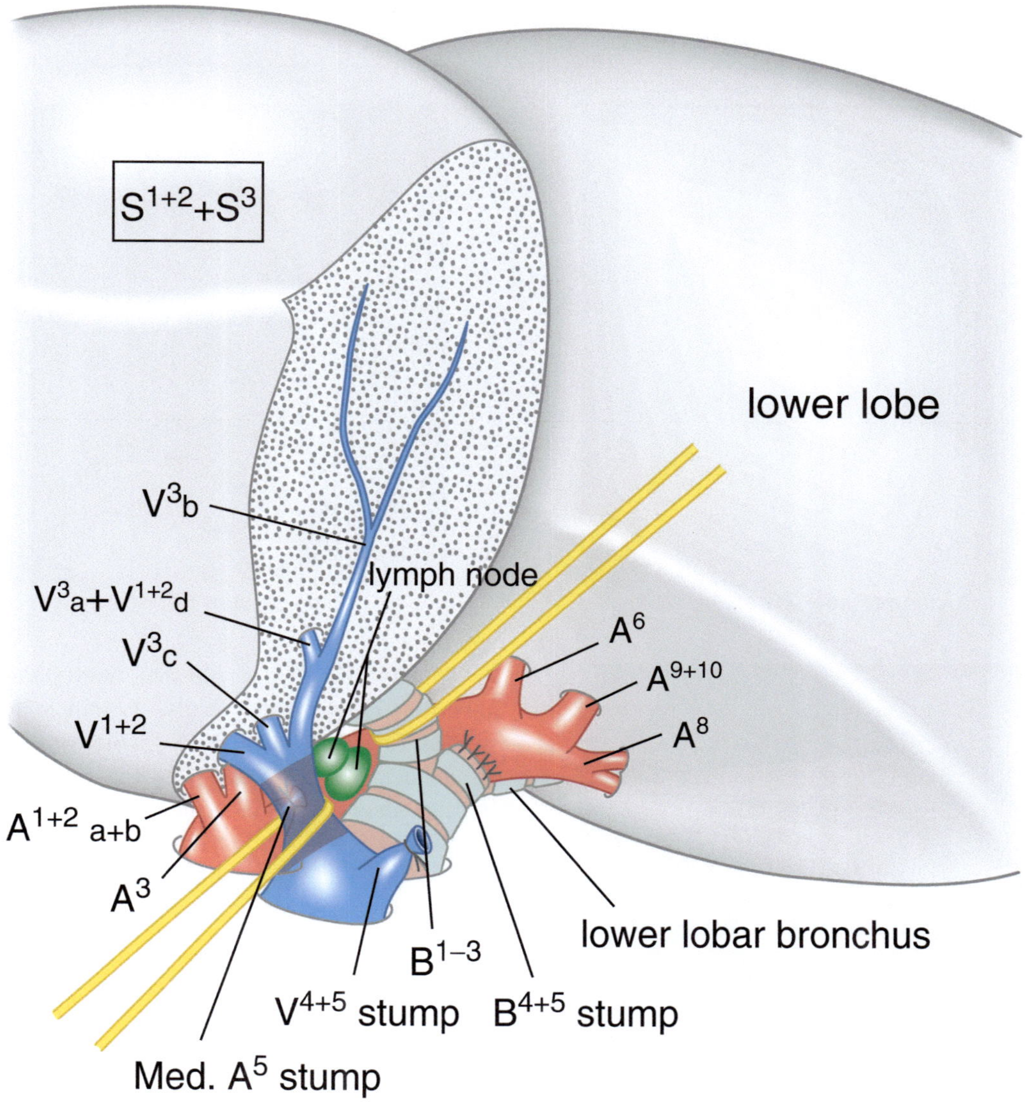

Fig. 5.4.9 Because the lymphatic flows from the lingular division goes into the root of the upper lobar bronchus, hilar lymph nodal dissection around B^{1-3} is important for the lingular division (S^4+S^5) segmentecotmy. The B^{1-3}, V^{1-3}, the truncus superior artery, and $A^{1+2}c$ are encircled with tape, and then the #12 lymph nodes around the B^{1-3} are dissected.

5.5 Left S^{1+2}+S^{3}c Segmentectomy

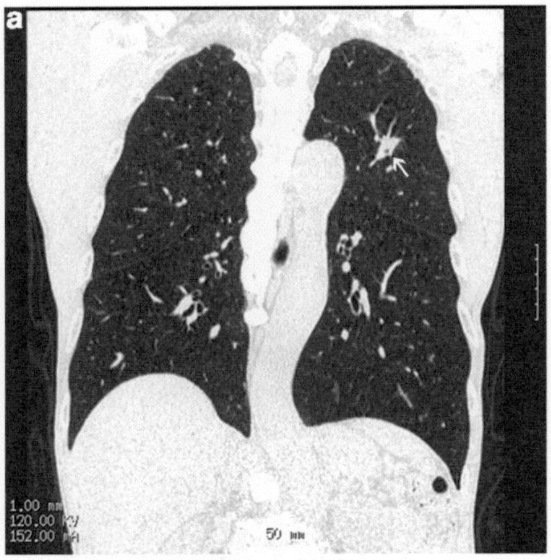

coronal view (CT scan)

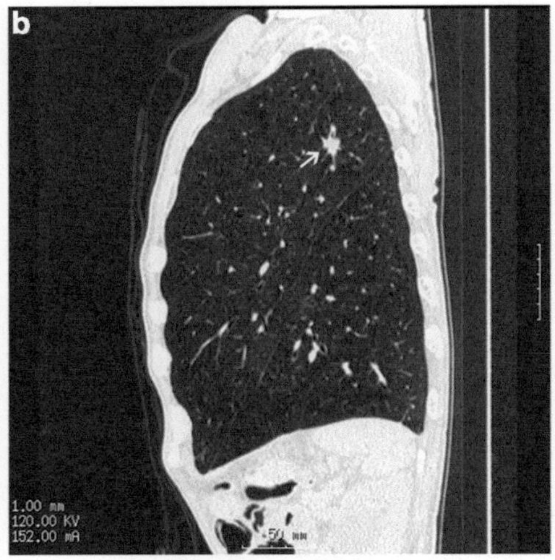

sagittal view (CT scan)

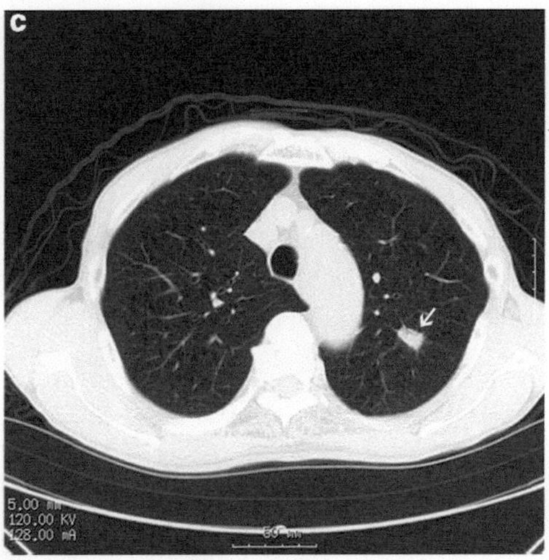

axial view (CT scan)

A CT scan of a 70-year-old male with poor pulmonary function revealed a solid 1.8-cm nodule with spicular formation in the left S^{1+2}b that was diagnosed as adenocarcinoma from a CT-guided needle biopsy. Because the tumor was located in the S^{1+2}a and near S^{3}c, the S^{1+2}+S^{3}c-segmentectomy was proceeded to take a sufficient surgical margin. The final pathological diagnosis was pT1aN0M0 papillary adenocarcinoma.

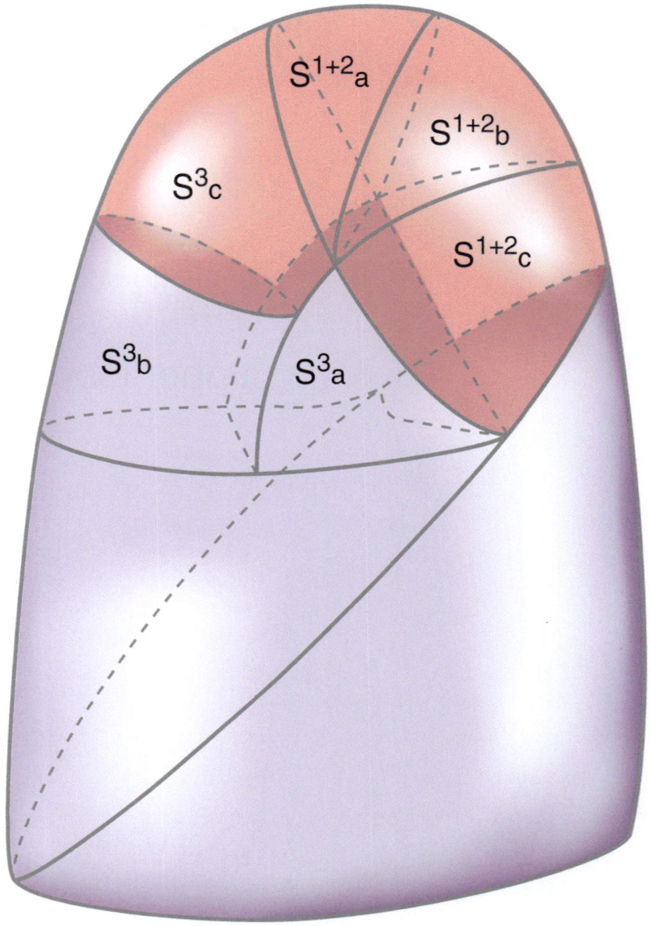

Fig. 5.5.1 This procedure is useful for resecting tumors located in $S^{1+2}a$ and also near to $S^{3}c$, because the upper division ($S^{1+2}+S^{3}$) segmentectomy which seriously damages pulmonary function of the left upper lobe can be avoided. Anatomical branching of the artery, vein, and bronchus is confirmed from axial, coronal, and sagittal views on HRCT. The branching pattern and sizes of B^{1+2} and B^{3} are further examined by bronchoscope after tracheal intubation. B^{3} frequently branches into $B^{3}a$ and $B^{3}b+c$.

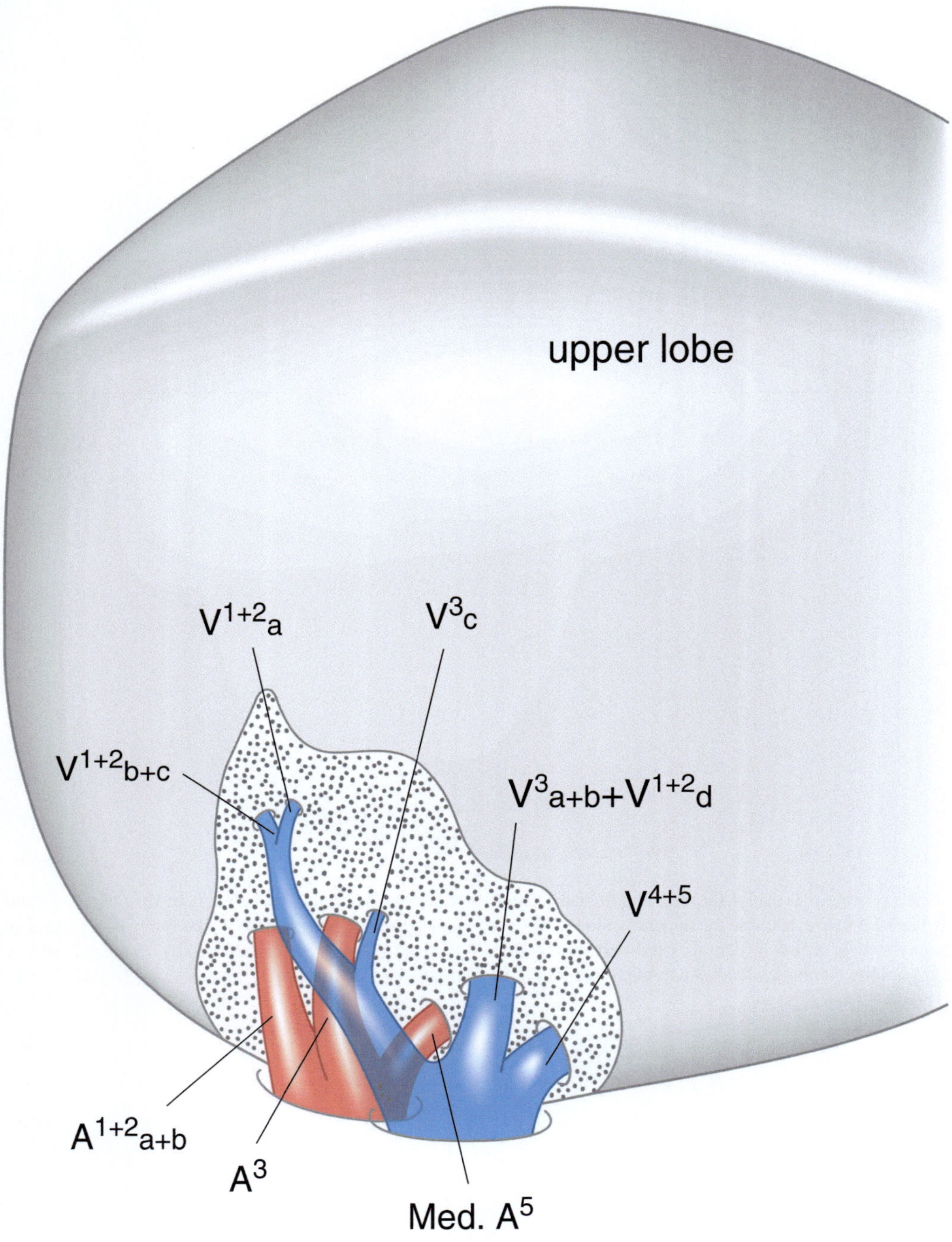

Fig. 5.5.2 The hilum of the left upper lobe is exposed from the ventral to the dorsal side to expose the superior pulmonary vein and arteries from left main to the proximal site of the interlobar artery. V^{1+2} is encircled with tape and exposed peripherally to reveal $V^{1+2}a$. The $V^{1+2}a$ runs towards the apex and near the surface layer between S^{1+2} and S^3. The $V^{1+2}b+c$ is not usually visible at this point. A thin V^{1+2} superior vein, which occasionally branches from proximal V^{1+2} and runs dorsally across A^{1+2}, is cut. By exposing the $V^{1+2}a$, A^{1+2} and A^3 can be identified, i.e. the former runs dorsal to the $V^{1+2}a$ and the latter runs ventral to it. The A^{1+2} branches into $A^{1+2}a+b$ and $A^{1+2}c$ in the figures of this session.

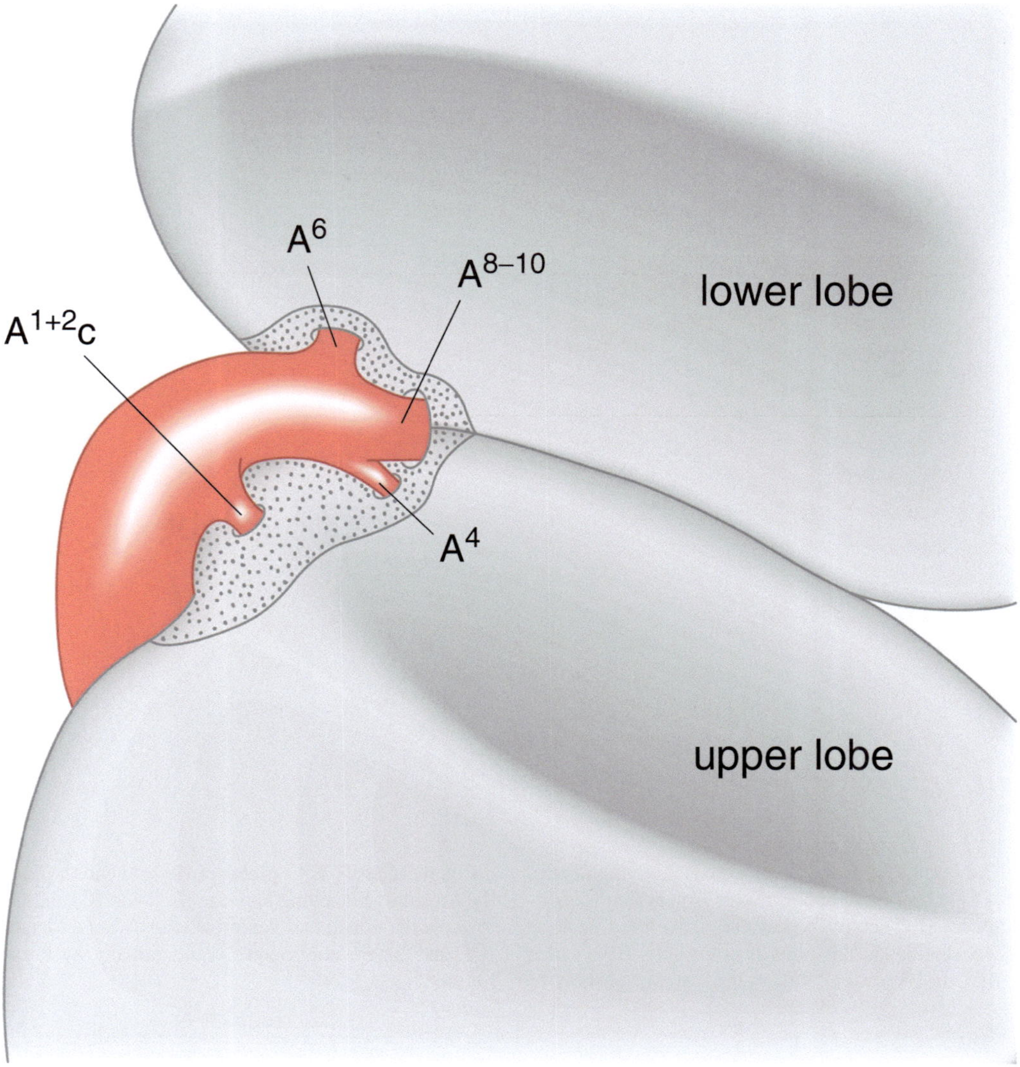

Fig. 5.5.3 The interlobar fissure is cut using electrocautery but not a stapler, because a staple line would impair later identification of the inflation–deflation line. The following procedure facilitates the fissure identification: a bronchoscope is inserted into B^{1+2} followed by jet ventilation, which forms an inflation-deflation line between the inflated S^{1+2} and deflated lower lobe. The fissure can be divided along the inflated-deflated line using electrocautery. A^{1+2}c branching from the truncus intermedius artery is identified at the dorsal side. A^{1+2}c sometimes branches near the level of A^6, which is difficult to differentiate from A^4. This unidentifiable branch is preserved at this point, which can be later identified after cutting B^{1+2}. That is, the A^{1+2} and A^4 run, respectively, towards and away from the distal stump of B^{1+2}.

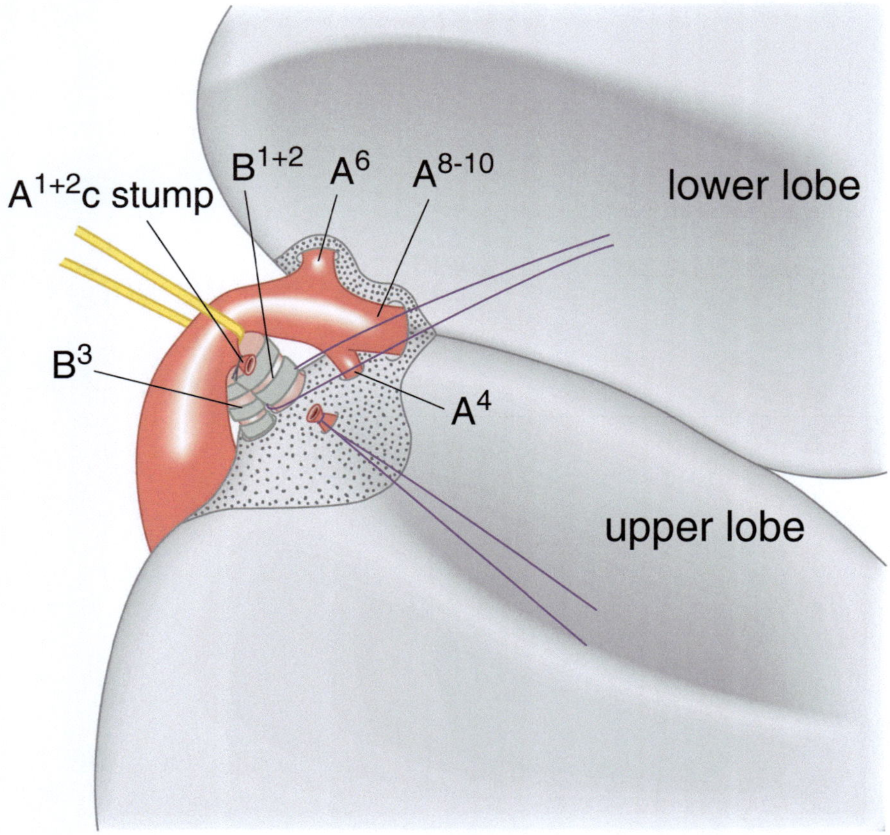

Fig. 5.5.4 Cutting $A^{1+2}a+b$ and $A^{1+2}c$ reveals the lymph nodes beside B^{1+2}. Dissecting these nodes reveals B^{1+2}, which is encircled with thread. B^{1+2} should be carefully identified because the bronchus visualized at this point is not usually B^{1+2}, which might be B^{1-3} or $B^{1+2}c$. The followings are important to correctly identify B^{1+2}: preoperative bronchoscopic findings of the bronchus branching and size; B^{1+2} and B^3 run, respectively, towards the dorsal and ventral side of A^3; and identification of B^{1+2} and B^3 are confirmed intraoperatively by bronchoscopic illumination.

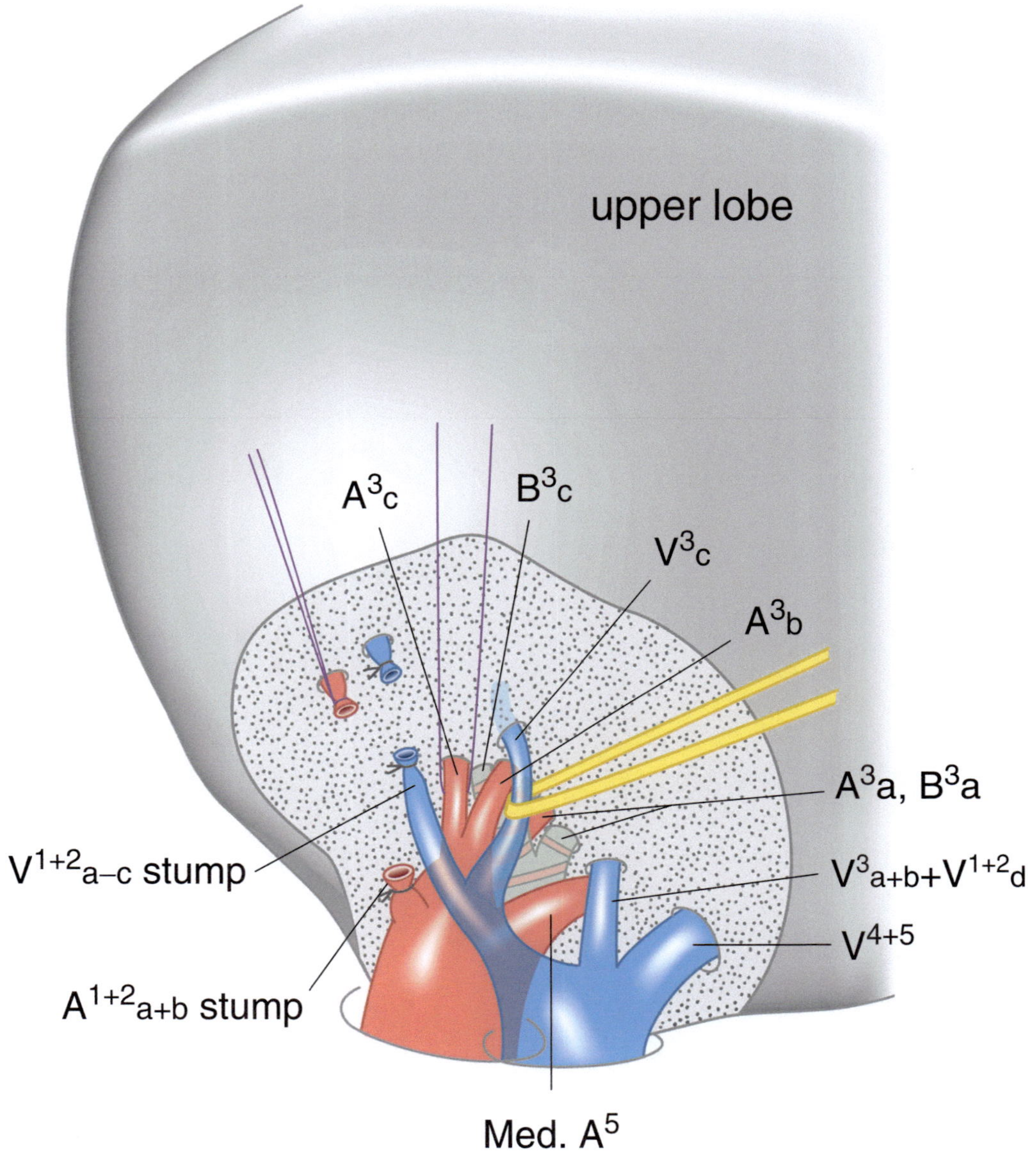

Fig. 5.5.5 At the ventral side, V^{1+2} is cut. A^3 is exposed peripherally to identify A^3c. This figure shows the pattern of A^3a and A^3b+c branching, of which frequency is 90 %. The A^3b+c runs near the surface and A^3a runs deeply into lung tissue. A^3c and A^3b run towards the cranial and ventral direction, respectively. Cutting A^3c exposes B^3c running behind A^3c. B^3c is encircled with thread.

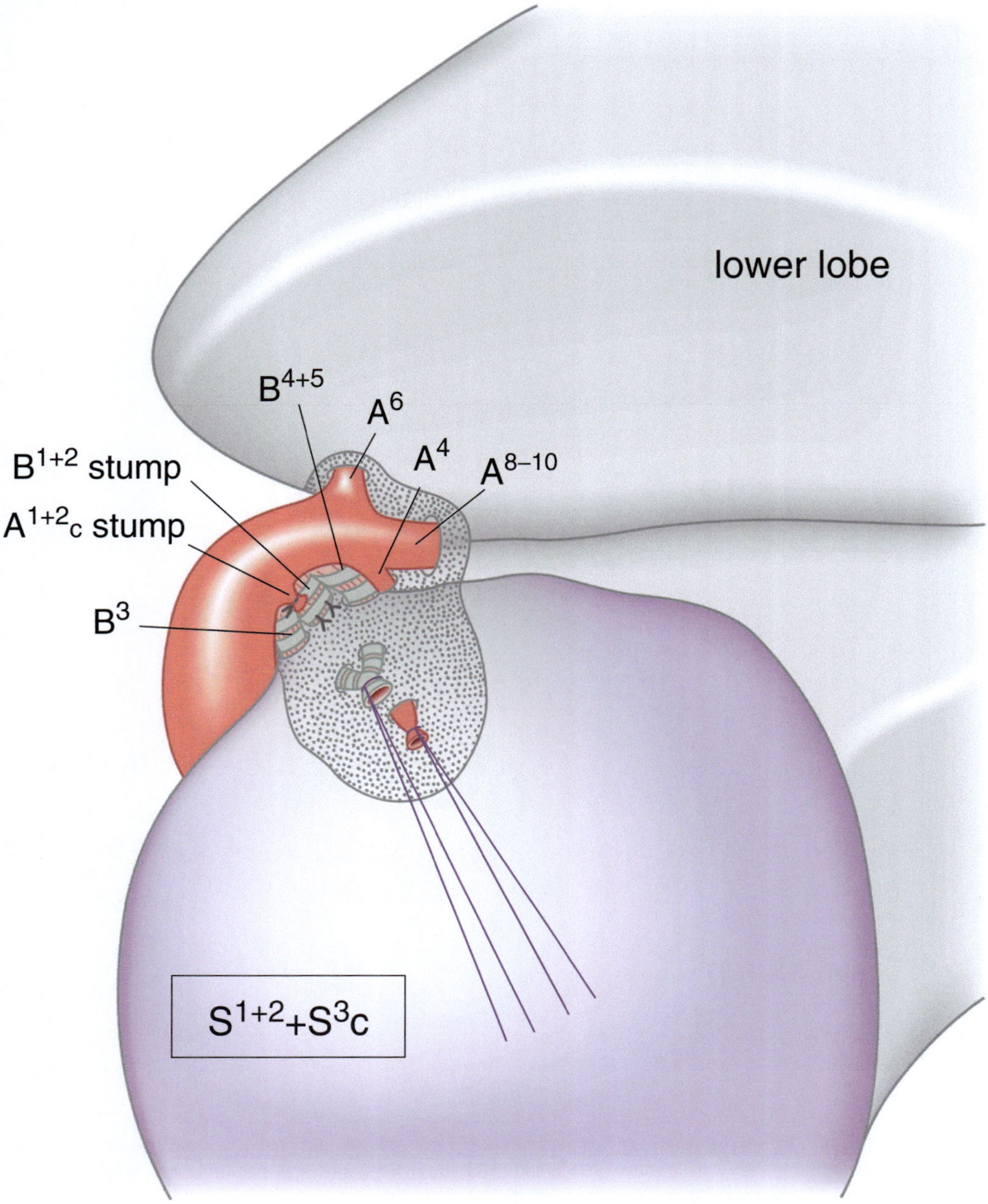

Fig. 5.5.6 S^{1+2} and S^3c are selectively inflated either by inserting a bronchoscope into B^{1+2} and B^3c followed by jet ventilation, or by cutting the B^{1+2} and B^3c and inserting a catheter into the peripheral stumps followed by air inflation. The distal stumps of B^{1+2} and B^3c are closed to trap air within S^{1+2} and S^3c. The proximal stumps are closed with suture or ligation. The distal bronchial stumps are lifted, and their back is denuded peripherally to move them away from the hilum. By lifting their distal stumps, the lung tissue at lateral side of the stumps is also elevated, which is cut toward the inflated–deflated line using an electrocautery.

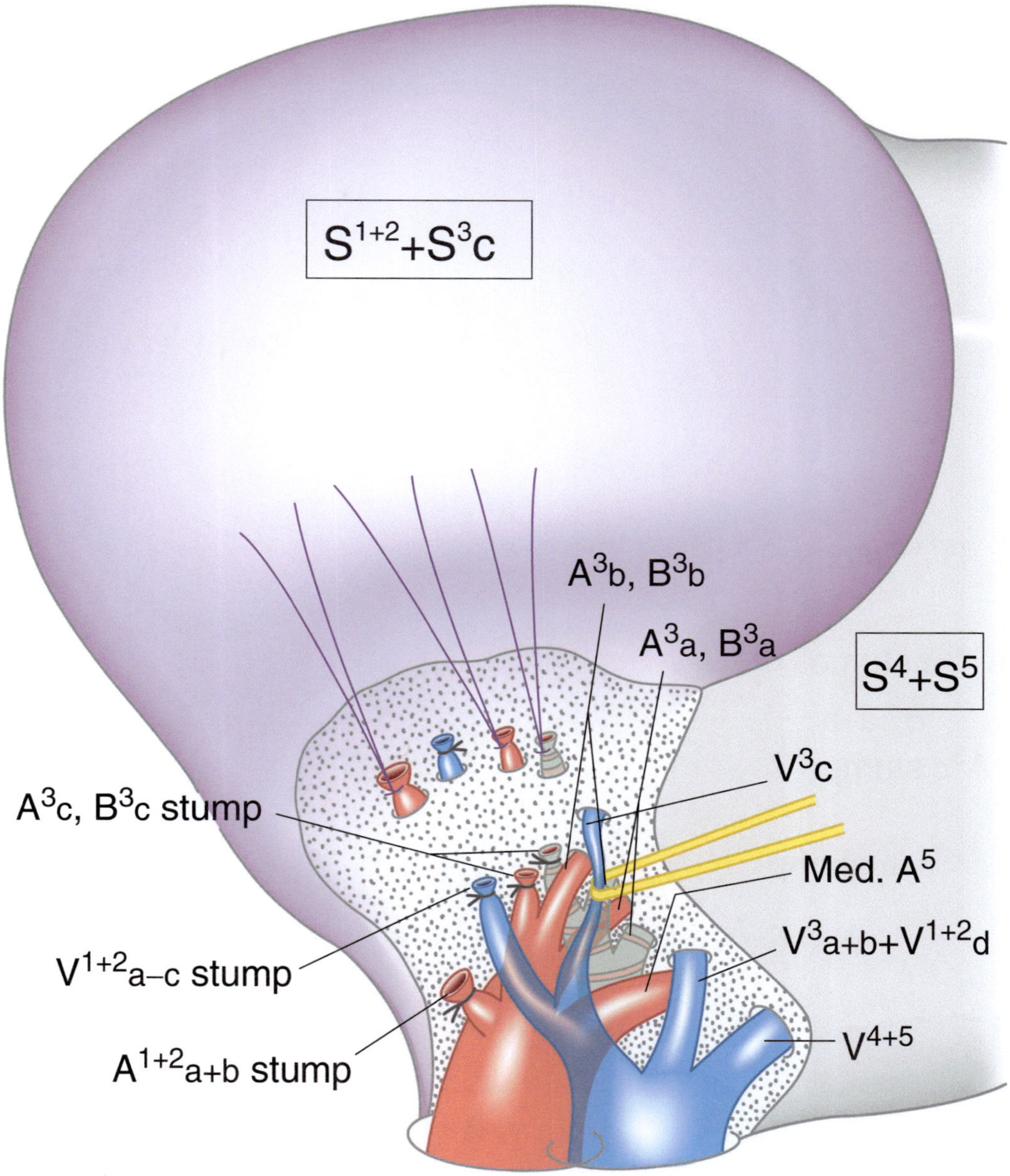

Fig. 5.5.7 V^3c (between S^3b and S^3c) and $V^{1+2}d$ (between $S^{1+2}c$ and S^3a), which can be seen along the inflation–deflation line while cutting lung tissue, are preserved if the surgical margin is sufficient.

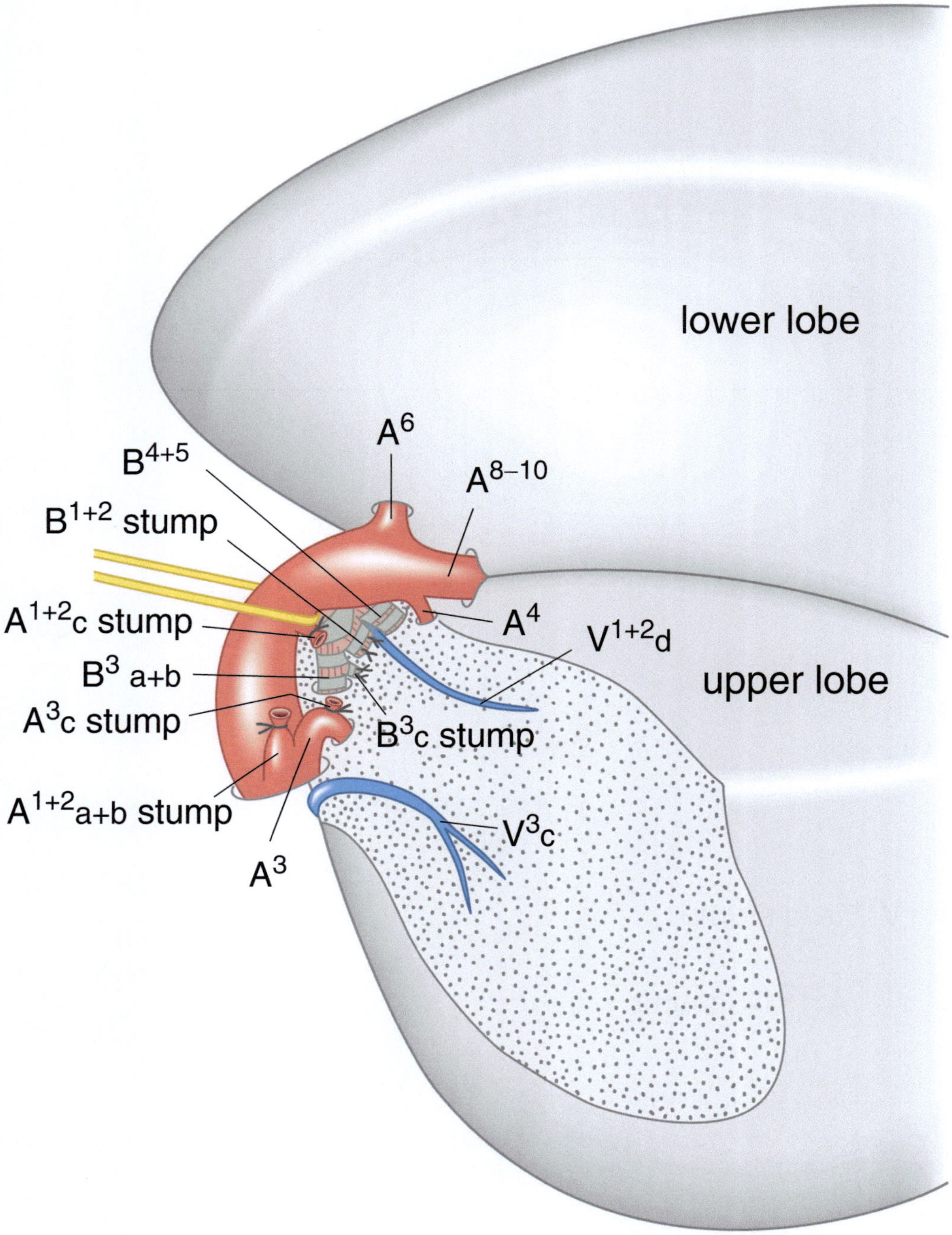

Fig. 5.5.8 After the segmental resection, $V^{1+2}d$ and $V^{3}c$ run on the intersegmental plane. With taping B^{3} and A^{3}, the #12u and #13 lymph nodes between B^{1-3} and B^{4+5} are exposed and dissected. For the dissection of #11, the interlobar fissure is sufficiently opened, and A^{4} or A^{5} is encircled with tape to facilitate simple and safe dissection.

5.6 Left S^{1+2}c + S^3a Segmentectomy

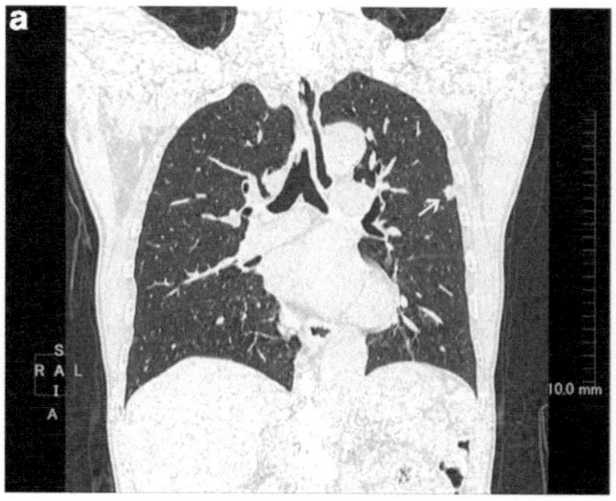

coronal view (CT scan)

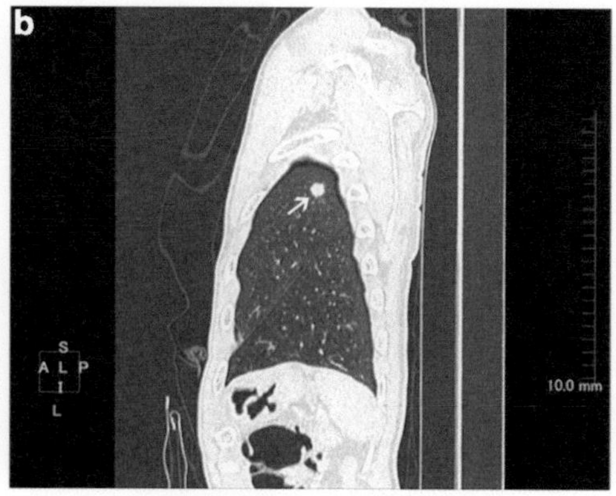

sagittal view (CT scan)

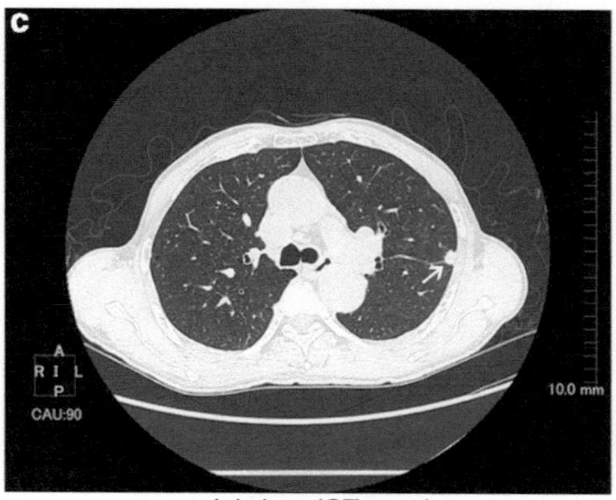

axial view (CT scan)

A CT scan of a 77-year-old male revealed a nodule at the left S^3a that had gradually increased. A CT scan 3 years later revealed a solid 1.3-cm nodule with spicular formation which was diagnosed as adenocarcinoma from a CT-guided needle biopsy specimen. The tumor involved V^{1+2}d, that is the border between S^{1+2}c and S^3a. Because the patient was not only elderly but also had poor pulmonary function, the resection of S^{1+2}c and S^3a were undertaken instead of upper division ($S^{1+2}+S^3$) segmentectomy, which could cause the major decrease of pulmonary function. The final pathological diagnosis was pT1aN0M0 papillary adenocarcinoma.

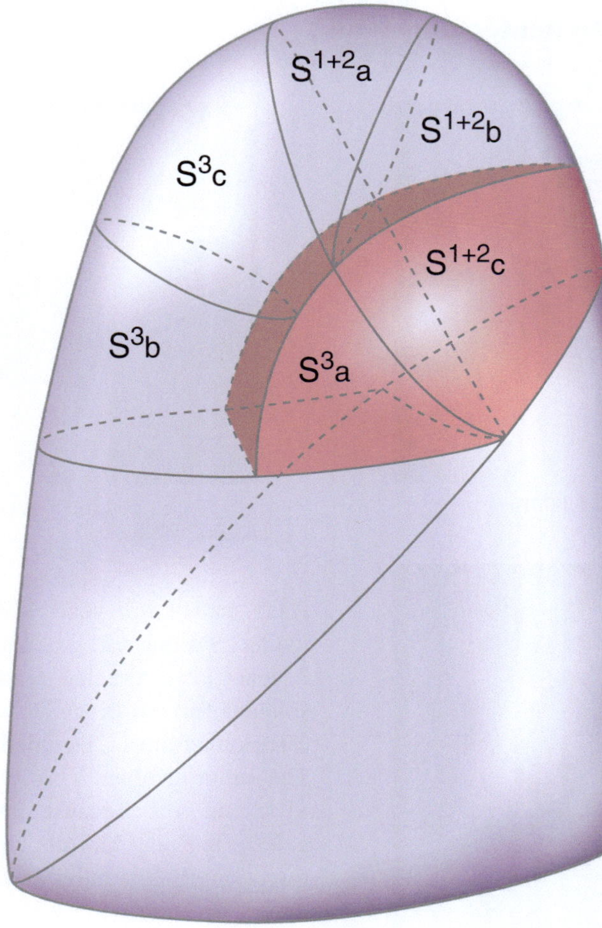

Fig. 5.6.1 This procedure could be indicated for small tumors or bronchioloalveolar carcinoma located deeply in lung tissue. It would be useful not only for curative resection but also for preserving pulmonary function rather than upper division ($S^{1+2}+S^{3}$) segmentectomy, which causes a major decrease in pulmonary function similar to right upper lobectomy. Branching pattern of segmental artery, vein, and bronchus is identified from axial, coronal, and sagittal views on HRCT. The branching pattern and sizes of B^{1+2} and B^{3} are reconfirmed by bronchoscope after tracheal intubation. The figures in this session show the most frequent type of branching, i.e. B^{1+2} branches into $B^{1+2}a+b$ and $B^{1+2}c$, and the B^{3} branches into $B^{3}a$ and $B^{3}b+c$.

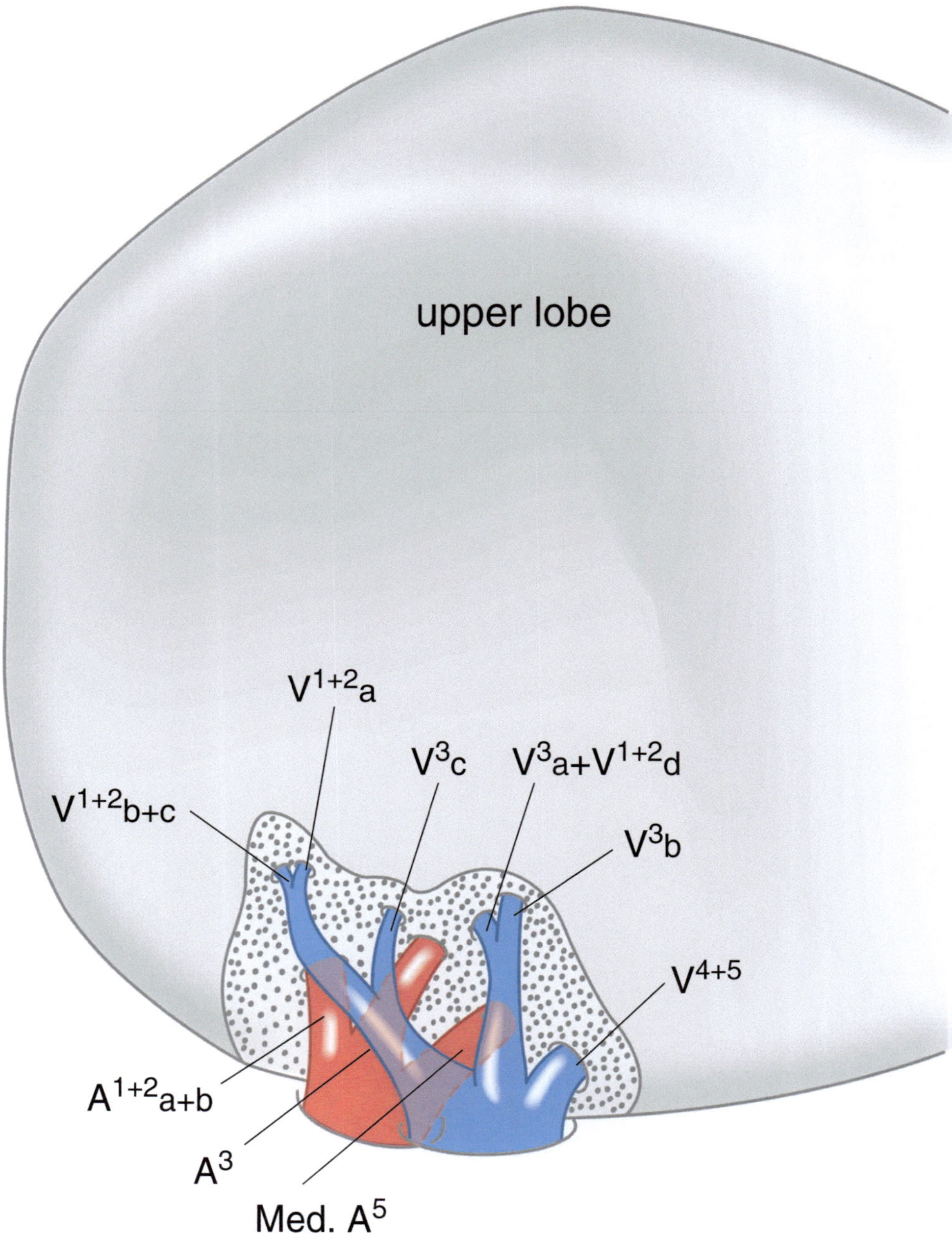

Fig. 5.6.2 The hilum of the left upper lobe is exposed from the ventral to the dorsal side to expose the superior pulmonary vein and arteries from left main to the proximal site of the interlobar artery. This figure shows a mediastinal A^{5}. V^{1+2} is encircled with tape and exposed peripherally to identify $V^{1+2}a$ running towards the apex and near the surface layer between S^{1+2} and S^{3}. Exposing $V^{1+2}a$ reveals A^{1+2} and A^{3}, which run dorsally and ventrally to $V^{1+2}a$, respectively. The $V^{3}b$ runs in the superficial layer at the ventral side. $V^{3}a$ and $V^{1+2}d$ usually form a common trunk and branch from the back of $V^{3}b$.

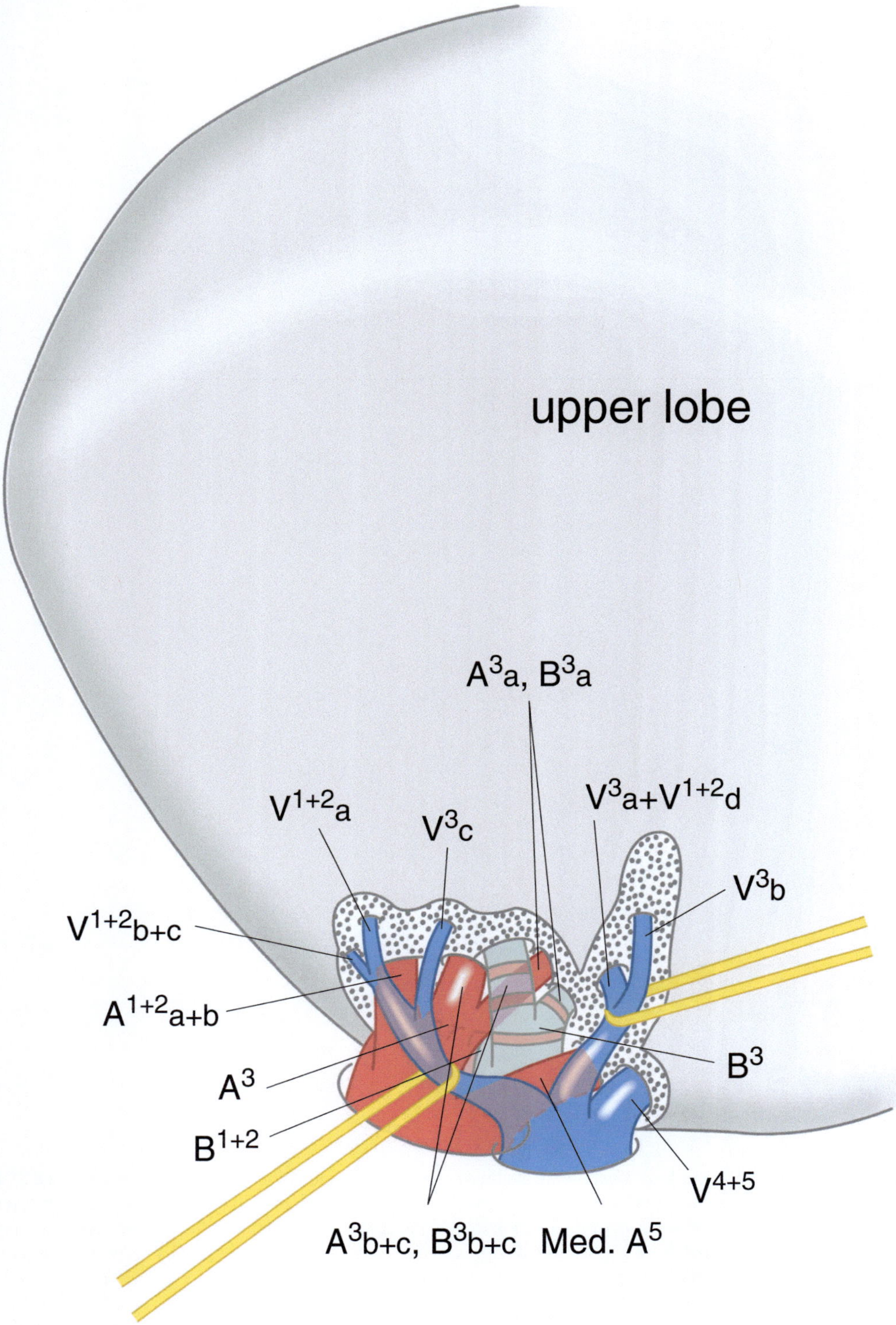

Fig. 5.6.3 A^3 is exposed peripherally to identify the branches of A^3a–c. The A^3b+c runs near the surface and A^3a runs deeply into the lung tissue. A^3a usually runs at the back of B^3b+c and along B^3a.

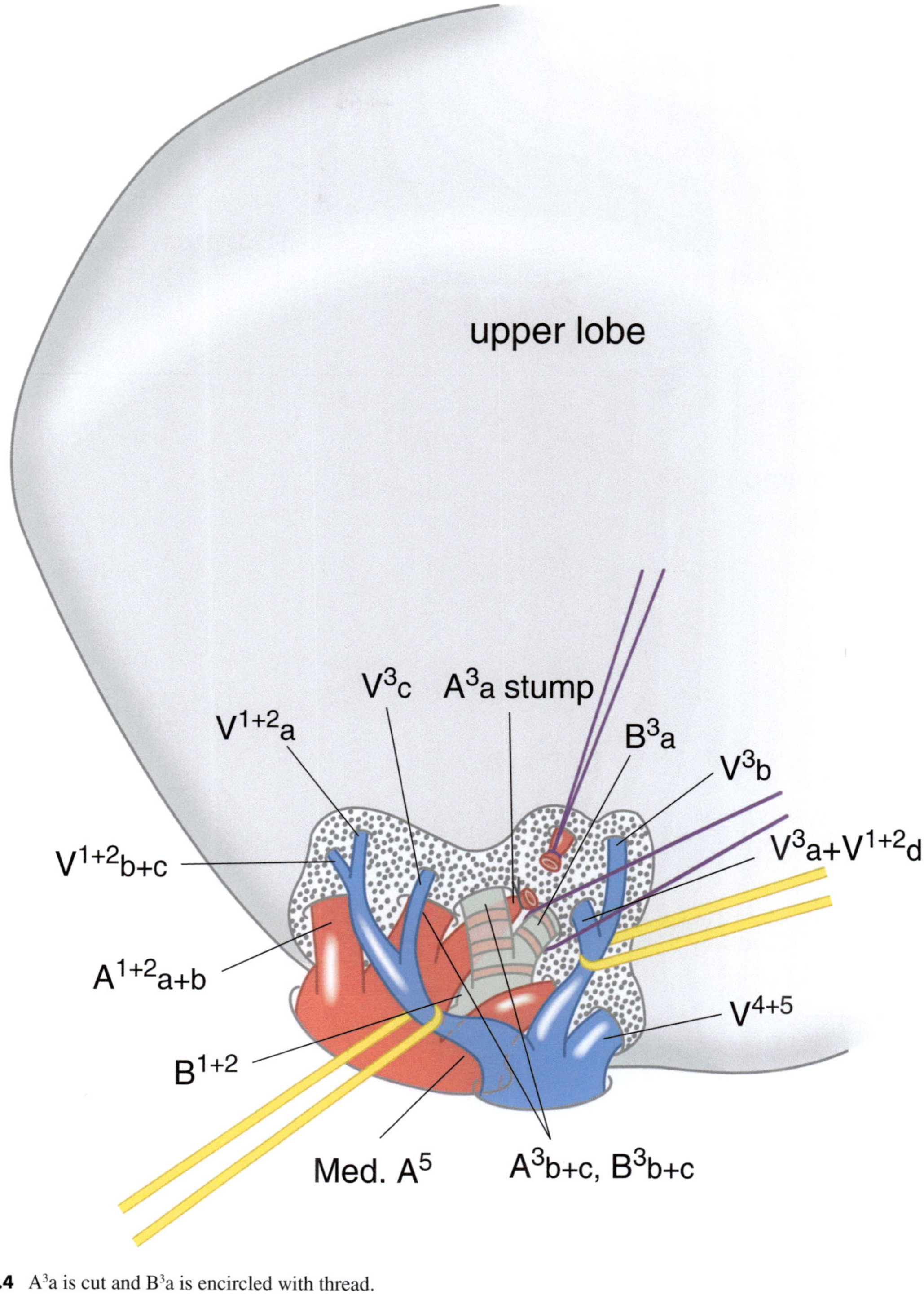

Fig. 5.6.4 $A^{3}a$ is cut and $B^{3}a$ is encircled with thread.

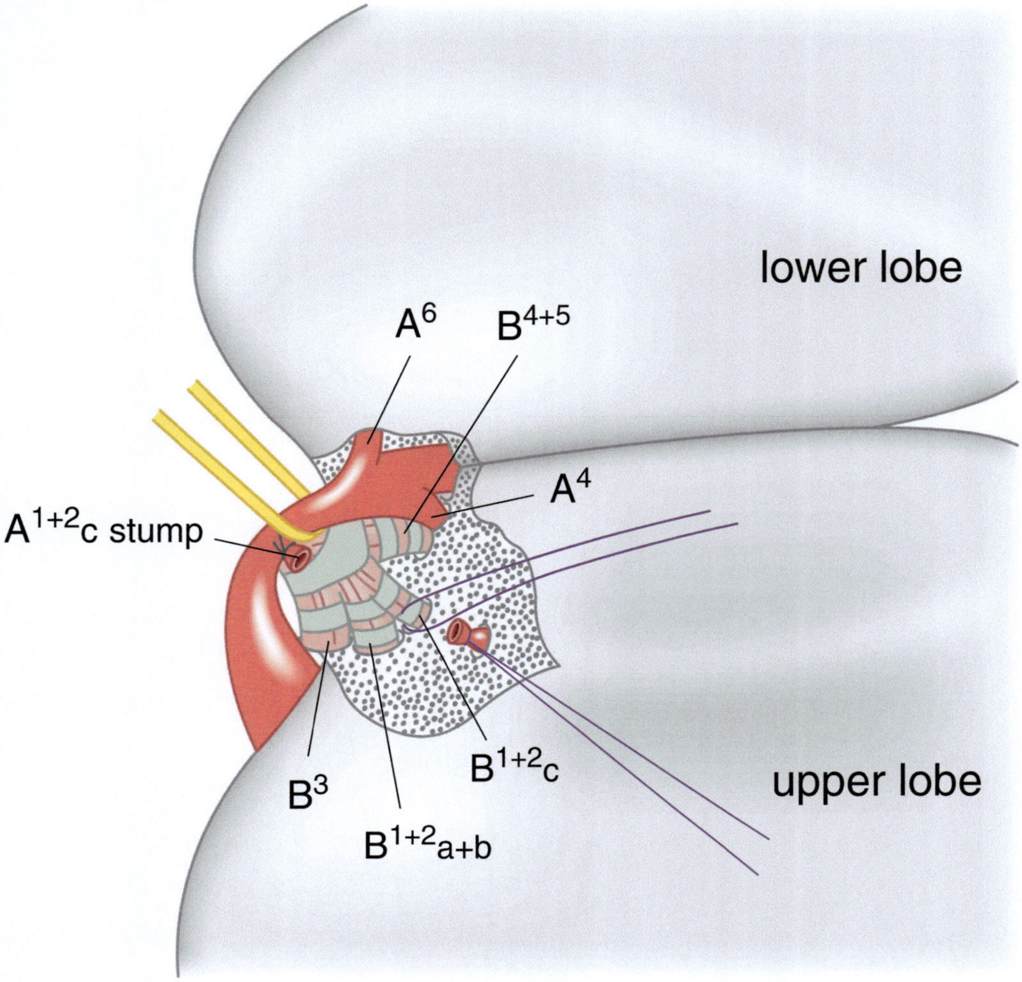

Fig. 5.6.5 $A^{1+2}c$ is cut and B^{1+2} is exposed peripherally to identify $B^{1+2}a+b$ and $B^{1+2}c$. From this view, $B^{1+2}c$ and $B^{1+2}a+b$ run the shallow and deep layers, respectively.

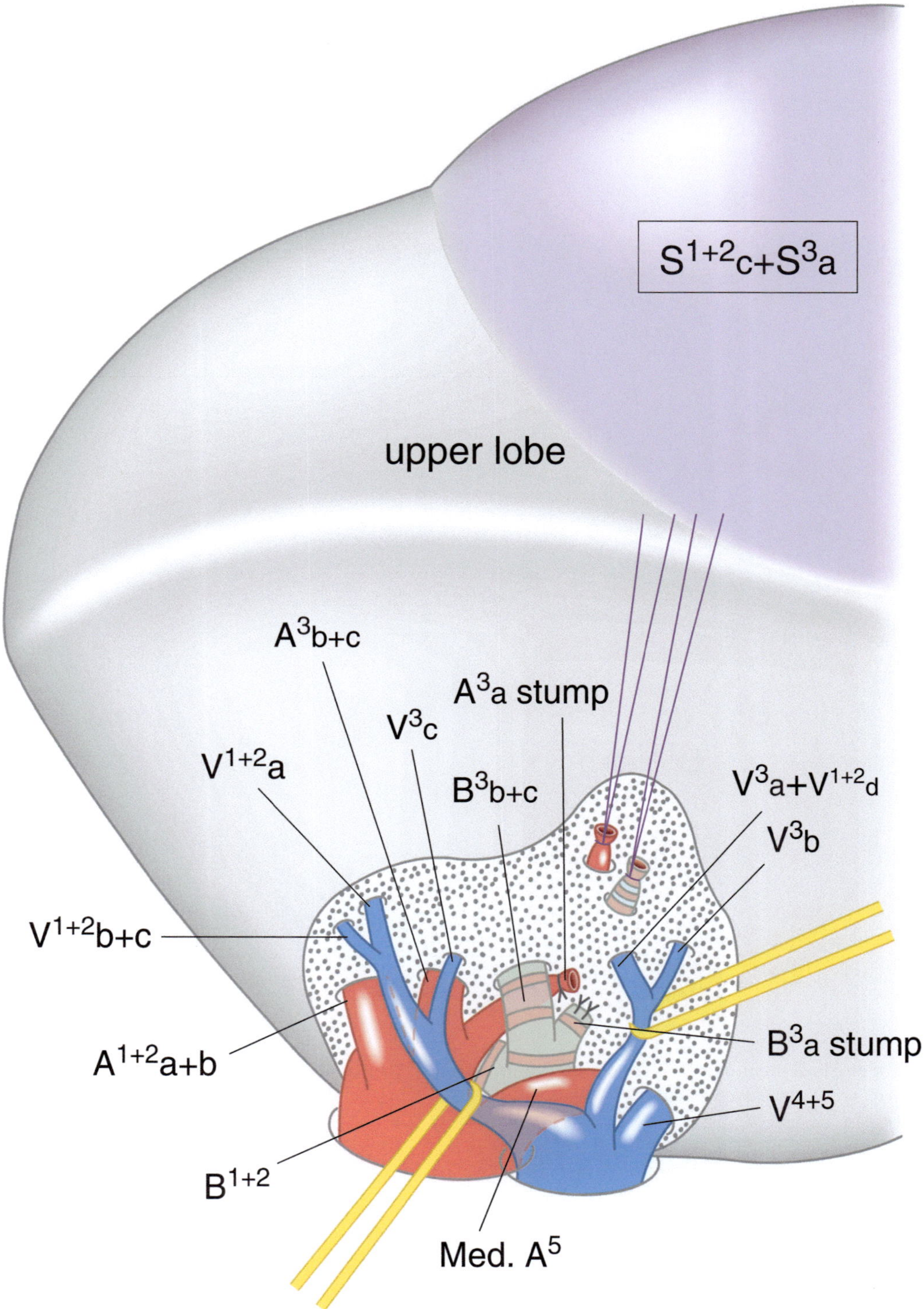

Fig. 5.6.6 The $S^{1+2}c$ and S^3a are selectively inflated either by inserting a bronchoscope into $B^{1+2}c$ and B^3a followed by jet ventilation, or by cutting the $B^{1+2}c$ and B^3a and inserting a catheter into the distal stumps followed by air inflation. The distal stumps are closed to trap air within $S^{1+2}c$ and S^3a. The proximal stump of B^3a is closed with suture or ligation. The distal stump of B^3a is lifted and denuded peripherally at the back to move it away from the hilum.

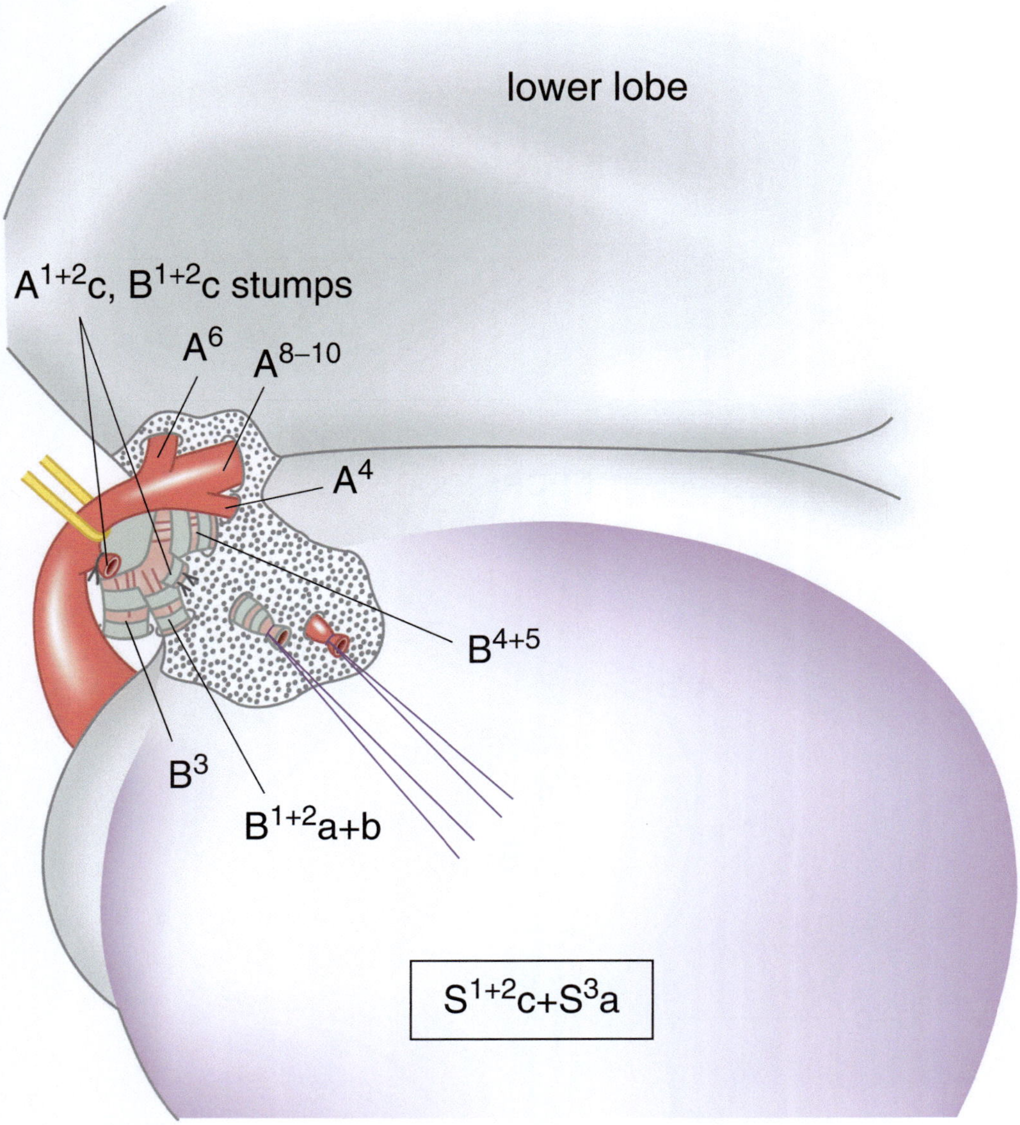

Fig. 5.6.7 The proximal stump of $B^{1+2}c$ is closed with suture or ligation. The distal stump of $B^{1+2}c$ is lifted and denuded peripherally at the back to move it away from the hilum.

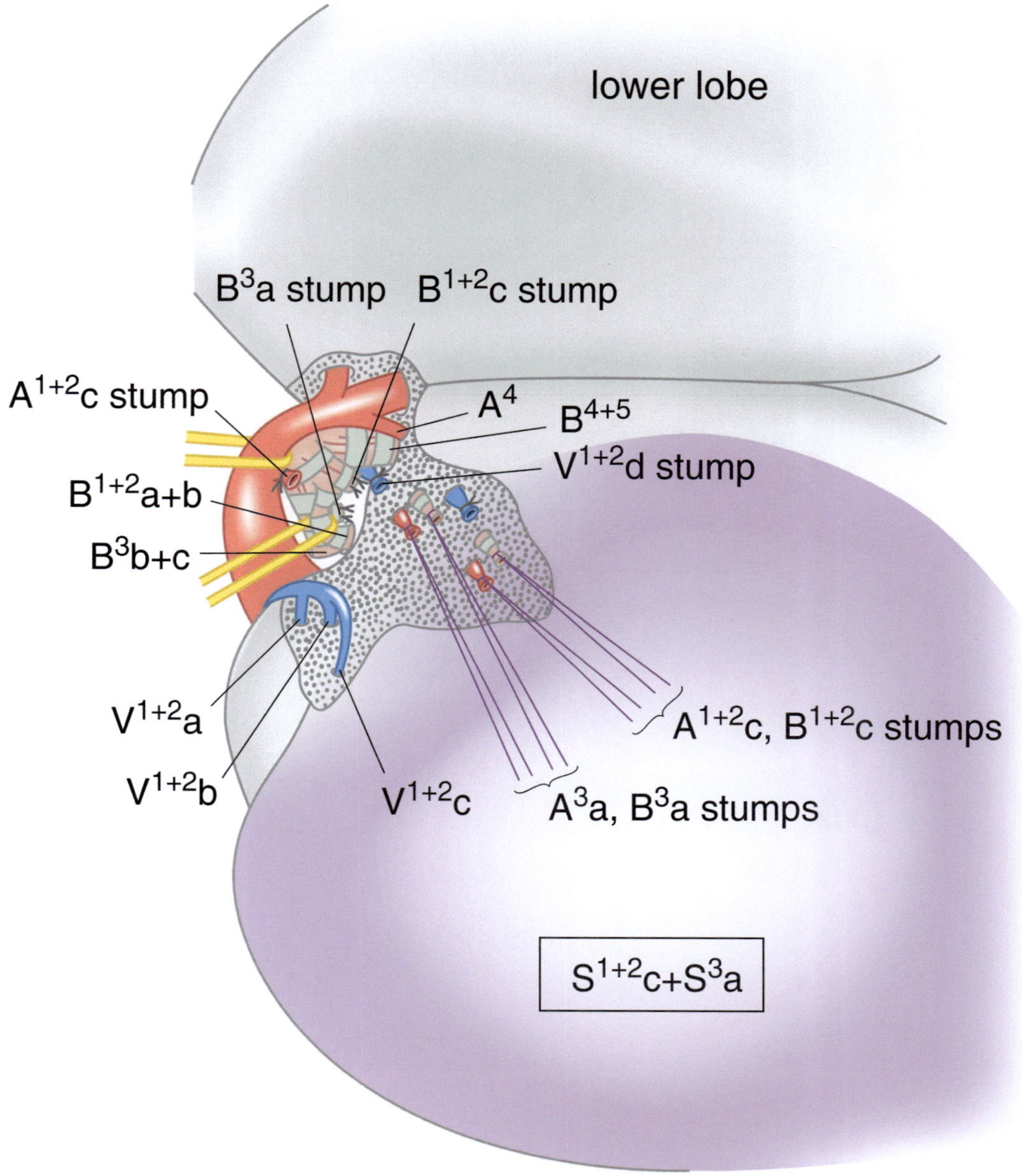

Fig. 5.6.8 The threads ligating the peripheral stumps of A^3a and B^3a are passed towards the backside, from where the peripheral stumps of A^3a, B^3a, $A^{1+2}c$ and $B^{1+2}c$ can be pulled together from the backside. Lung tissue is cut along the inflation–deflation line, which reveals $V^{1+2}d$ running between the $B^{1+2}c$ and B^3a. The $V^{1+2}d$ is cut. The intersegmental plane is cut from various directions to facilitate simple and accurate intersegmental cutting.

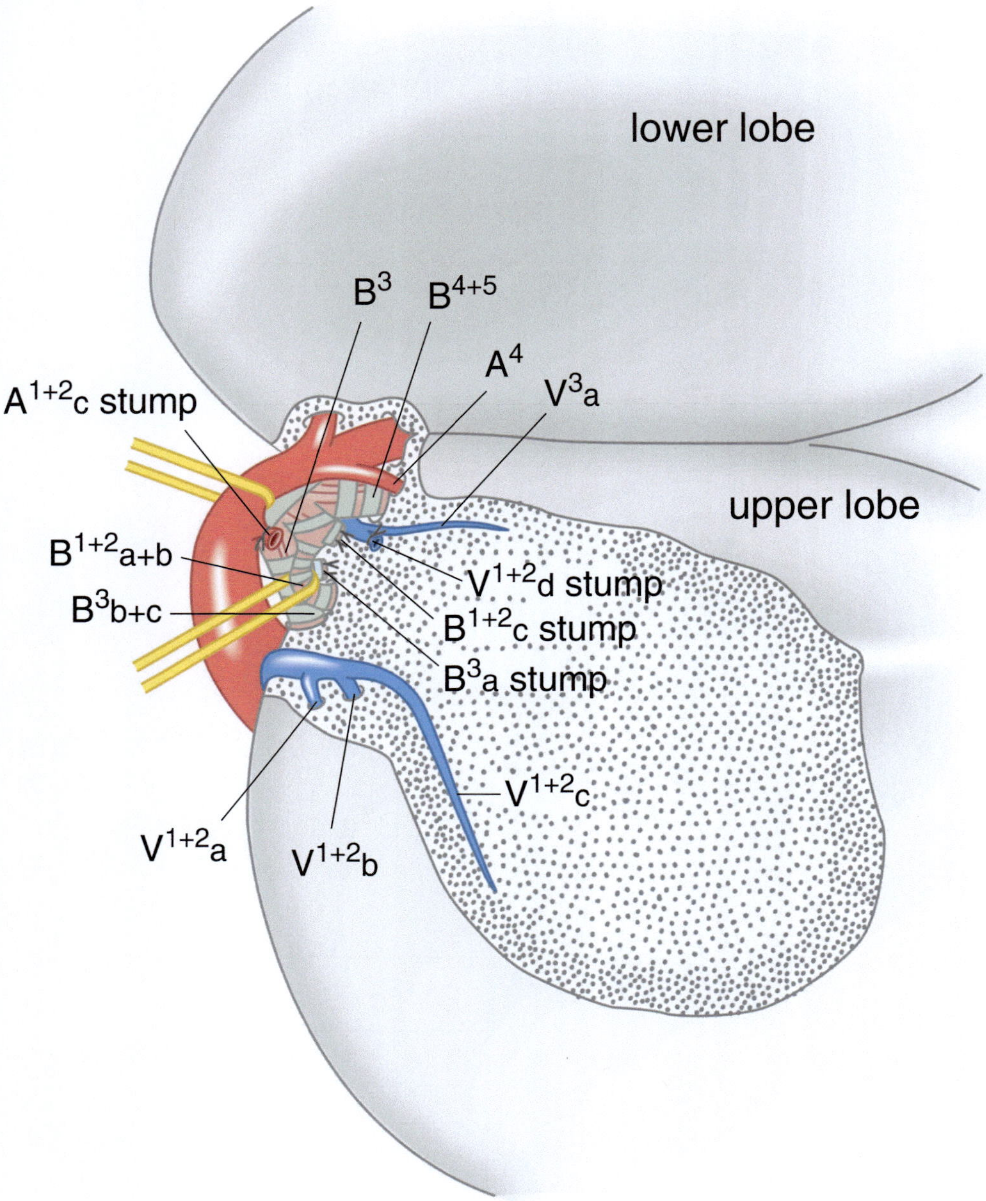

Fig. 5.6.9 The cut plane results in being located only on the backside of the upper lobe. $V^{1+2}c$ (between $S^{1+2}b$ and $S^{1+2}c$) and $V^{3}a$ (between $S^{3}a$ and $S^{3}b$) are preserved on the segmental plane.

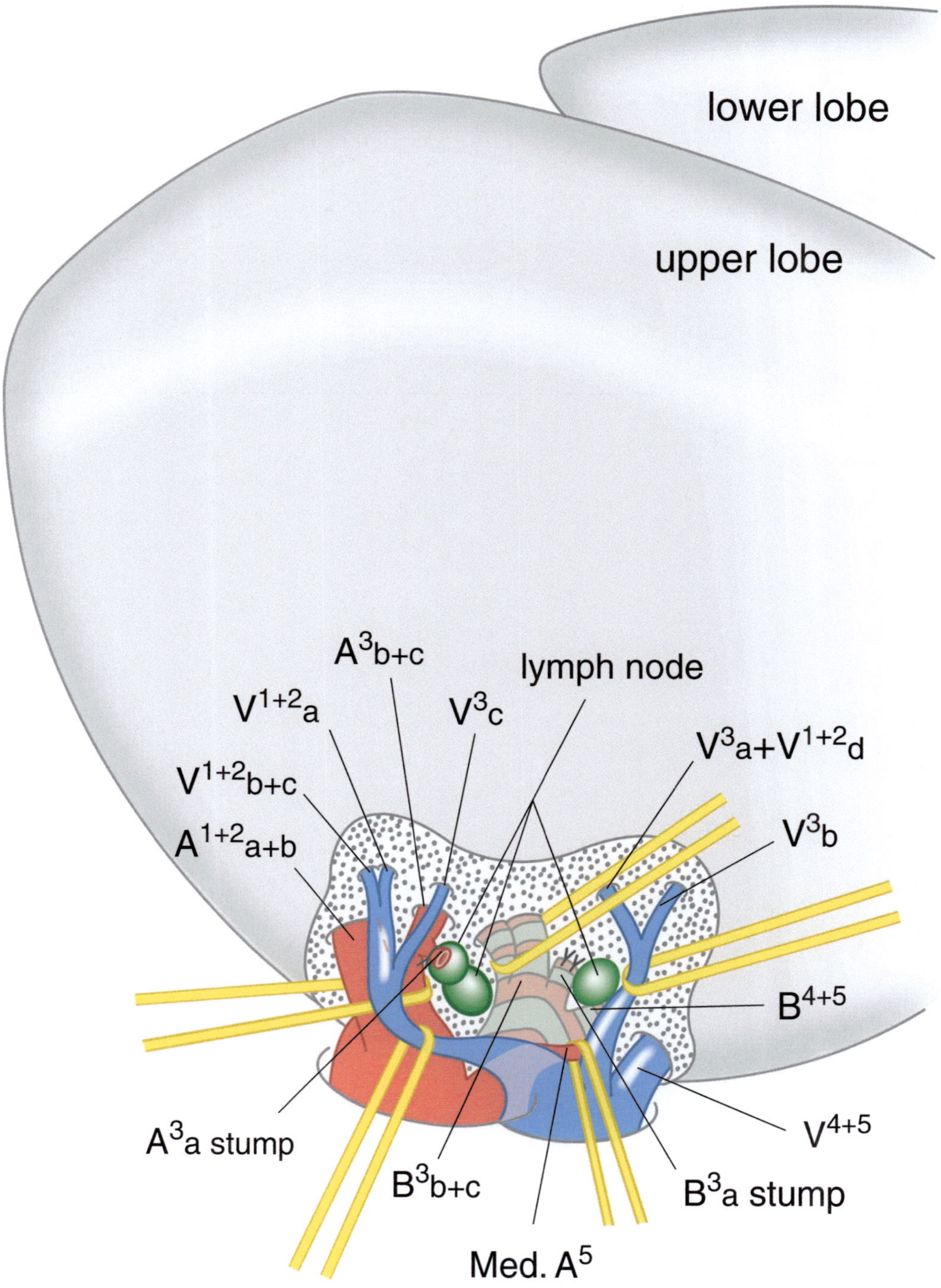

Fig. 5.6.10 The #12 and #13 lymph nodes are dissected from both the ventral and dorsal sides with taping B^{1-3}, V^{1+2}, and the truncus superior artery. When dissecting the #13 lymph node between B^{1-3} and B^{4+5} from the ventral side, care is required to avoid damaging the truncus intermedius artery, which is adjacent to the lymph nodes.

6 Segmentectomy of the Left Lower Lobe

The segmental vessels, particularly the segmental vein vary more in the lower than in the upper lobe. However, unlike the upper lobe, the segmental vein does not need to be identified for segmentectomy of the lower lobe, in which the segmental arteries are identified and cut first, followed by cutting the segmental bronchus. Next, the segmental veins running towards the segment scheduled for resection are cut, which does not require their identification. Instead, the segmental arteries should be identified accurately from both MDCT and intraoperative findings during segmentectomy of the lower lobe. Like this, anatomical segmentectomy of a lower lobe depends on precise identification of the segmental arteries.

Branching profile			Frequency (%)
Bronchus	B^6	B^6a+c and B^6b	18
		B^6a+b and B^6c	54
		B^6a and B^6b and B^6c	6
		B^6a and B^6b+c	22
	B^{8-10}	B^8 and B^{9+10}	80
		B^{8+9} and B^{10}	4
		B^8 and B^9 and B^{10}	16
	B^*		4
Segmental artery	A^6	One branch	80
		Two branches	20
	A^{8-10}	A^8 and A^{9+10}	74
		A^{8+9} and A^{10}	16
		A^8 and A^9 and A^{10}	10
	A^*		4
Vein	Inferior pulmonary vein	V^6 and common basal vein	88
		V^6 and superior and inferior basal vein	12
	Basal vein	V^{8+9} and V^{9+10}	30
		V^{8+9+10} and V^{10}	6
		V^8, V^{8+9+10}	4
		V^{8+9} and V^{10}	28
		V^8 and V^{9+10}	24
		V^8 and V^9 and V^{10}	8

H. Nomori and M. Okada, *Illustrated Anatomical Segmentectomy for Lung Cancer*,
DOI 10.1007/978-4-431-54144-8_6, © Springer Japan 2012

6.1 Left S⁶ Segmentectomy

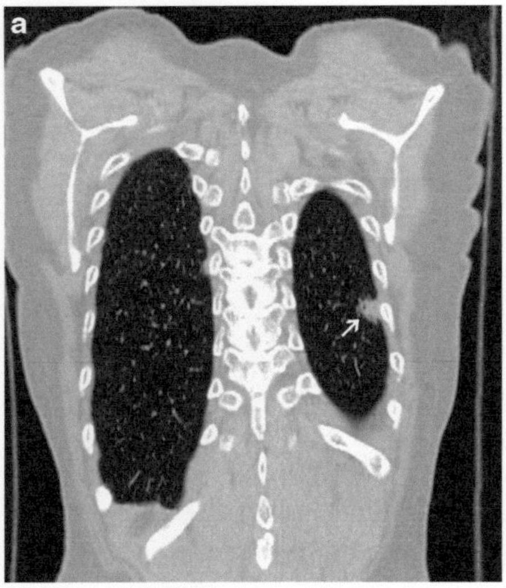

coronal view (CT scan)

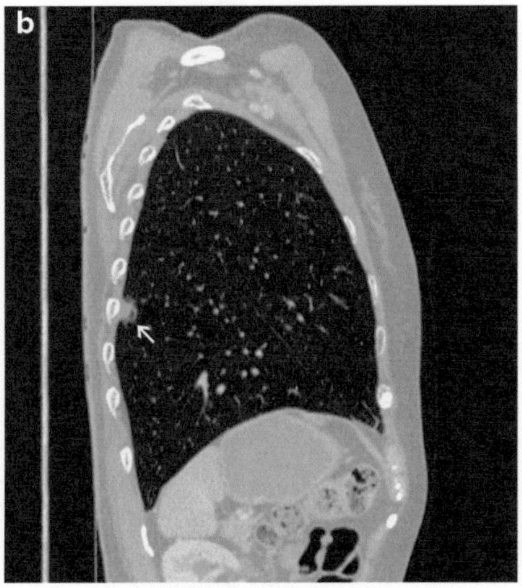

sagittal view (CT scan)

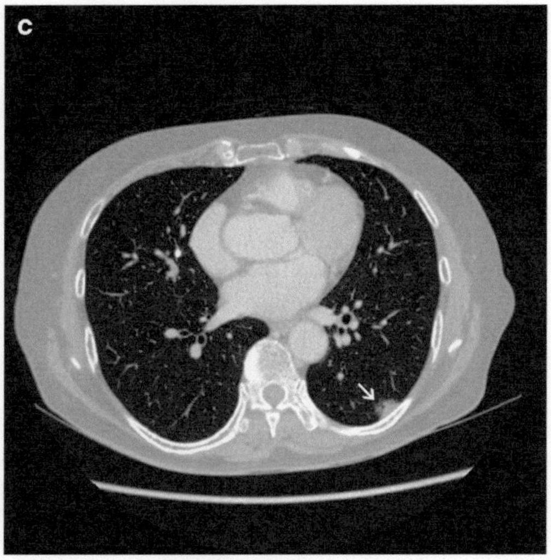

axial view (CT scan)

A CT scan of a 72-year-old female at a medical examination revealed a solid 1.5-cm nodule located at the left S^6 and near V^6c at the border between S^6c and $S^{10}a$. S^6-segmentectomy was proceeded with partial resection of $S^{10}a$. The final pathological diagnosis was pT1aN0M0 papillary adenocarcinoma.

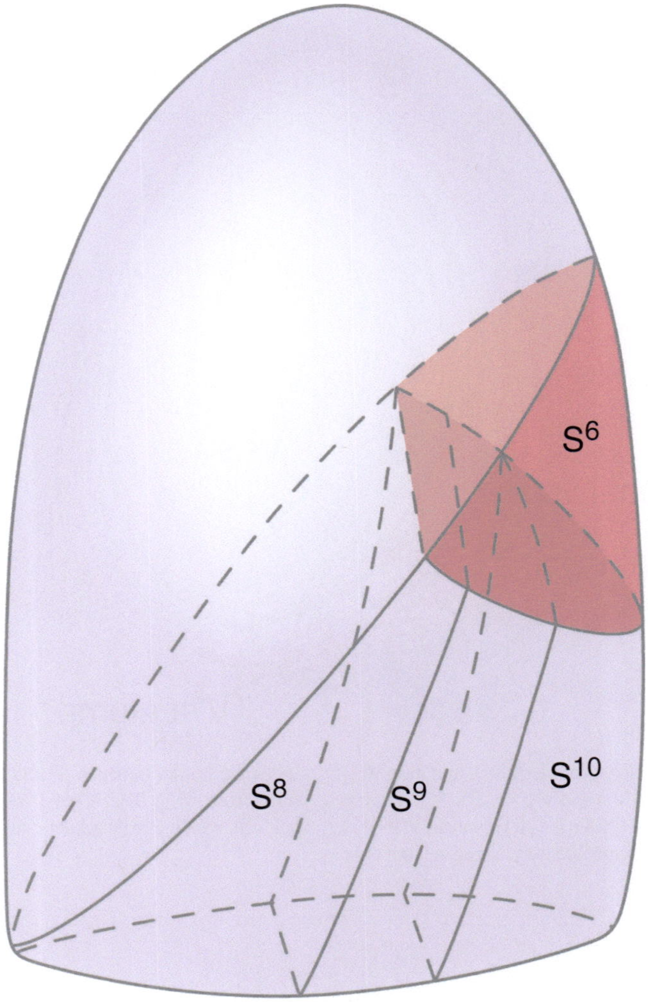

Fig. 6.1.1 The anatomical branching of A^6 and V^6 is confirmed from axial, coronal, and sagittal views on HRCT. The size and branching of B^6 are further examined using bronchoscope after tracheal intubation. S^6-segmentectomy is the simplest in all types of segmentectomy, because A^6 and B^6 are easy to be identified. The presence of B* branching from the basal bronchus caudal to B^6 is checked by either HRCT or preoperative bronchoscope. Lateral thoracotomy at the fifth intercostal space is usually optimal for S^6-segmentectomy.

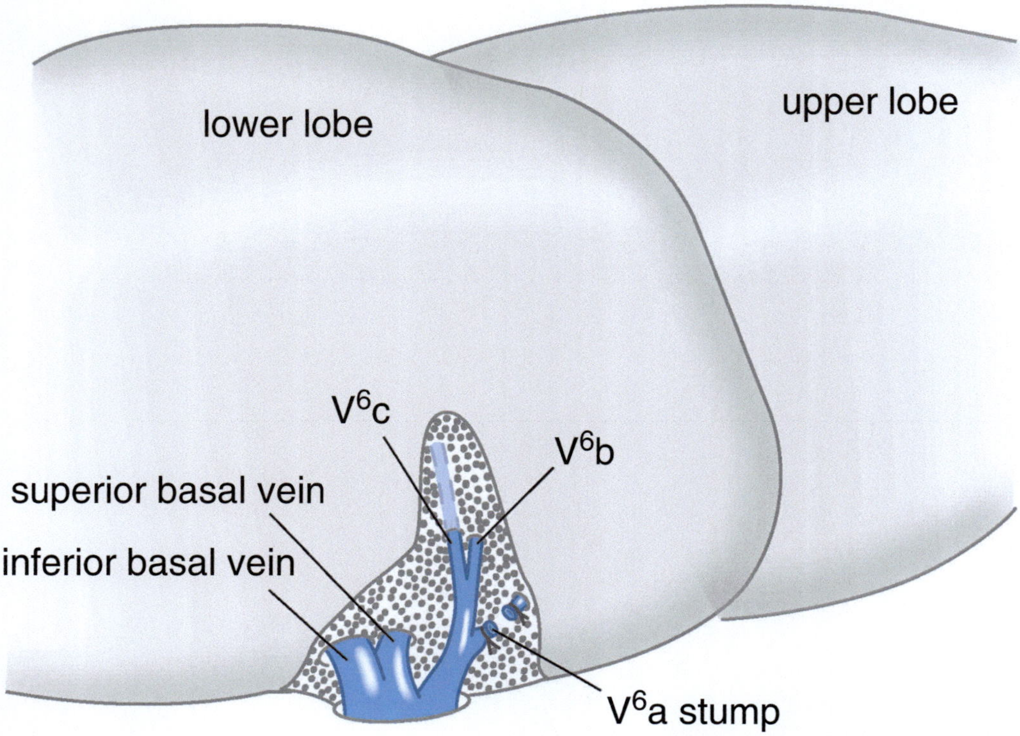

Fig. 6.1.2 The inferior pulmonary vein is exposed, and then V^6 is identified. V^6 usually branches to V^6a and V^6b+c. The V^6a running along the border between S^6a and S^6b+c is cut. However, V^6b+c is preserved in principle in the S^6-segmentectomy, because it not only guides the border between S^6 and S^{8-10} but also preserves venous return from S^{8-10}. The V^6b+c is exposed peripherally from the backside, which can help later cutting between S^6 and S^{10}.

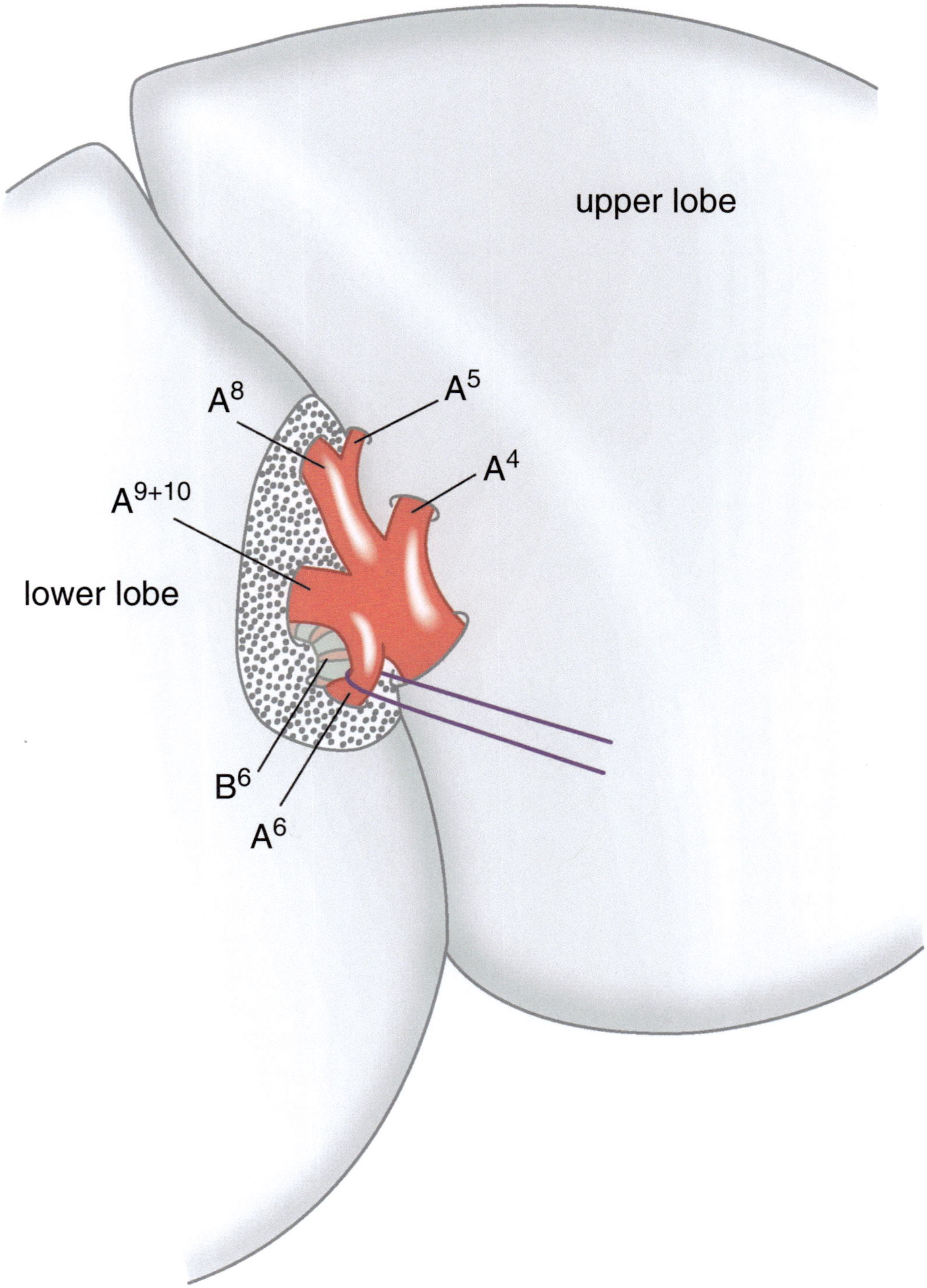

Fig. 6.1.3 Here, the operator is positioned at the dorsal side of the patient. The fissure between S^{1+2} and S^6 can be cut with a stapler because the staple line usually does not disturb the identification of the intersegmental plane during S^6-segmentectomy. However, the fissure can be also cut by using electrocautery without difficulty. A^6 and A^{8-10} are exposed. This figure shows a single A^6 branch, of which frequency is 78%.

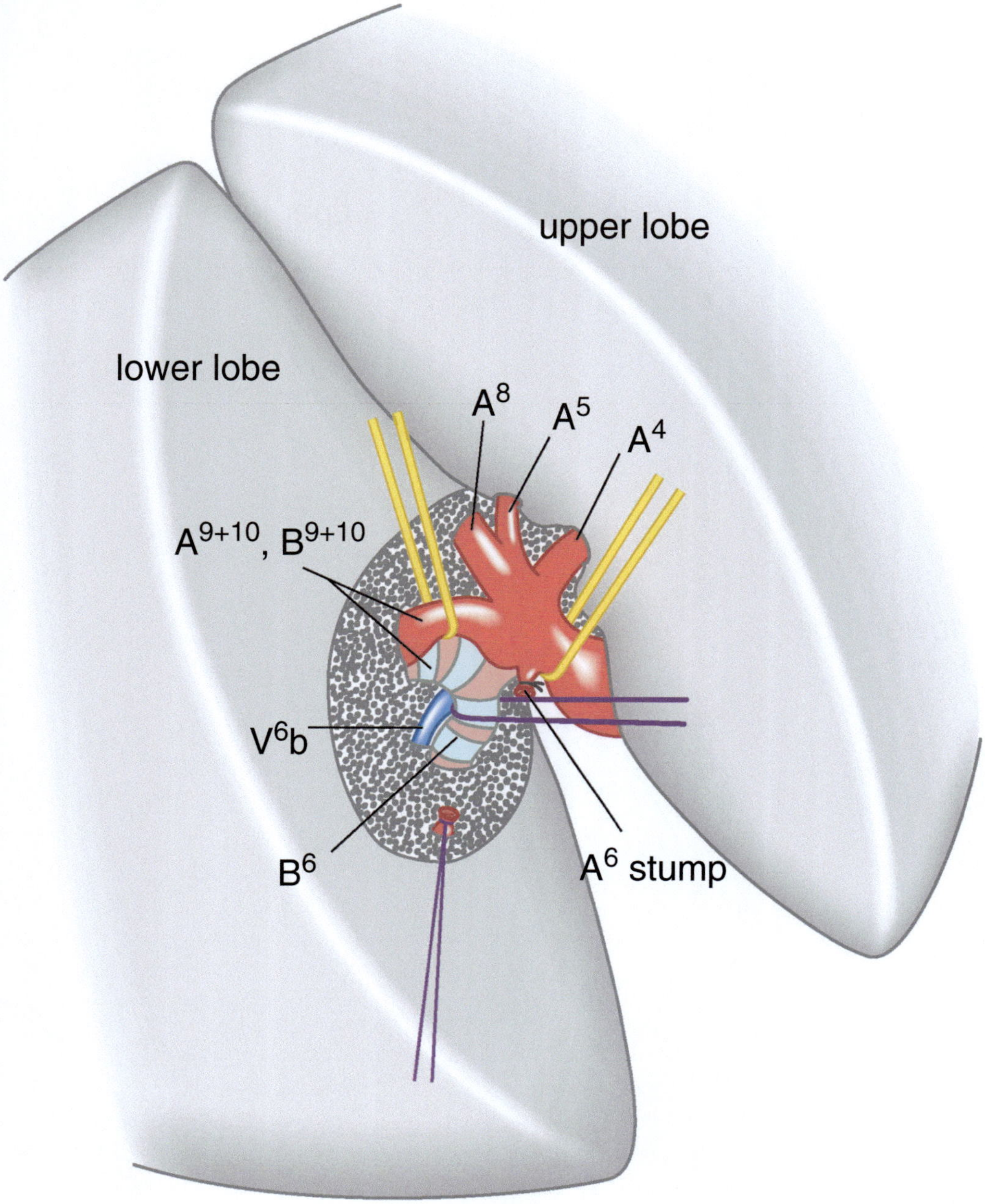

Fig. 6.1.4 A^6 is cut which exposes B^6 running caudally and behind A^6. The B^6 is carefully encircled with thread to avoid damage to V^6b, which runs at the back of B^6.

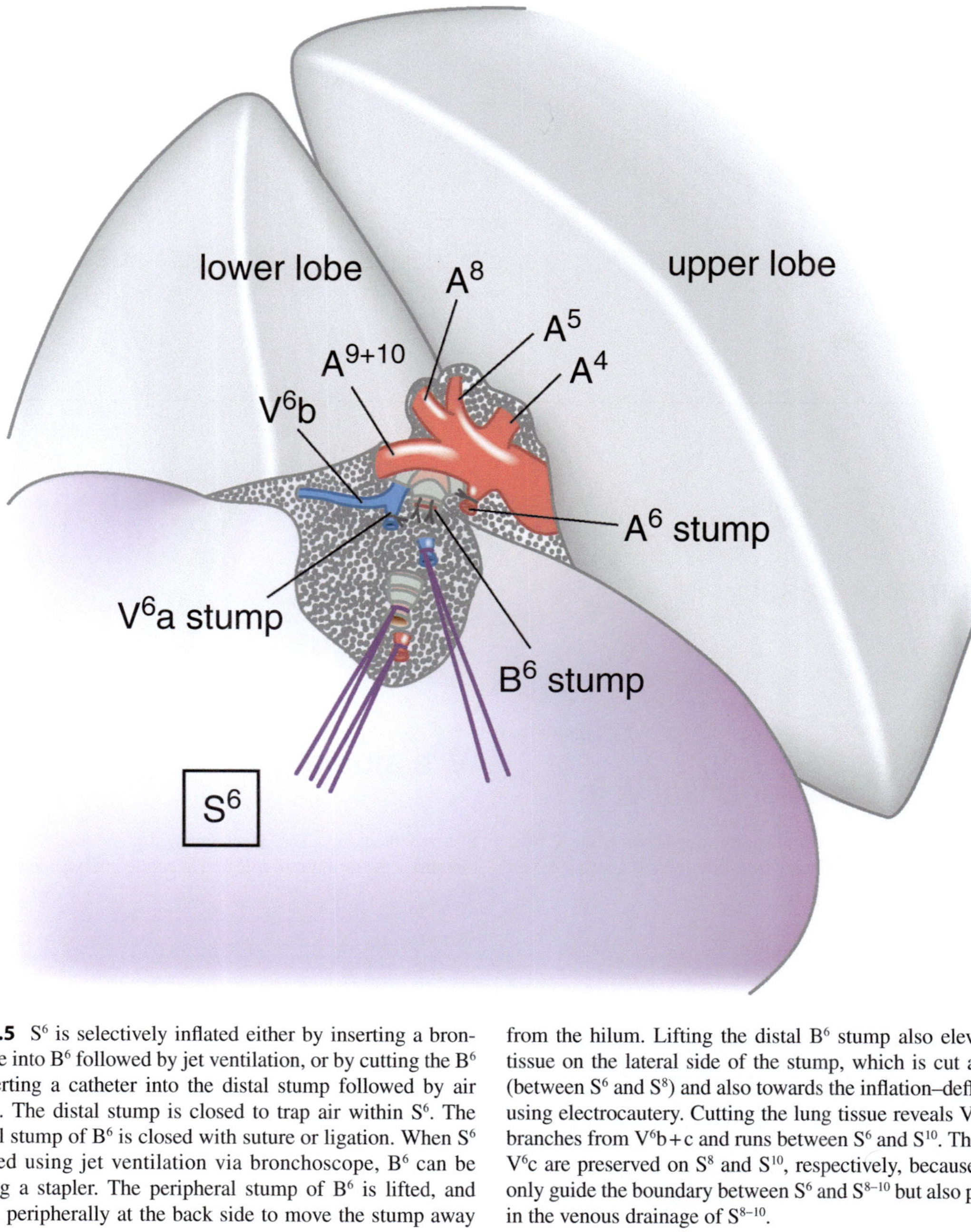

Fig. 6.1.5 S^6 is selectively inflated either by inserting a bronchoscope into B^6 followed by jet ventilation, or by cutting the B^6 and inserting a catheter into the distal stump followed by air inflation. The distal stump is closed to trap air within S^6. The proximal stump of B^6 is closed with suture or ligation. When S^6 is inflated using jet ventilation via bronchoscope, B^6 can be cut using a stapler. The peripheral stump of B^6 is lifted, and denuded peripherally at the back side to move the stump away from the hilum. Lifting the distal B^6 stump also elevates lung tissue on the lateral side of the stump, which is cut along V^6b (between S^6 and S^8) and also towards the inflation–deflation line using electrocautery. Cutting the lung tissue reveals V^6c, which branches from V^6b+c and runs between S^6 and S^{10}. The V^6b and V^6c are preserved on S^8 and S^{10}, respectively, because they not only guide the boundary between S^6 and S^{8-10} but also play a role in the venous drainage of S^{8-10}.

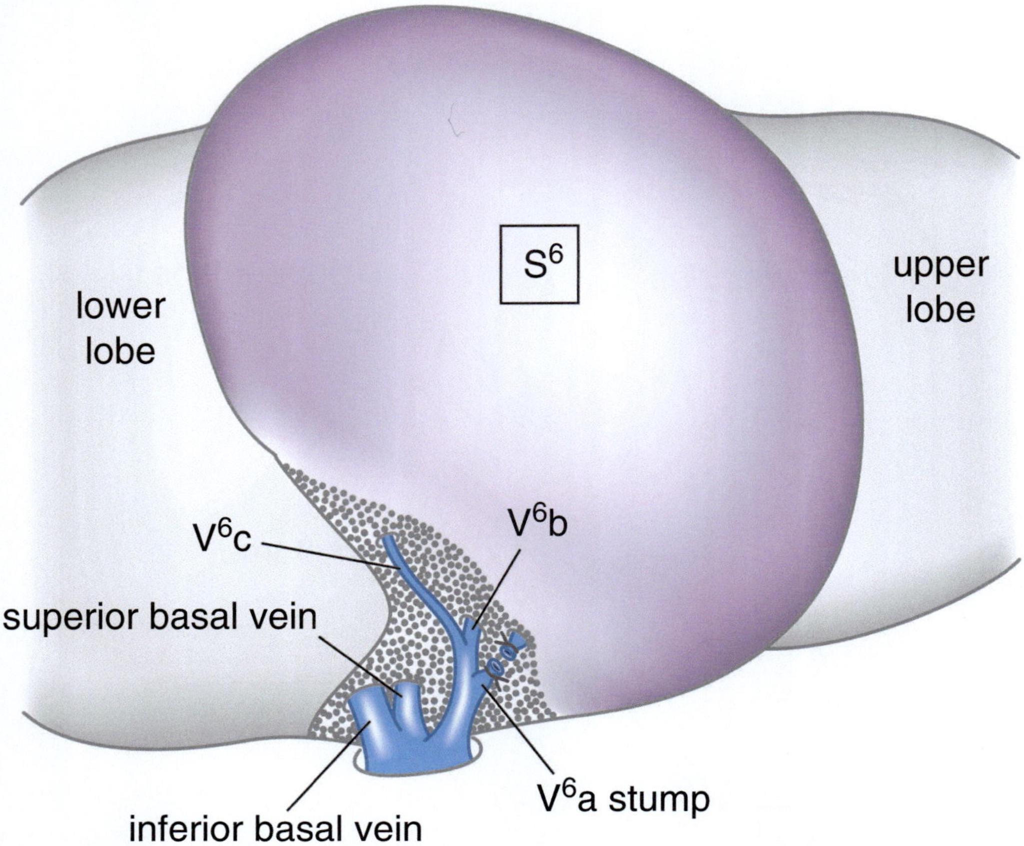

Fig. 6.1.6 The lung tissue is cut from the dorsal site along V^6b+c and also along the inflation–deflation line, which completes the S^6-segmentectomy. The intersegmental plane is cut from various directions to facilitate simple and accurate intersegmental cutting.

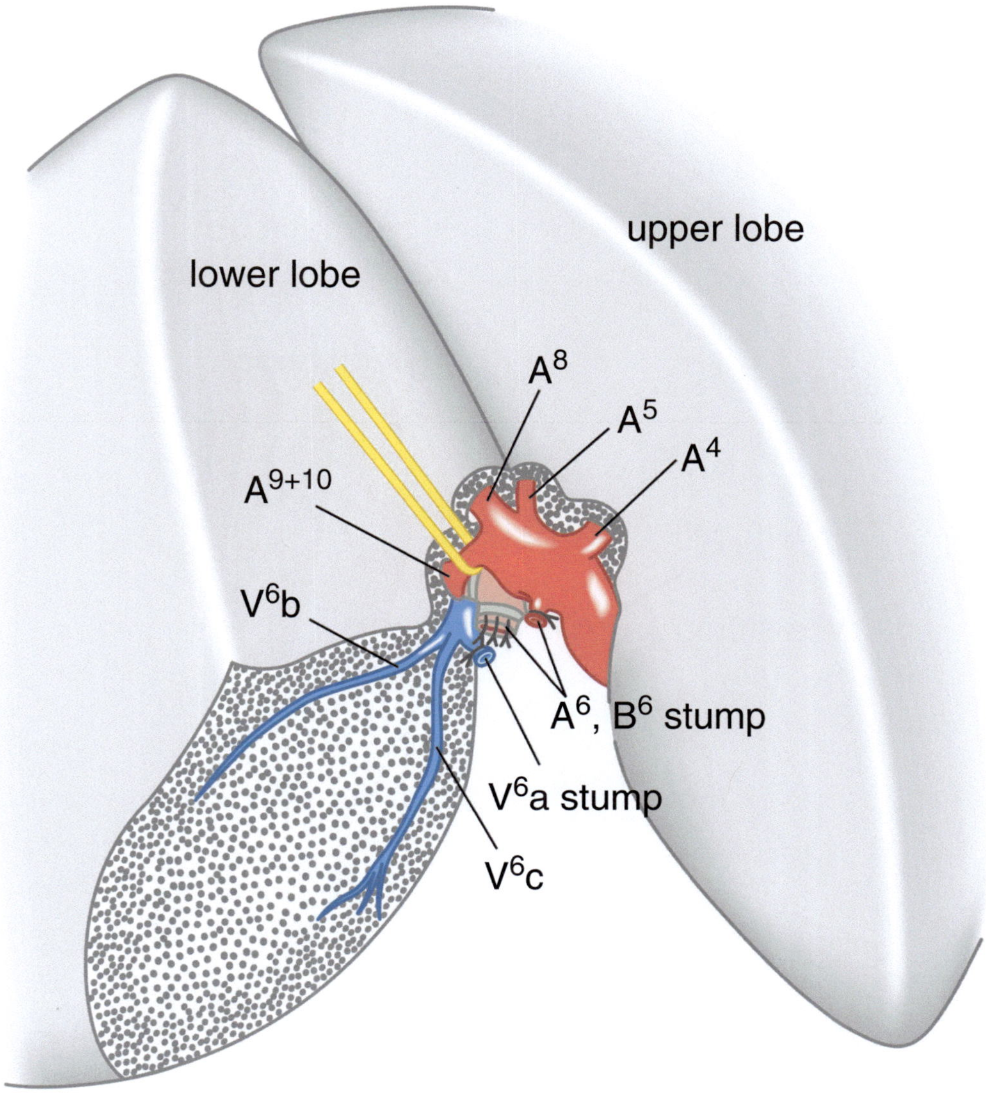

Fig. 6.1.7 After resection of S^6, V^6b (between S^6b and S^8) and V^6c (between S^6c and $S^{10}a$) are seen on S^{8-10}.

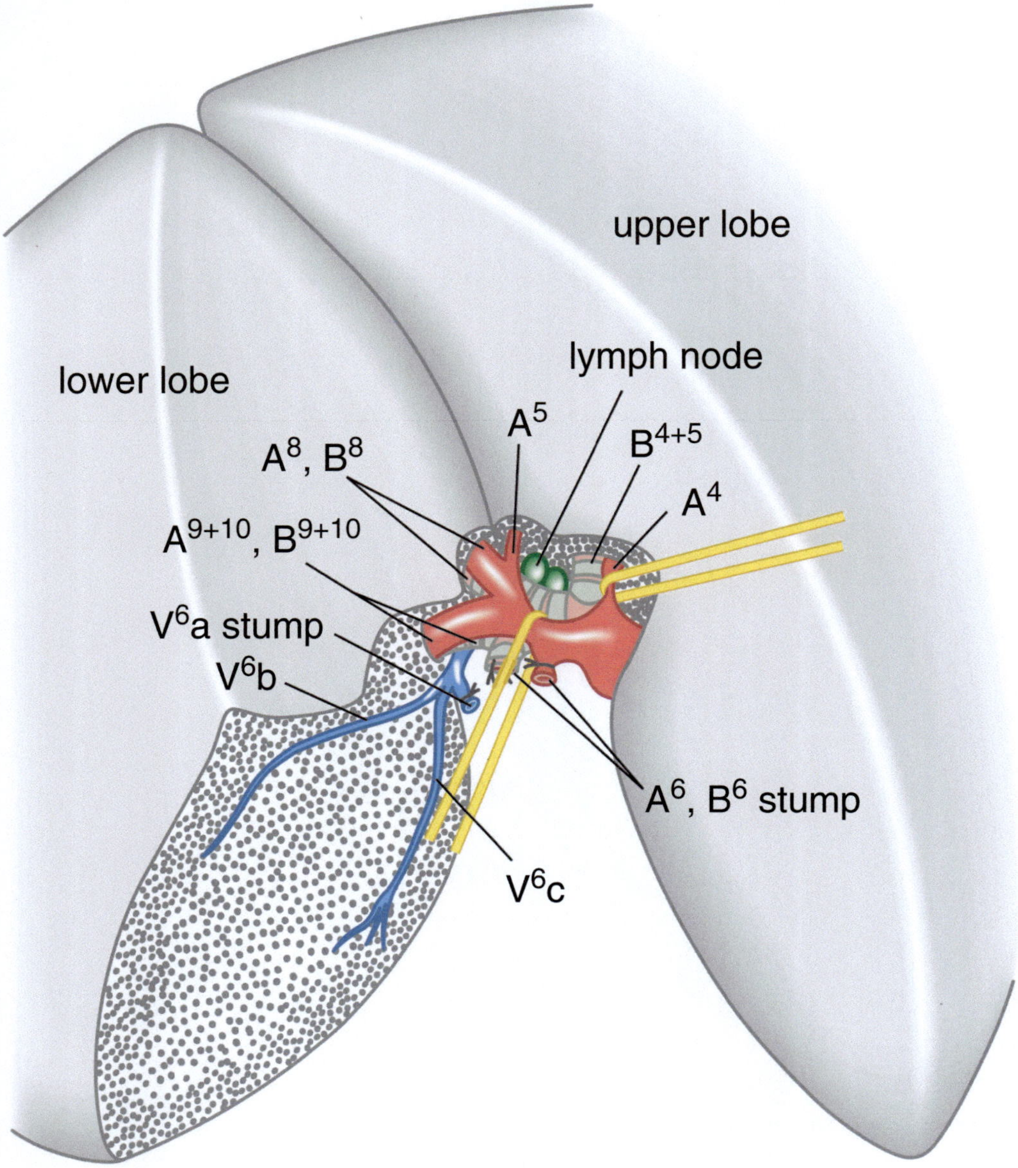

Fig. 6.1.8 The interlobar pulmonary arterial and A^4 are encircled with tape for hilar lymph node dissection. The #11 and the anterior #12l nodes located between the upper lobar bronchus and lower lobar bronchus are dissected.

6.2 Left S^8 Segmentectomy

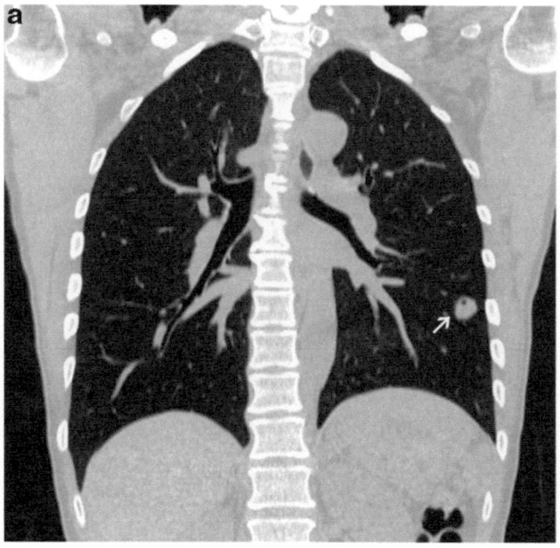

coronal view (CT scan)

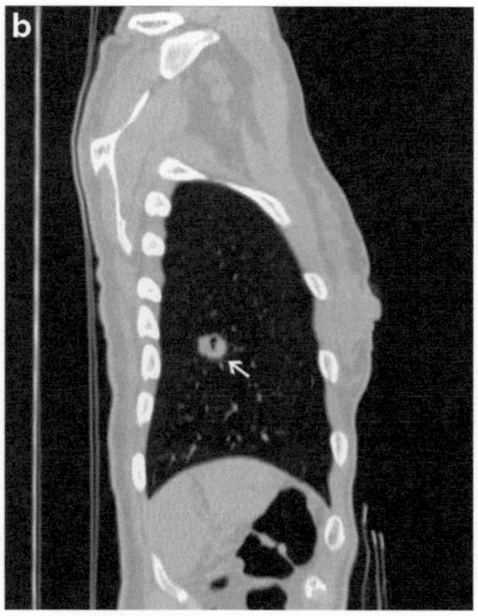

sagittal view (CT scan)

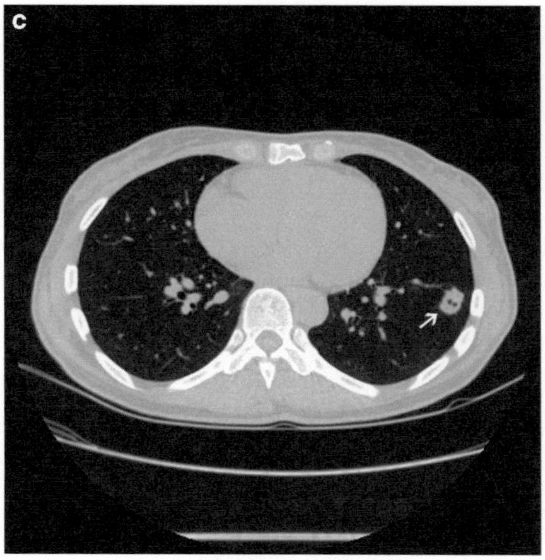

axial view (CT scan)

A medical examination uncovered an abnormal shadow in the left lower lung field of a 54-year-old female smoker. The CT revealed a 2-cm solid nodule with a cavity at S^8a that was diagnosed as squamous cell carcinoma from a CT-guided needle biopsy specimen. S^8-segmentectomy was proceeded, and the final pathological diagnosis was T1aN0M0 squamous cell carcinoma.

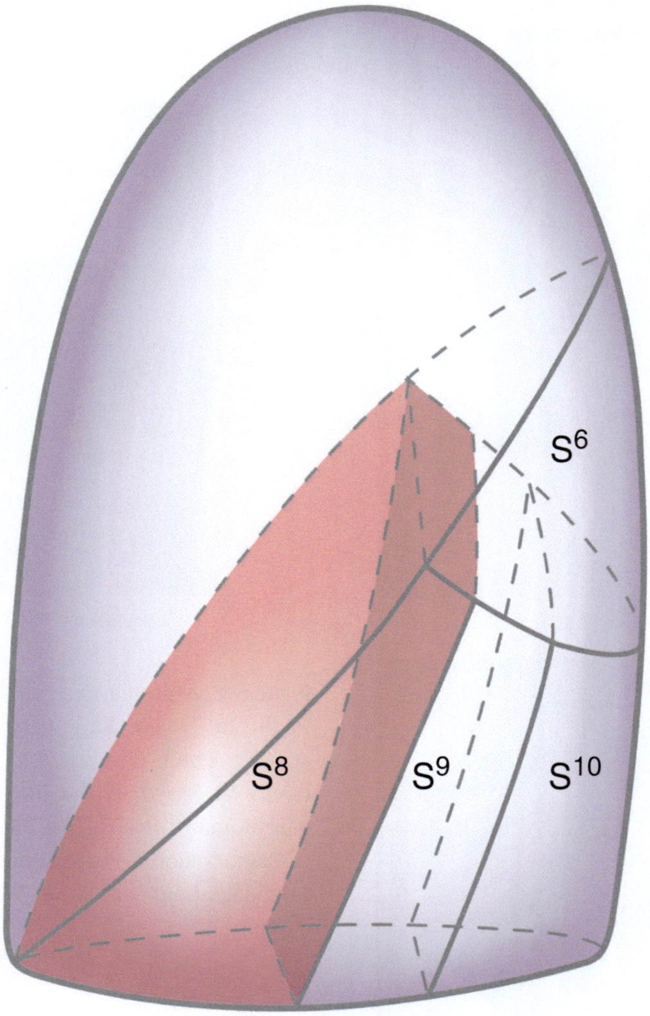

Fig. 6.2.1 The segmental arteries (A^{8-10}) and bronchi (B^{8-10}) are identified from axial, coronal, and sagittal views on HRCT. The anatomical branching and sizes of B^8, B^9, and B^{10} are further checked by bronchoscope after tracheal intubation. Lateral thoracotomy at the fifth intercostal space is usually optimal for S^8-segmentectomy. The figures in this session show the most frequent types of bronchial and arterial branching, i.e. B^8 and B^{9+10}, and A^8 and A^{9+10}, respectively.

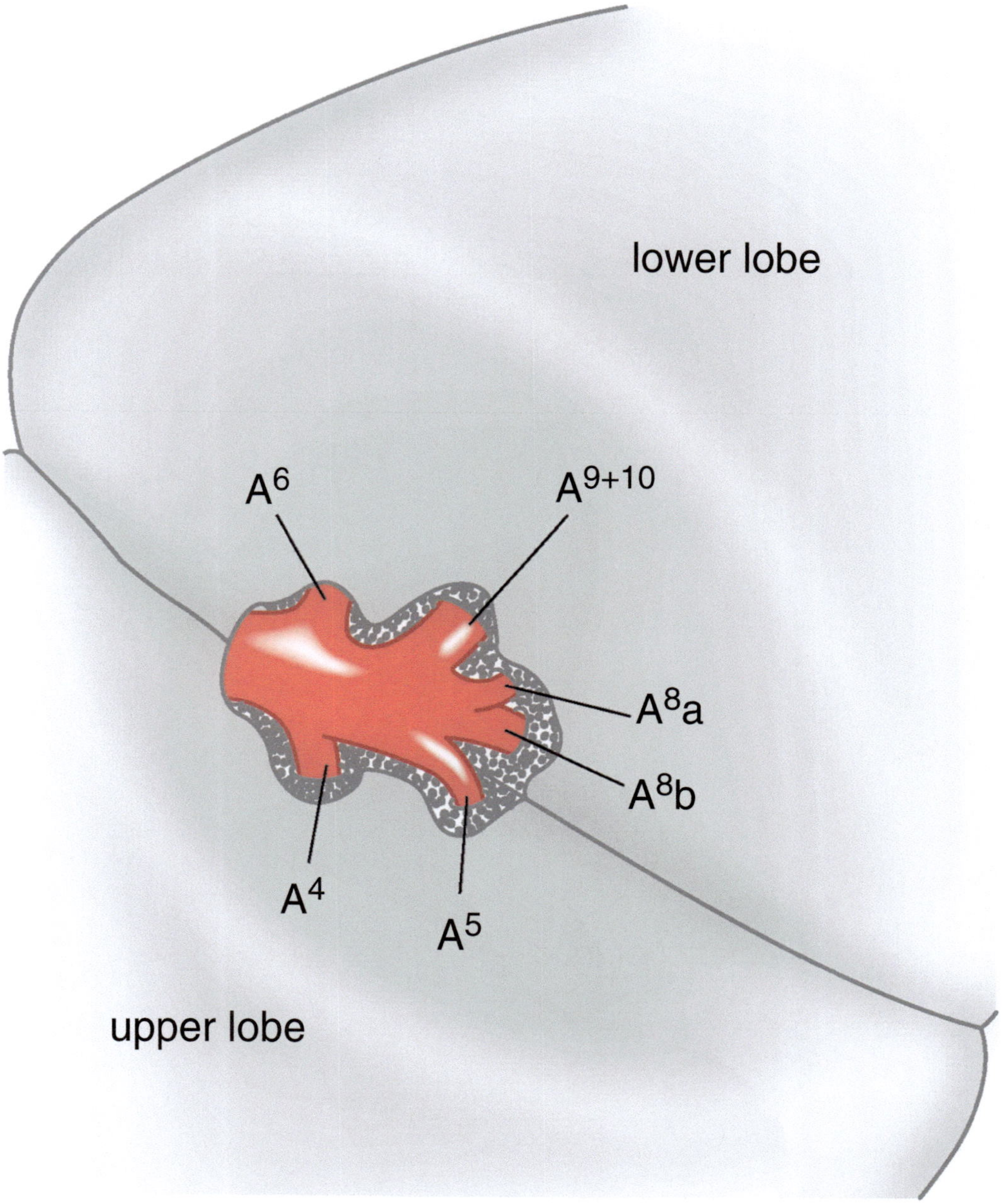

Fig. 6.2.2 S^8-segmentectomy does not require exposure of the inferior pulmonary vein. In addition, superior basal pulmonary vein should not be cut, because V^8 is usually not identical to a superior basal pulmonary vein. Besides, the exposure of inferior pulmonary vein does not help the identification of segmental vein. In the segmentectomy for S^8, S^9, and S^{10}, the exposure of all branches of A^6, A^8, and A^{9+10} is important, not to mistake the identification of these arterial branches. The branching of A^8a and A^9a is sometimes complicated, such as A^8a branching from A^{9+10} and A^9a from A^8. To identify them accurately, A^8 is sufficiently exposed towards the peripheral direction. If A^8a or A^9a is still difficult to be defined, only the ventral branch of A^8 is cut first, which must not be A^9a. After cutting B^8, the remaining arterial branches can be easily identified, i.e. A^8-branch runs closely to the distal stump of B^8, whereas A^9-branch runs away from it.

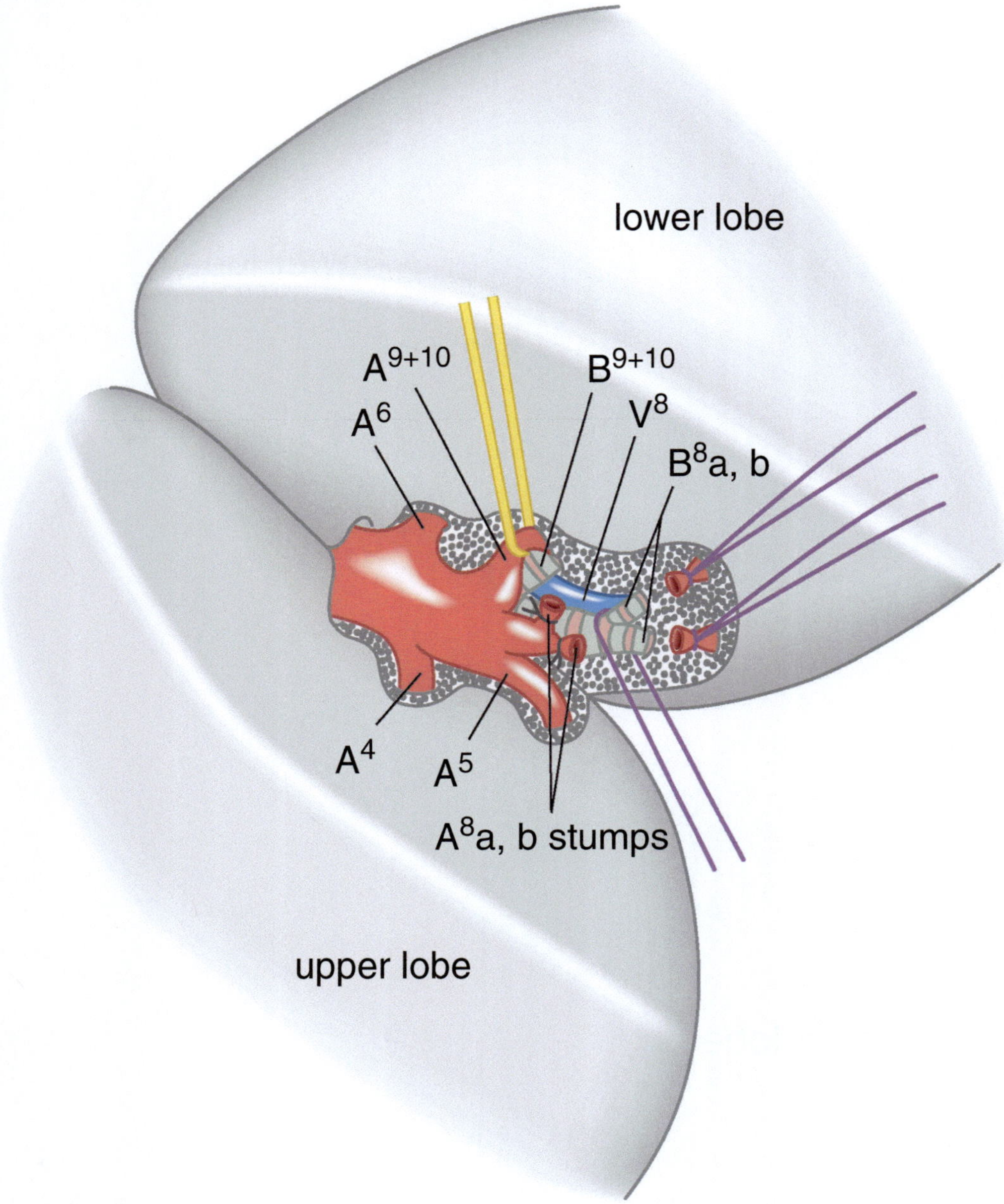

Fig. 6.2.3 Cutting A^8 reveals B^8 which runs behind A^8. The B^8 is carefully encircled with thread to avoid damaging V^8 running behind it. If B^8 cannot be identified with certainty, illumination from a bronchoscope inserted into B^8, B^9, and B^{10} can help the identification.

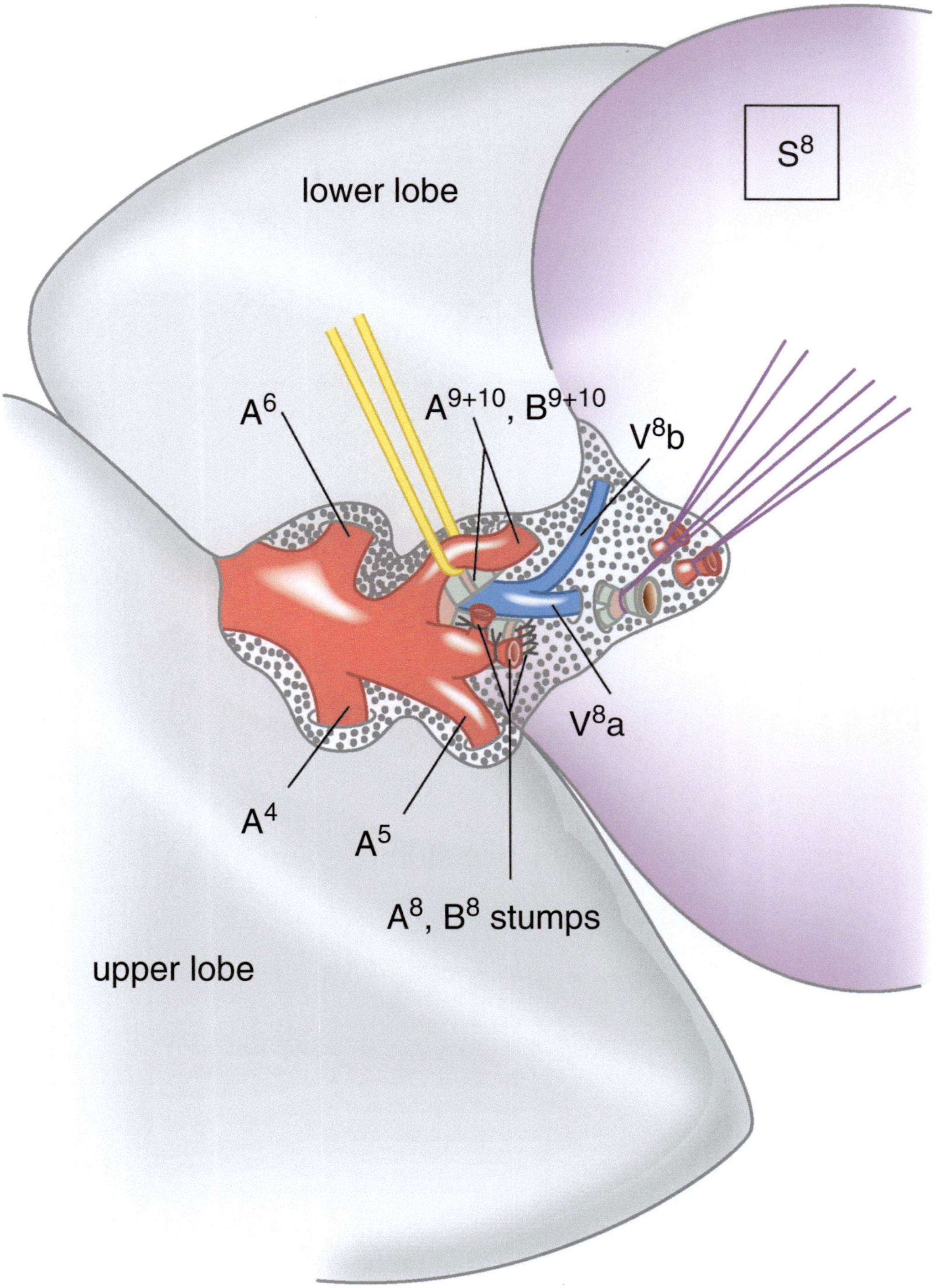

Fig. 6.2.4 S^8 is selectively inflated by either inserting a bronchoscope into B^8 followed by jet ventilation, or by cutting the B^8 and inserting a catheter into the distal stump followed by air inflation. The distal stump is closed to trap air within S^8. The proximal stump of B^8 is closed with suture or ligation. When S^8 is inflated using jet ventilation via bronchoscope, B^8 can be cut using a stapler. The distal stump of B^8 is lifted and denuded at the backside to move it away from the hilum. Lifting the distal B^8 stump exposes V^8a (between S^8a and S^8b) running towards the stump. Cutting V^8a further elevates the stump of B^8 together with lung tissue around it, which is cut along V^8b (between S^8 and S^9) and also towards the inflation–deflation line using electrocautery. V^8b is preserved to conserve the venous return of S^9 and also to be used as a landmark for cutting the segmental plane if the surgical margin is sufficient. The intersegmental plane is cut from various directions, which can make the intersegmental cutting easy and accurate.

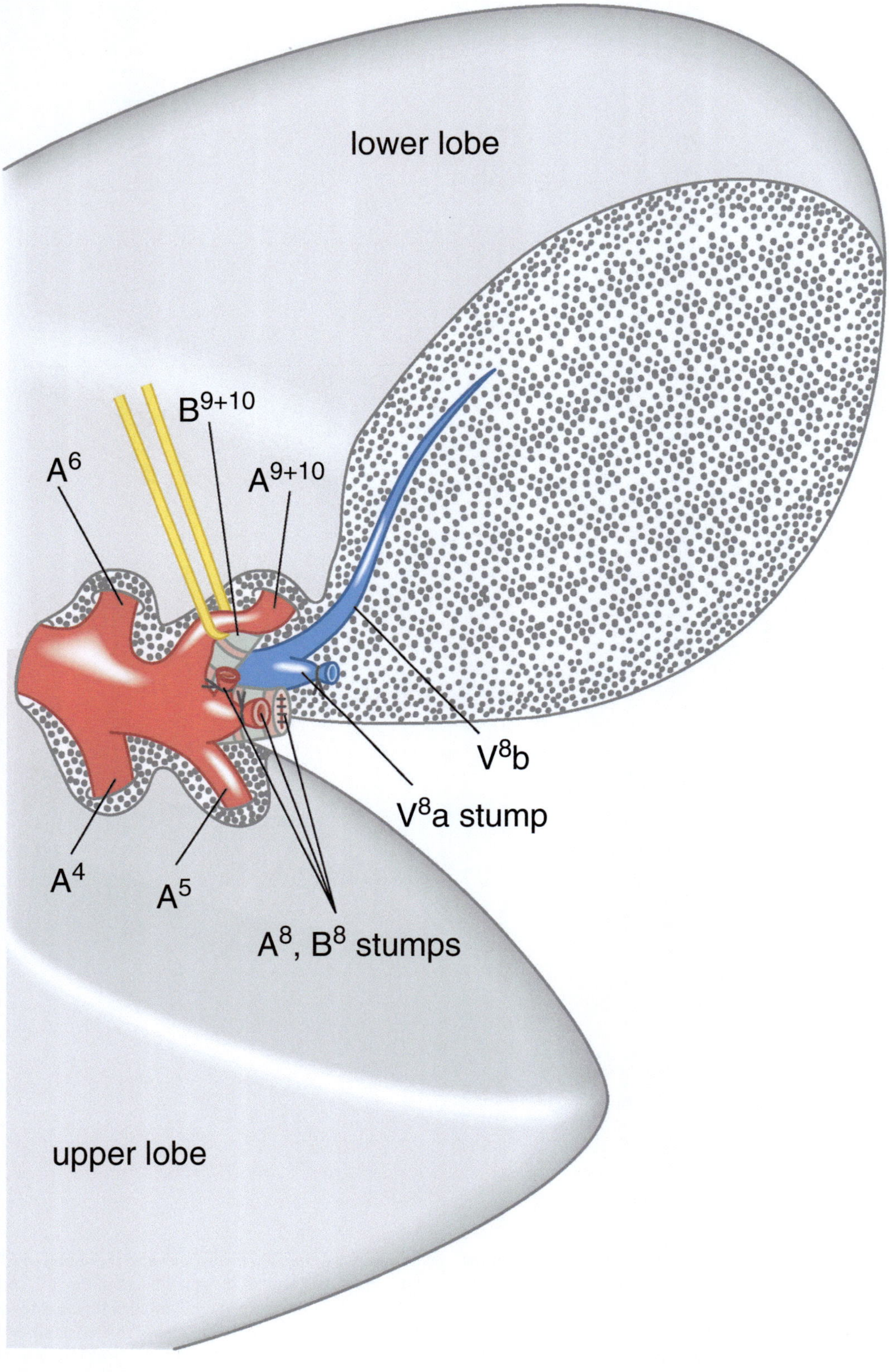

Fig. 6.2.5 After S^8 resection, V^8b (between S^8 and S^9) is revealed on S^9. The B^6, A^6, and the interlobar pulmonary artery are encircled with tape, followed by dissection of the #12l and #13 (around B^6) lymph nodes, which lie along the lymphatic chain from S^8 towards #7 node. The #11 lymph node can be dissected with taping the A^{8-10} and A^{4+5}, which can expose it sufficiently.

6.3 Left S^9 Segmentectomy

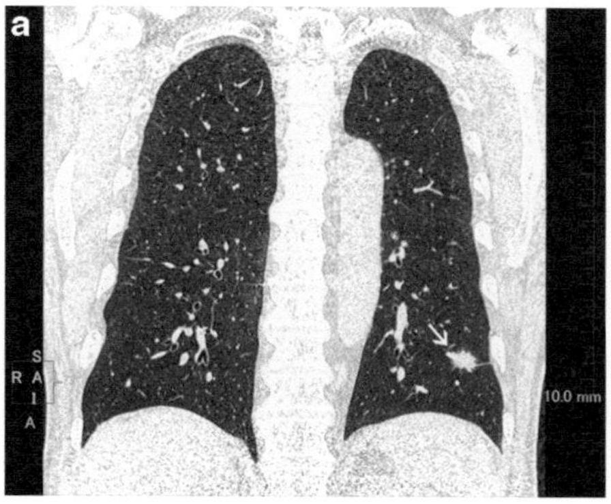

coronal view (CT scan)

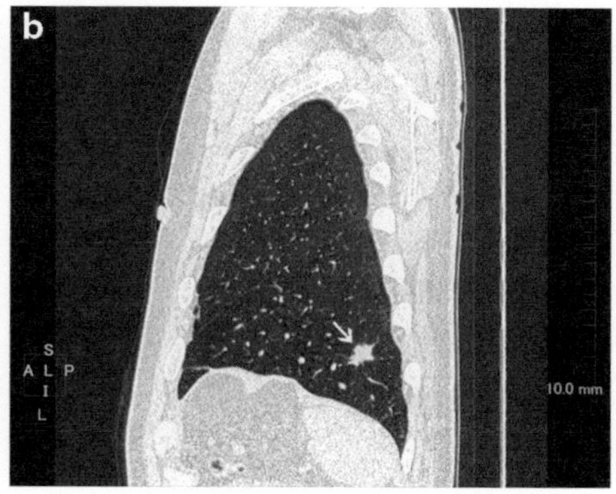

sagittal view (CT scan)

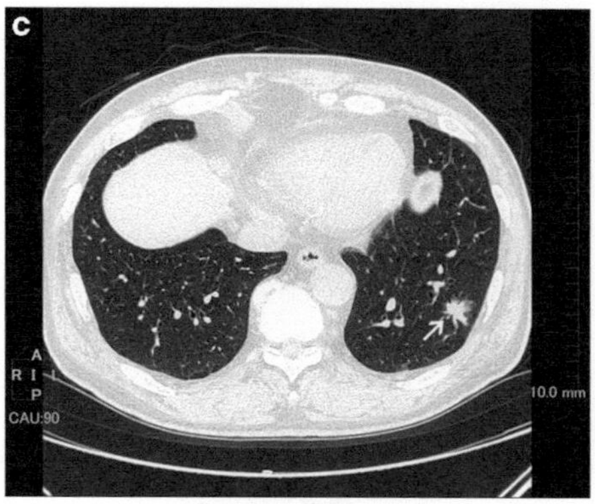

axial view (CT scan)

A CT scan of a 71-year-old male at a medical examination uncovered a mixed GGO nodule at the left S^9. Follow-up CT showed that the nodule had increased and had formed a solid area. Two years later, CT revealed a solid 1.6-cm nodule with spicular formation and pleural indentation that was diagnosed as adenocarcinoma from a CT-guided needle biopsy specimen. S^9-segmentectomy was proceeded. The final pathological diagnosis was pT1aN0M0 papillary adenocarcinoma.

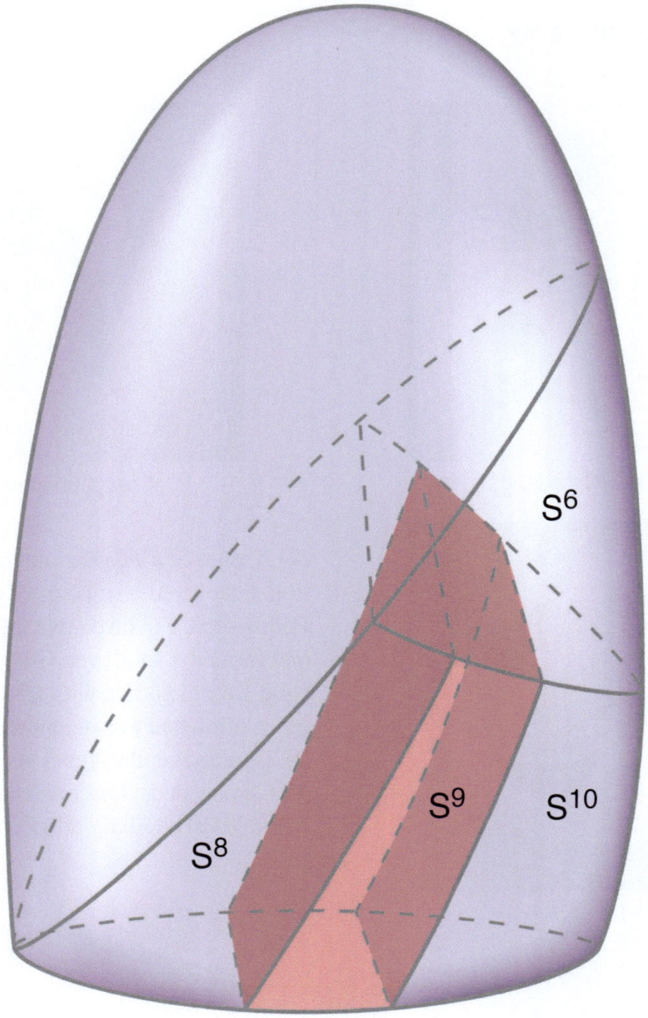

Fig. 6.3.1 The segmental arteries (A^{8-10}) and bronchi (B^{8-10}) are identified from axial, coronal, and sagittal views on HRCT. The branching profiles and size of B^8, B^9, and B^{10} are further checked by bronchoscope after tracheal intubation. Lateral thoracotomy at the fifth intercostal space is generally appropriate for S^9-segmentectomy. The branching pattern of bronchus and artery in the figures of this session is the most frequent manner, i.e. B^8 and B^{9+10}, and A^8 and A^{9+10}.

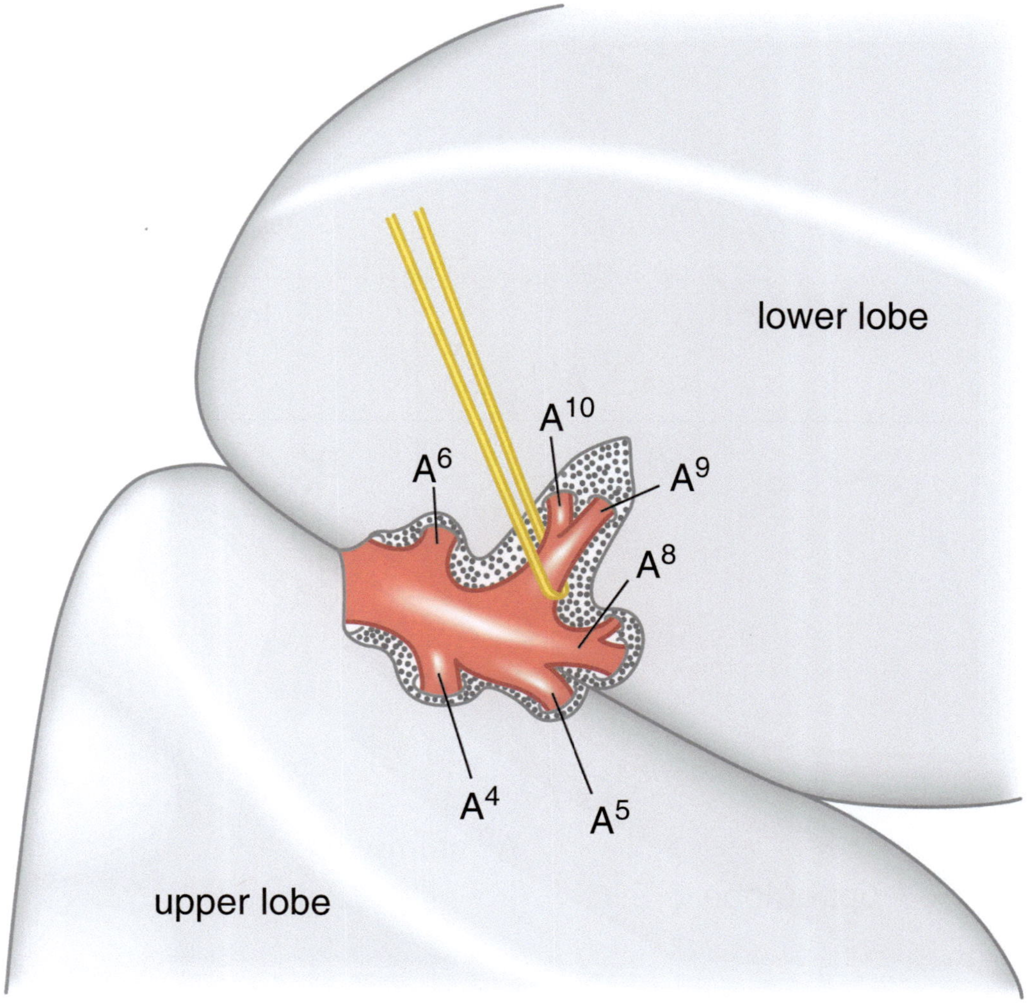

Fig. 6.3.2 The interlobar pulmonary artery is exposed, followed by exposing A^6, A^8, and A^{9+10}. The inferior pulmonary vein does not need to be exposed for S^9-segmentectomy, because V^9 is usually impossible to be identified from the root of the inferior pulmonary vein. The peripheral side of A^{9+10} is exposed after encircling with tape. When preoperative bronchoscopy reveals a long common trunk of B^{9+10}, that of A^{9+10} is usually also long. The S^6 and S^8 face the interlobar fissure, whereas both S^9 and S^{10} do not, and this should be taken into consideration at this point. Namely, to reach the S^9, the border between S^6 and S^8 should be cut from the interlobar fissure, which has no landmark however and therefore is not always simple. Exposing the peripheral side of A^{9+10} reveals that A^9 and A^{10} run to the lateral and dorsal sides, respectively. A^8a and A^9a branching has some variations, such as A^8a arising from A^{9+10} and A^9a arising from A^8. When identifying A^9 and A^{10} is difficult, the most ventral branch of A^{9+10} should be cut first, because it must not be the A^{10}-branch. Cutting the most ventral arterial branch reveals B^9 behind it, which is cut. After cutting the B^9, the A^9- and A^{10} branches can be identified easily, because the former runs towards the distal stump of B^9, whereas the latter runs away from it.

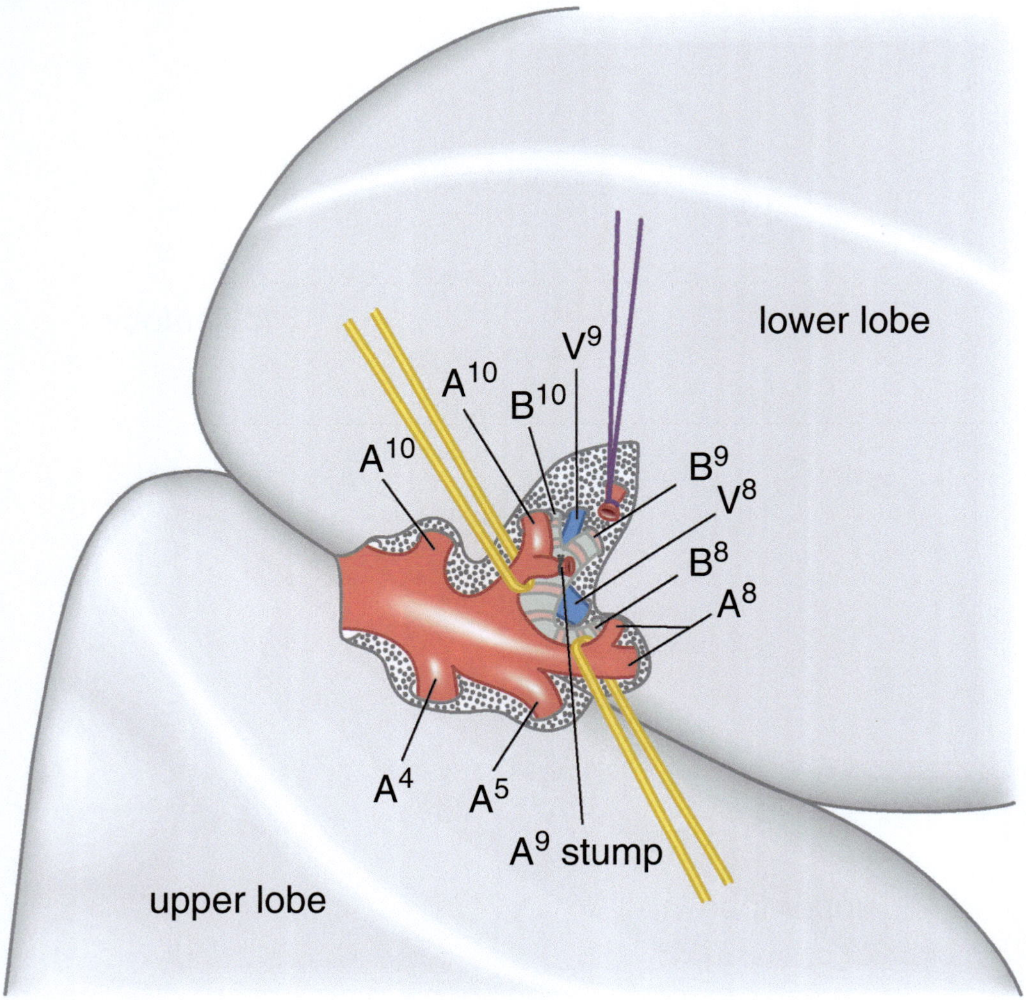

Fig. 6.3.3 Because V^8 and V^9 run behind B^9, B^9 is carefully encircled with thread to avoid damage of V^8 and V^9. The identification of B^9 can be also confirmed by illumination from a bronchoscope inserted into B^9 and B^{10}.

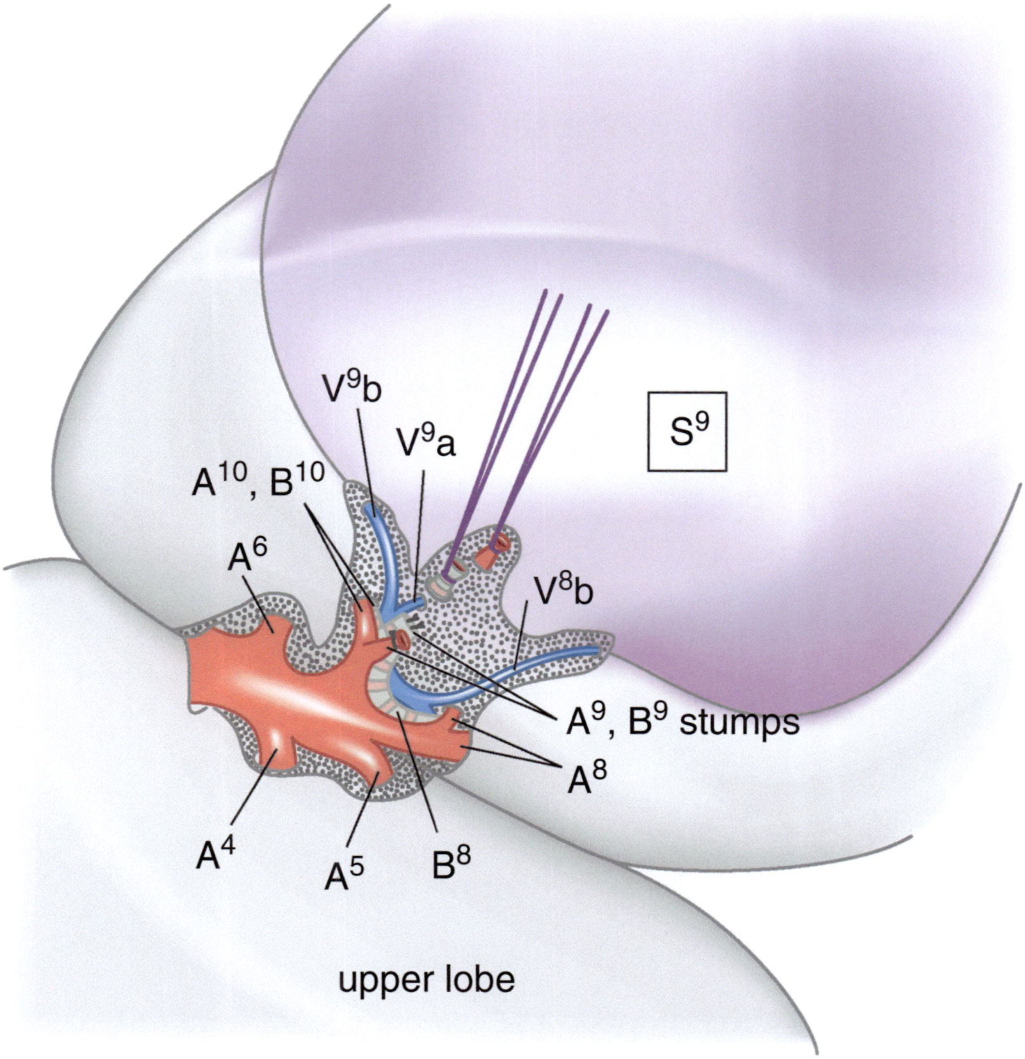

Fig. 6.3.4 S^9 is selectively inflated either by inserting a bronchoscope into B^9 followed by jet ventilation, or by cutting the B^9 and inserting a catheter into the distal stump followed by air inflation. The distal stump is closed to trap air within S^9. The proximal stump of B^9 is closed with suture or ligation. The distal stump of B^9 is lifted and denuded peripherally at the back to move it away from the hilum. Lifting the distal B^9 stump reveals V^9a (between S^9a and S^9b) running toward the stump, which is cut. Cutting V^9a further elevates the peripheral stump of B^9 together with lung tissue on its both sides, which is cut along V^8b (between S^8 and S^9) and V^9b (between S^9 and S^{10}) and also towards the inflation–deflation line using electrocautery. V^8b and V^9b are preserved on S^8 and S^{10}, respectively, because they can not only guide the intersegmental plane and but also make a role for venous return from S^8 and S^{10}. The intersegmental plane is cut from various directions to facilitate simple and accurate intersegmental cutting.

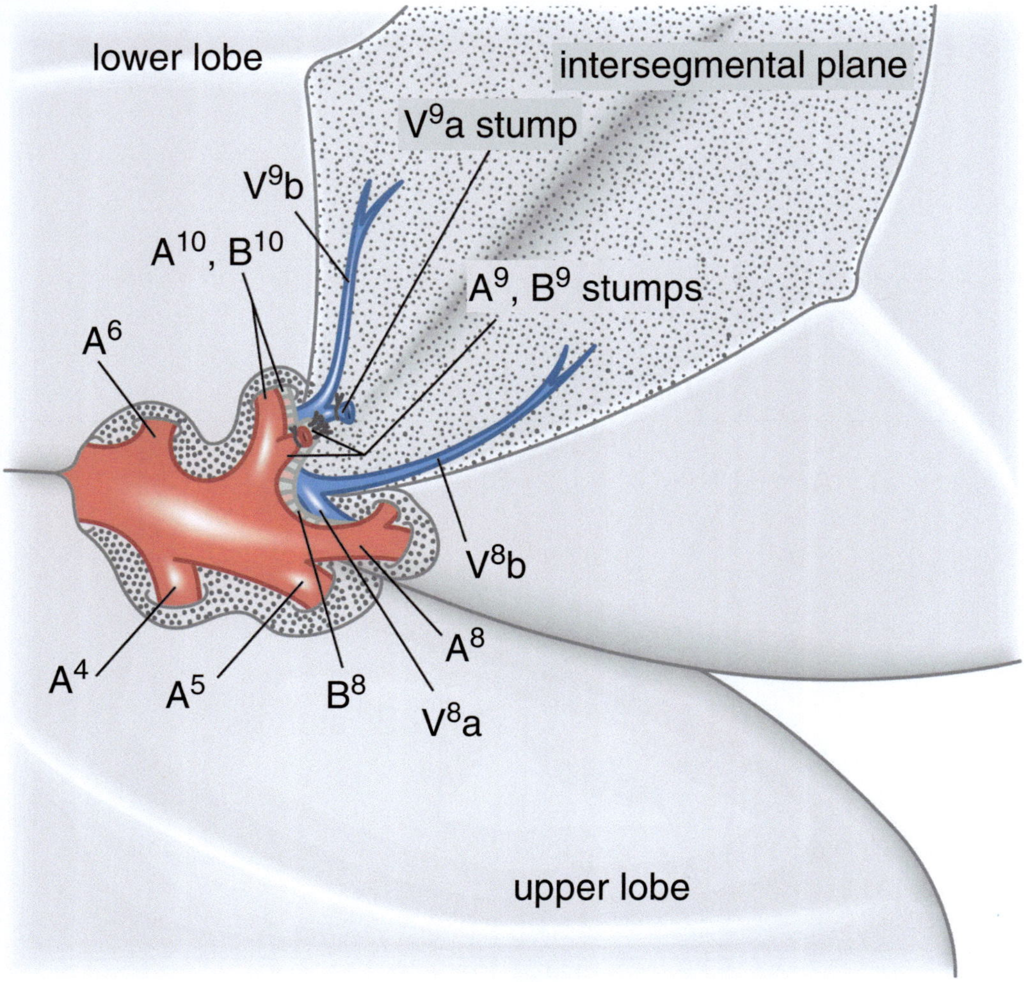

Fig. 6.3.5 V^8b (between S^8b and S^9b) and V^9b (between S^9b and $S^{10}b$) are preserved on the intersegmental plane.

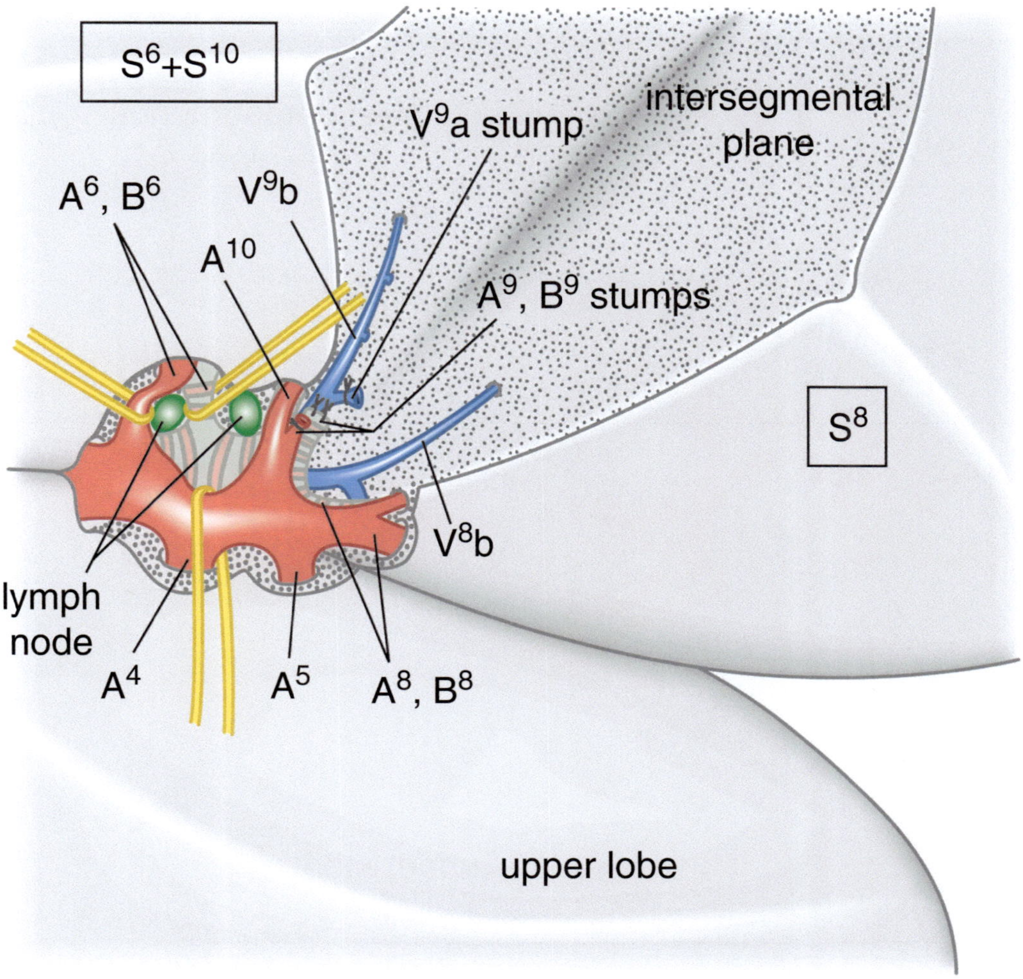

Fig. 6.3.6 B^6, A^6, and the interlobar pulmonary artery are encircled with tape for dissection of the posterior #12l and #13 (around B^6) nodes, which lie along the lymphatic chain from S^9 towards #7 node.

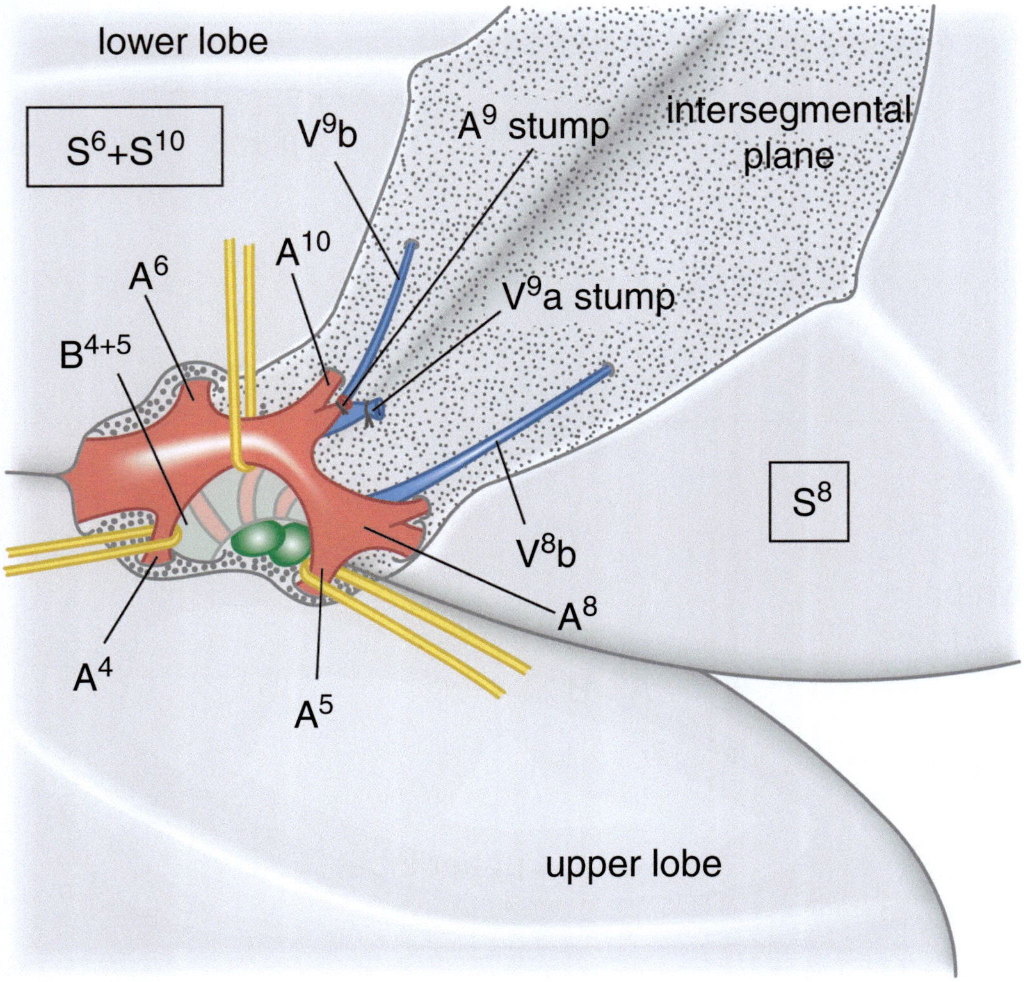

Fig. 6.3.7 A^4, A^5, and the interlobar pulmonary artery are encircled with tape and then the #11 lymph node is dissected.

6.4 Left S^{10} Segmentectomy

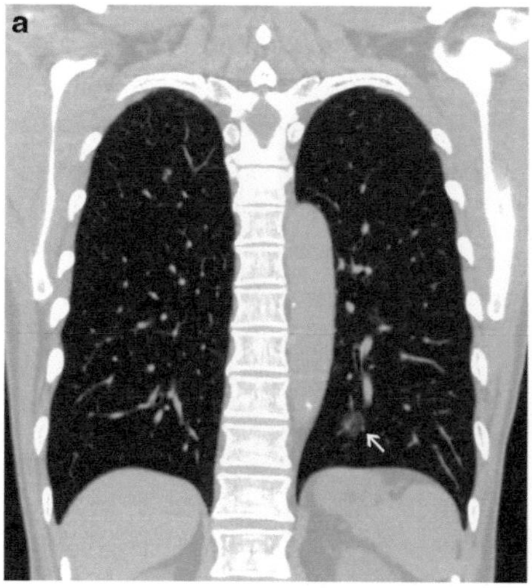

coronal view (CT scan)

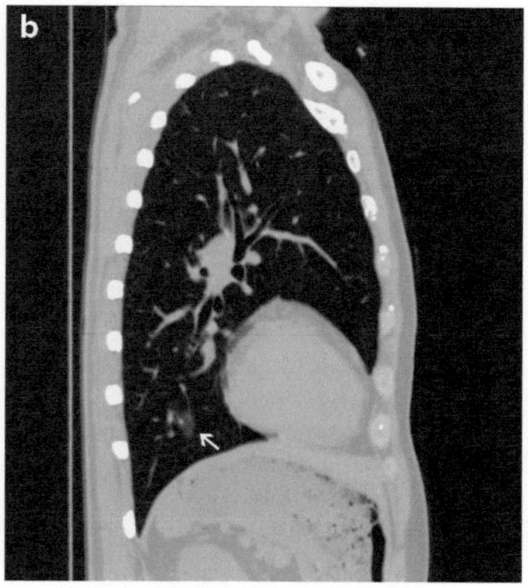

sagittal view (CT scan)

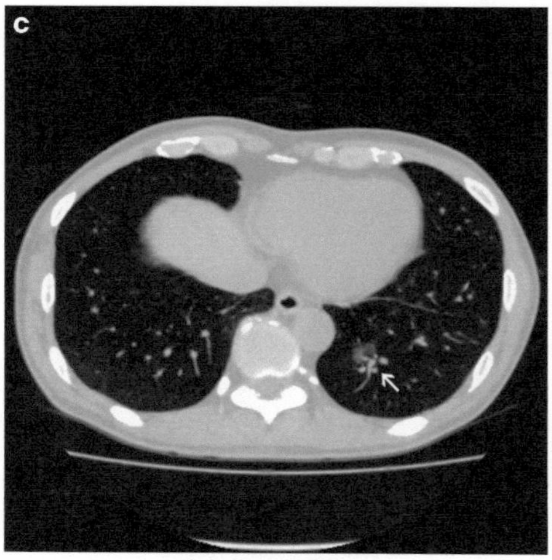

axial view (CT scan)

A CT scan of a 69-year-old male at a medical examination had uncovered a pure GGO nodule, which had been followed up. A CT scan 5 years later revealed a denser 1.8-cm nodule to with GGO findings located near the hilum of S^{10}. The nodule was diagnosed as bronchioloalveolar carcinoma from a CT-guided needle biopsy specimen. Because the nodule was located near the hilum, it was marked with lipiodol as described in the session of "General Knack". The marked nodule was grasped with a ring-shaped forceps to take a sufficient surgical margin during the S^{10}-segmentectomy. The final pathological diagnosis was pT1aN0M0 bronchioloalveolar carcinoma.

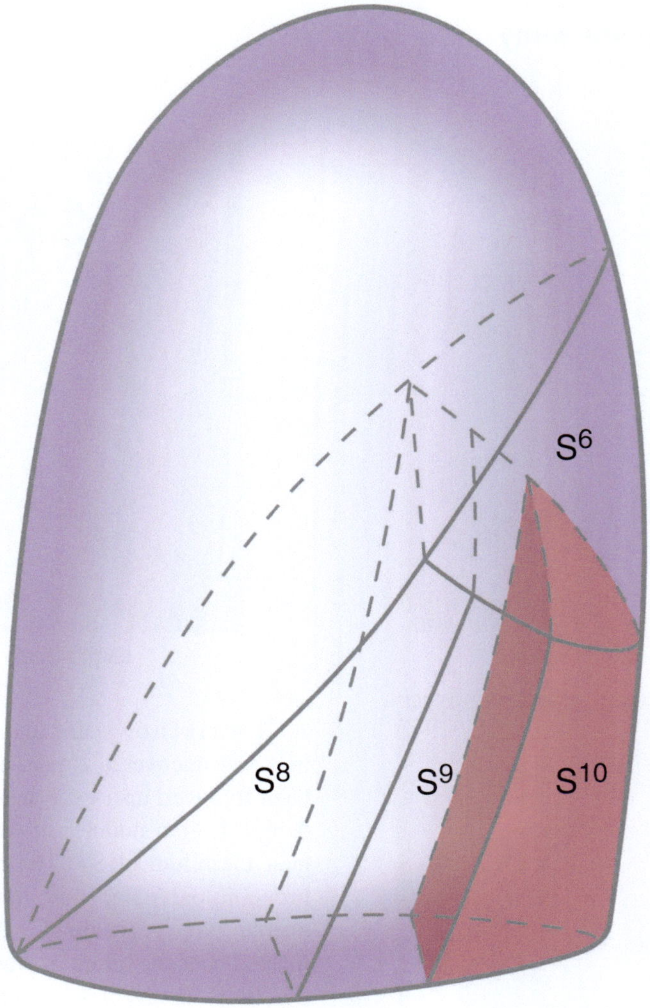

Fig. 6.4.1 S^{10}-segmentectomy is one of the most difficult procedures in segmentectomy, of which reasons are as follows: (1) because S^{10} does not face interlobar fissure, the border between the S^6 and S^8 should be divided from the interlobar fissure to reach the S^{10}, which is always not easy, because there is no landmark of the border; (2) because A^{10} branches from the A^{9+10} to the dorsal direction and goes far away from the thoracotomy site, it is always not easy to be identified. Before segmentectomy, the segmental arteries (A^{8-10}) and bronchi (B^{8-10}) are identified from axial, coronal, and sagittal views on HRCT. The branching profiles of B^8, B^9, and B^{10} are further checked by bronchoscope after tracheal intubation. When S* is present, A^{10}a and A* and B^{10}a and B* should be carefully differentiated. The figures in this session show the most frequent branching pattern, i.e. two branches with B^8 and B^{9+10}. The thoracotomy site is usually at the lateral fifth or sixth intercostal space, but the sixth intercostal space is preferable for obtaining the branches of A^9 and A^{10}, which is the point of S^{10}-segmentectomy.

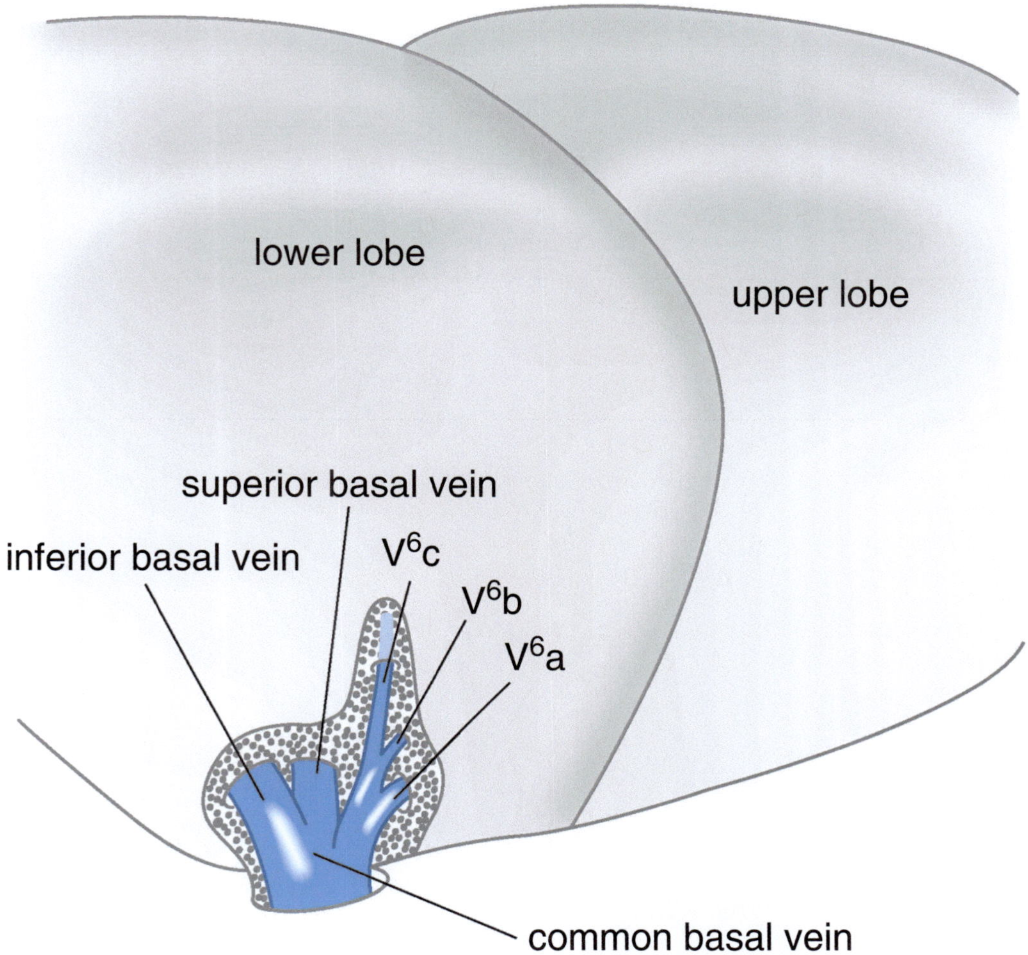

Fig. 6.4.2 The inferior pulmonary ligament is divided to expose the inferior pulmonary vein. The inferior pulmonary vein is exposed for S^{10}-segmentectomy, whereas which is not necessary during either S^8- or S^9-segmentectomy, because S^{10} usually faces the inferior pulmonary vein. Cutting the inferior pulmonary ligament exposes the root of V^6 and common basal pulmonary vein. V^6b+c is exposed peripherally to serve as a landmark for later cutting between S^6 and S^{10}.

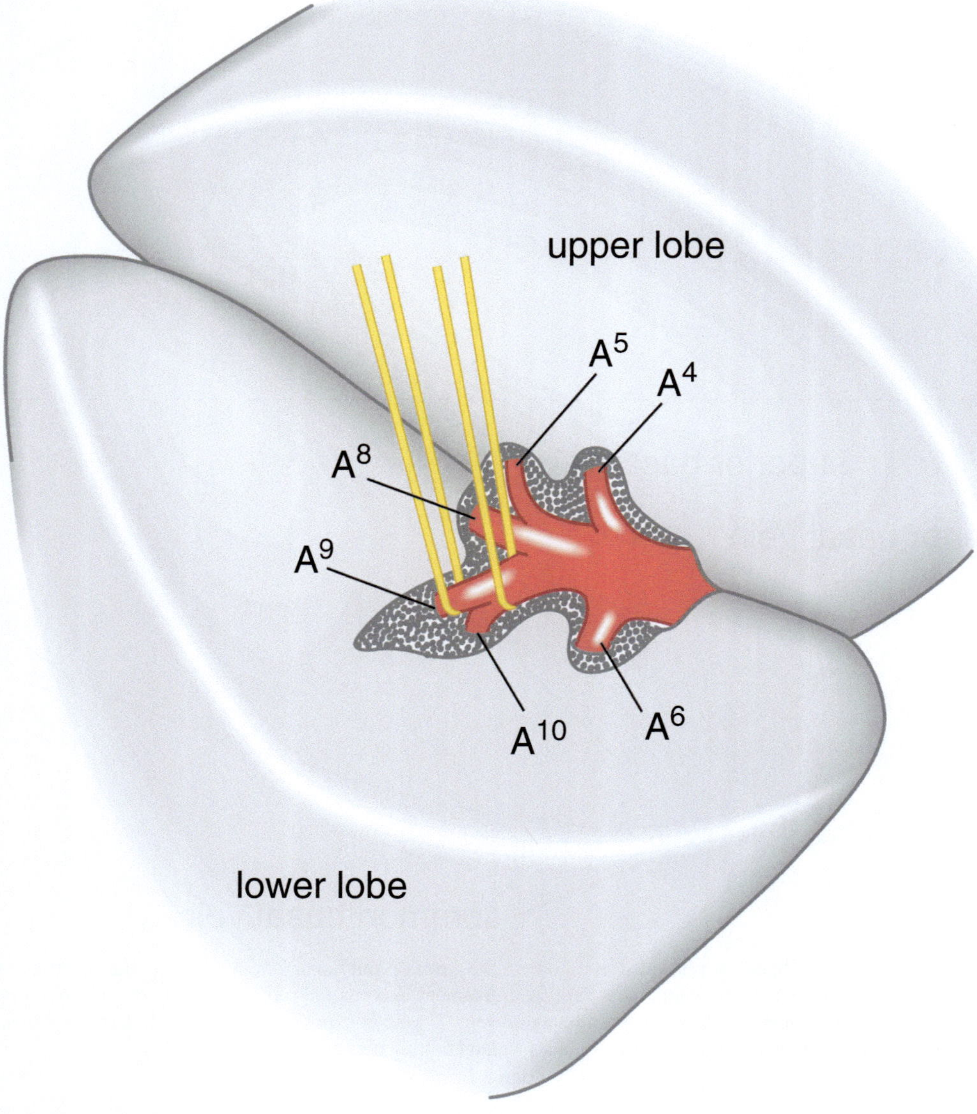

Fig. 6.4.3 The operator stands on the dorsal side of the patient, because A^{10} is easily visualized from this position. The A^6, A^8, and A^{9+10} branches are exposed. A^{9+10} is sometimes composed of A^9a, A^9b and A^{10} branches. When bronchoscopy reveals a long common truncus of B^{9+10}, that of A^{9+10} is also long. When cutting lung tissue covering the A^{9+10}, the border between S^6 and S^8 should be cut, whereas there is no landmark for the border, which is one of the reasons for the difficulty of S^{10}-segmentectomy.

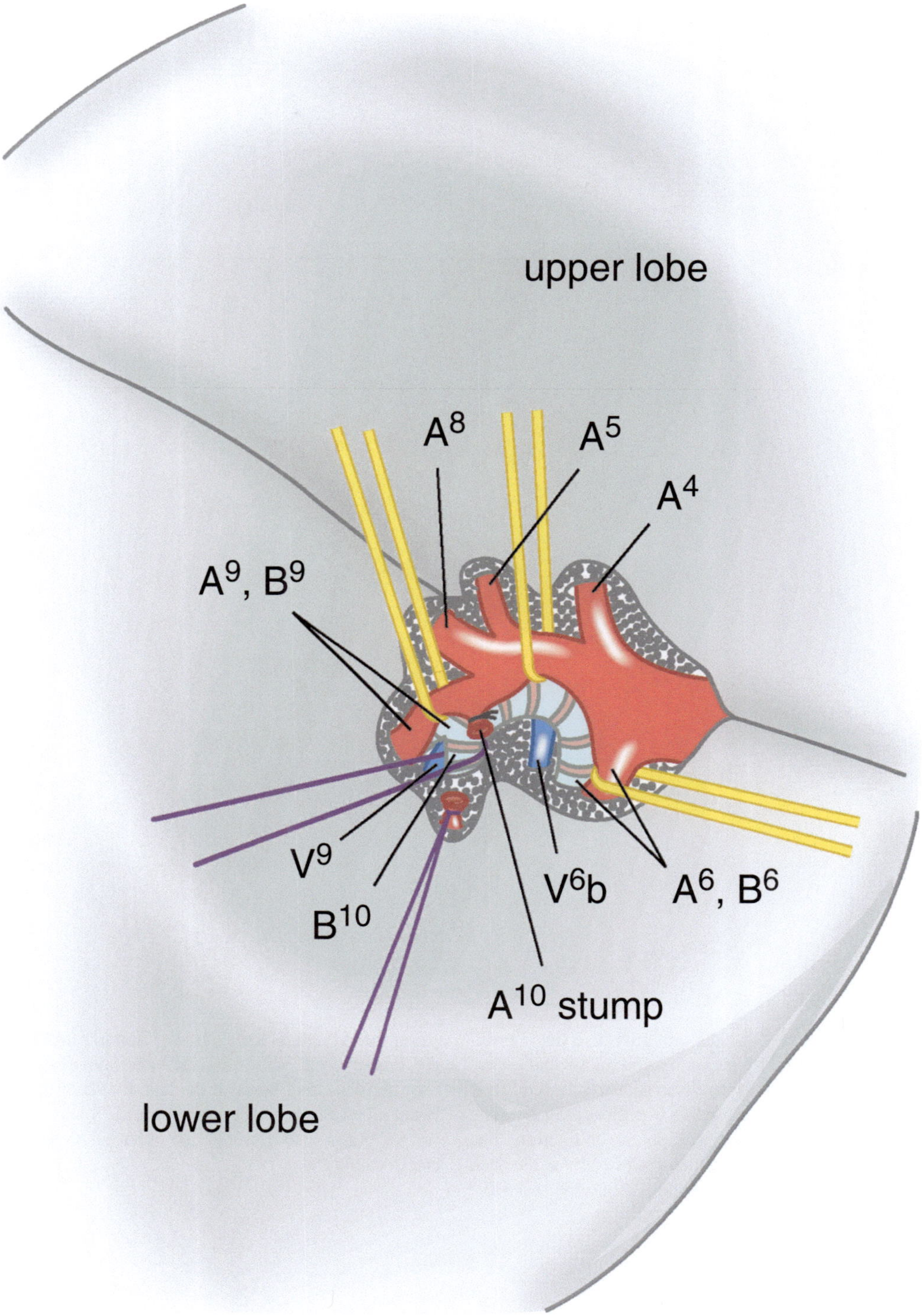

Fig. 6.4.4 A^9 and A^{10} run towards the lateral and dorsal directions, respectively. When A^{10} is difficult to be differentiated from A^9, the most dorsal branch is cut first, because it must be A^{10} or its branch, but not A^9-branch. Cutting the most dorsal arterial branch reveals B^{10} behind, which is cut. After cutting B^{10}, the remaining arterial branches can be easily identified, i.e. the branches run away from the distal stump of B^{10} are A^9-branch, whereas those run toward it are A^{10}-branch. The B^{10} is carefully encircled with thread to avoid damaging V^9 and V^{10} which runs behind the B^{10}. The identification of B^{10} can be also confirmed by illumination from a bronchoscope inserted into B^9 and B^{10}.

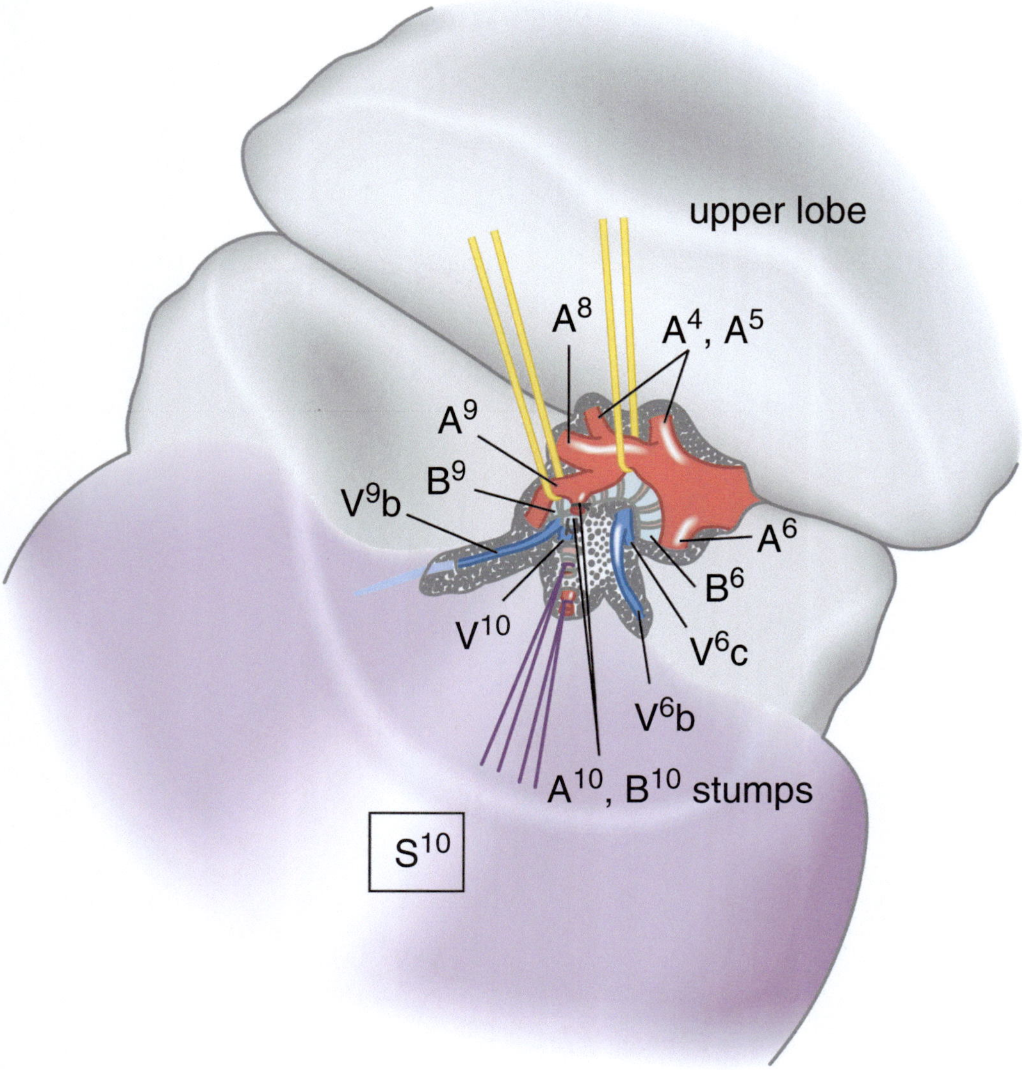

Fig. 6.4.5 S^{10} is selectively inflated either by inserting a bronchoscope into B^{10} followed by jet ventilation, or by cutting the B^{10} and inserting a catheter into the distal stump followed by air inflation. The distal stump is closed to trap air within S^{10}. The proximal stump of B^{10} is closed with suture or ligation. The distal stump of B^{10} is lifted and denuded peripherally at the back to move the stump away from the hilum. Lifting the distal B^{10} stump reveals the branches of V^{10} running into the S^{10}. Cutting the branches of V^{10} further elevates the distal stump of B^{10} together with lung tissue at the lateral side of the stump, which is cut along the $V^{6}c$ (between S^{6} and S^{10}) and $V^{9}b$ (between S^{9} and S^{10}) and also towards the inflation–deflation line using electrocautery.

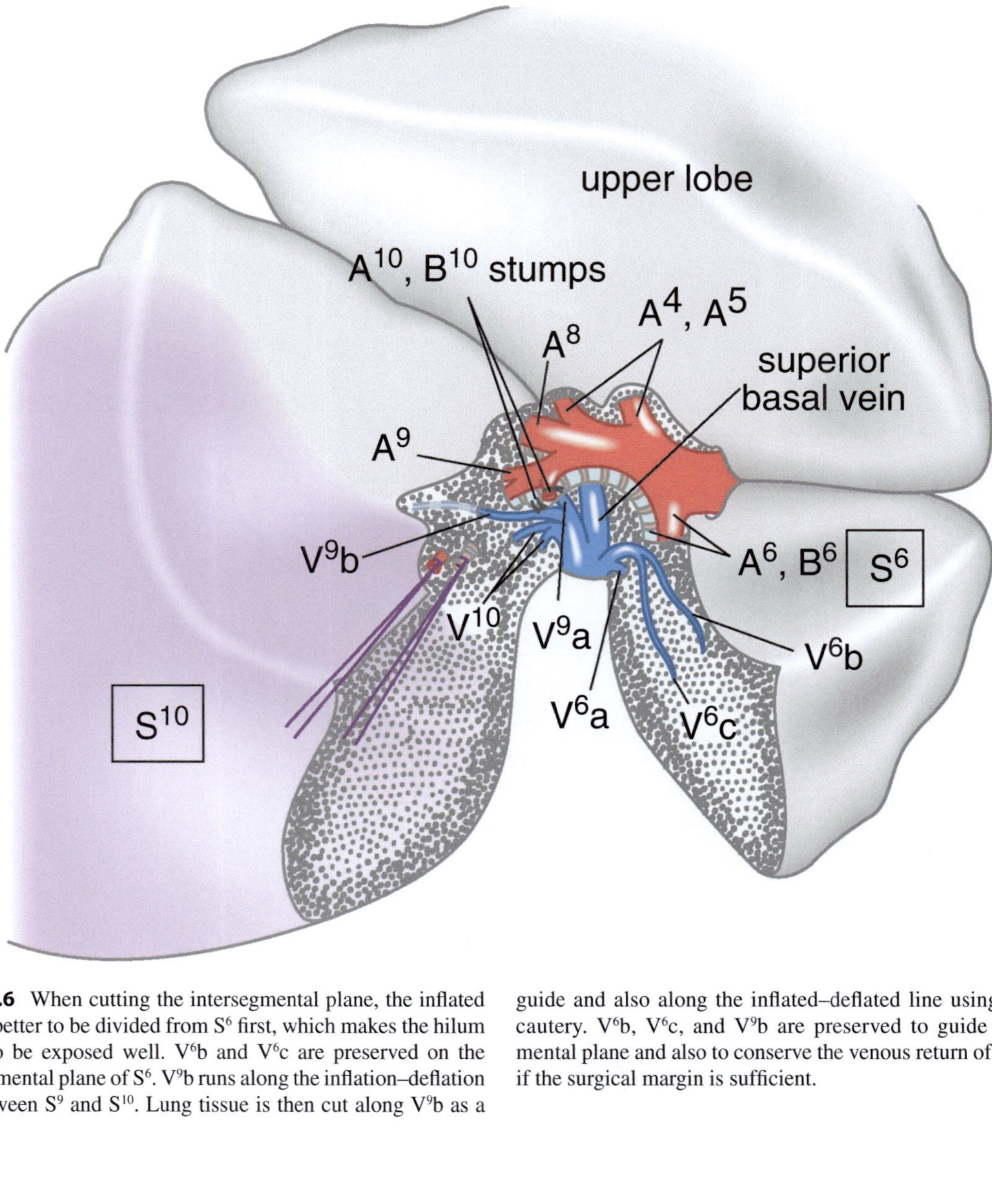

Fig. 6.4.6 When cutting the intersegmental plane, the inflated S^{10} had better to be divided from S^6 first, which makes the hilum of S^{10} to be exposed well. V^6b and V^6c are preserved on the intersegmental plane of S^6. V^9b runs along the inflation–deflation line between S^9 and S^{10}. Lung tissue is then cut along V^9b as a guide and also along the inflated–deflated line using electrocautery. V^6b, V^6c, and V^9b are preserved to guide intersegmental plane and also to conserve the venous return of S^6 and S^9 if the surgical margin is sufficient.

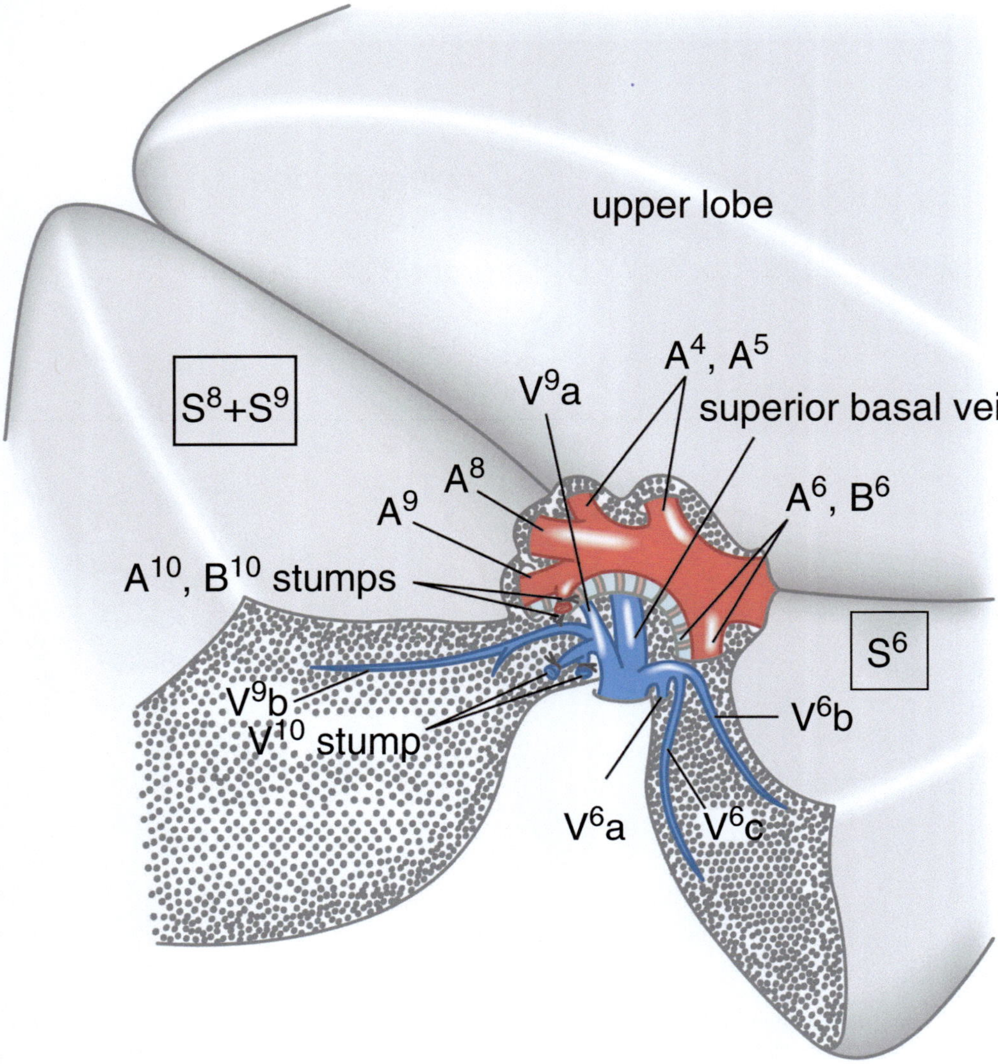

Fig. 6.4.7 After S^{10}-segmentectomy, S^6 and S^8+S^9 are completely separated. V^6b and V^6c are preserved on S^6, and V^9b is preserved on S^9.

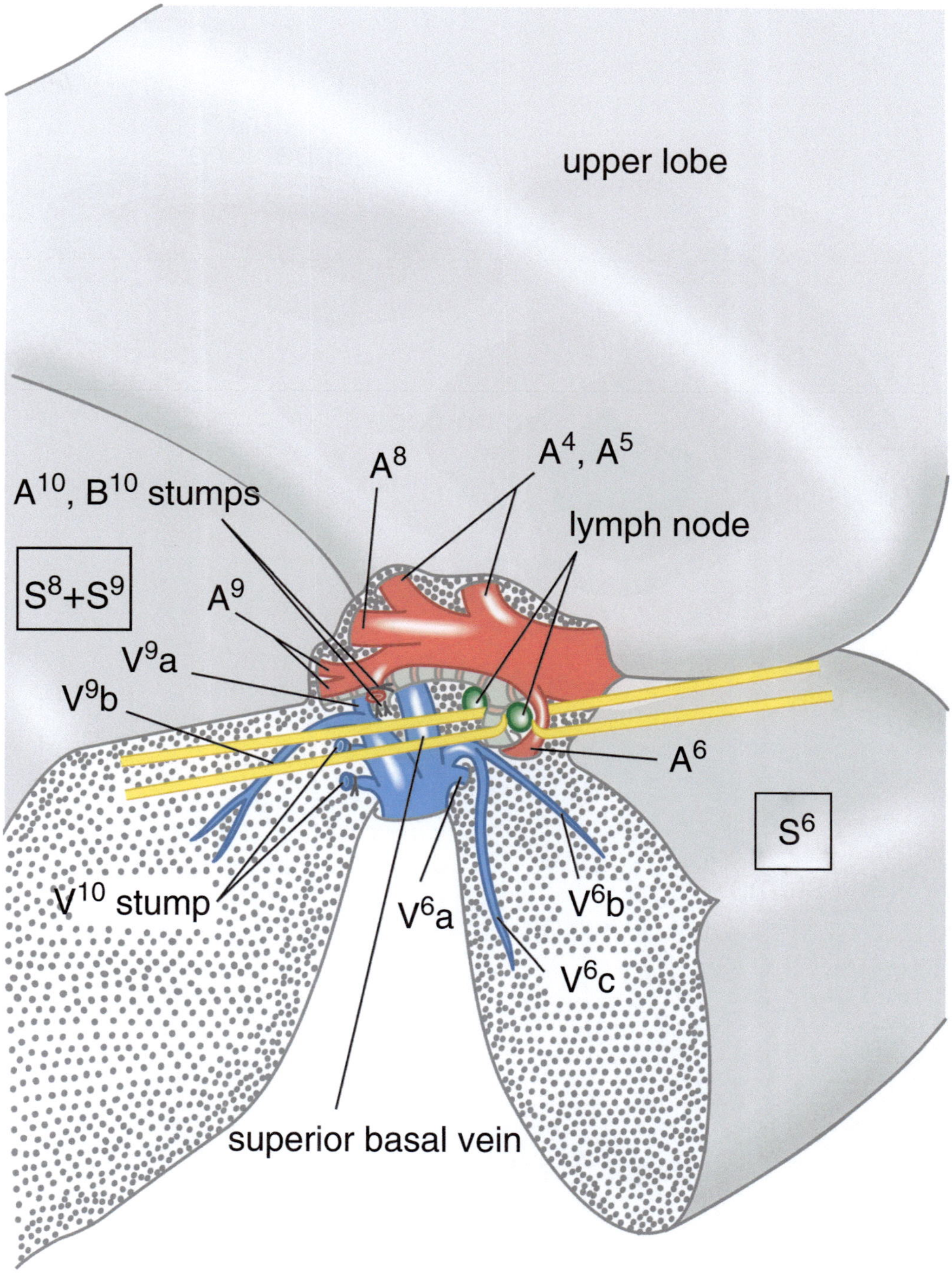

Fig. 6.4.8 B^6, A^6 and A^{8-10} are encircled with tape for dissection of the #12l and #13 (around B^6) nodes, which lie along the lymphatic chain from S^{10} towards the #7 node.

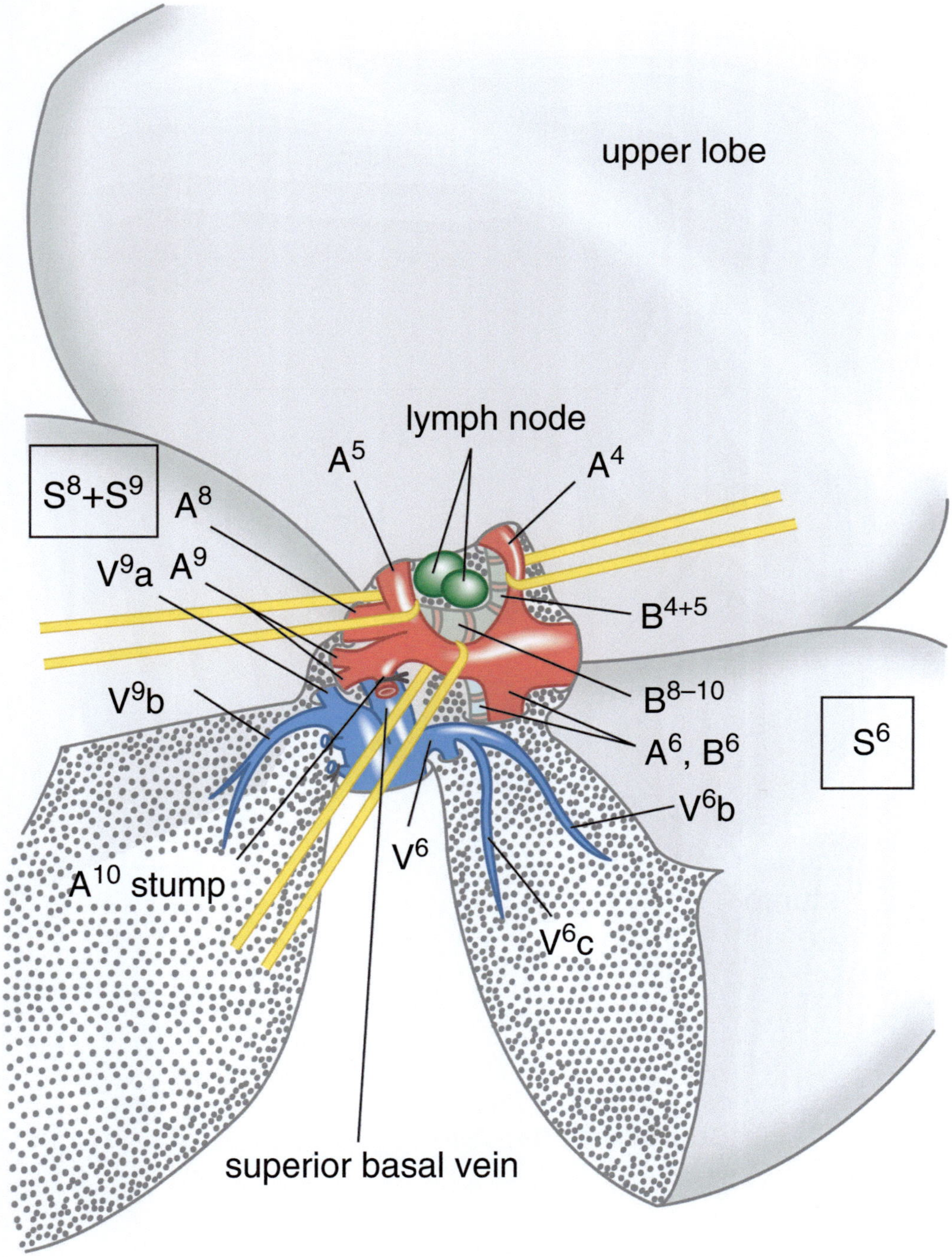

Fig. 6.4.9 The #11 lymph nodes between B^{4+5} and the lower lobar bronchus are dissected with taping $A^{4+5}$and $A^{8\text{-}10}$.

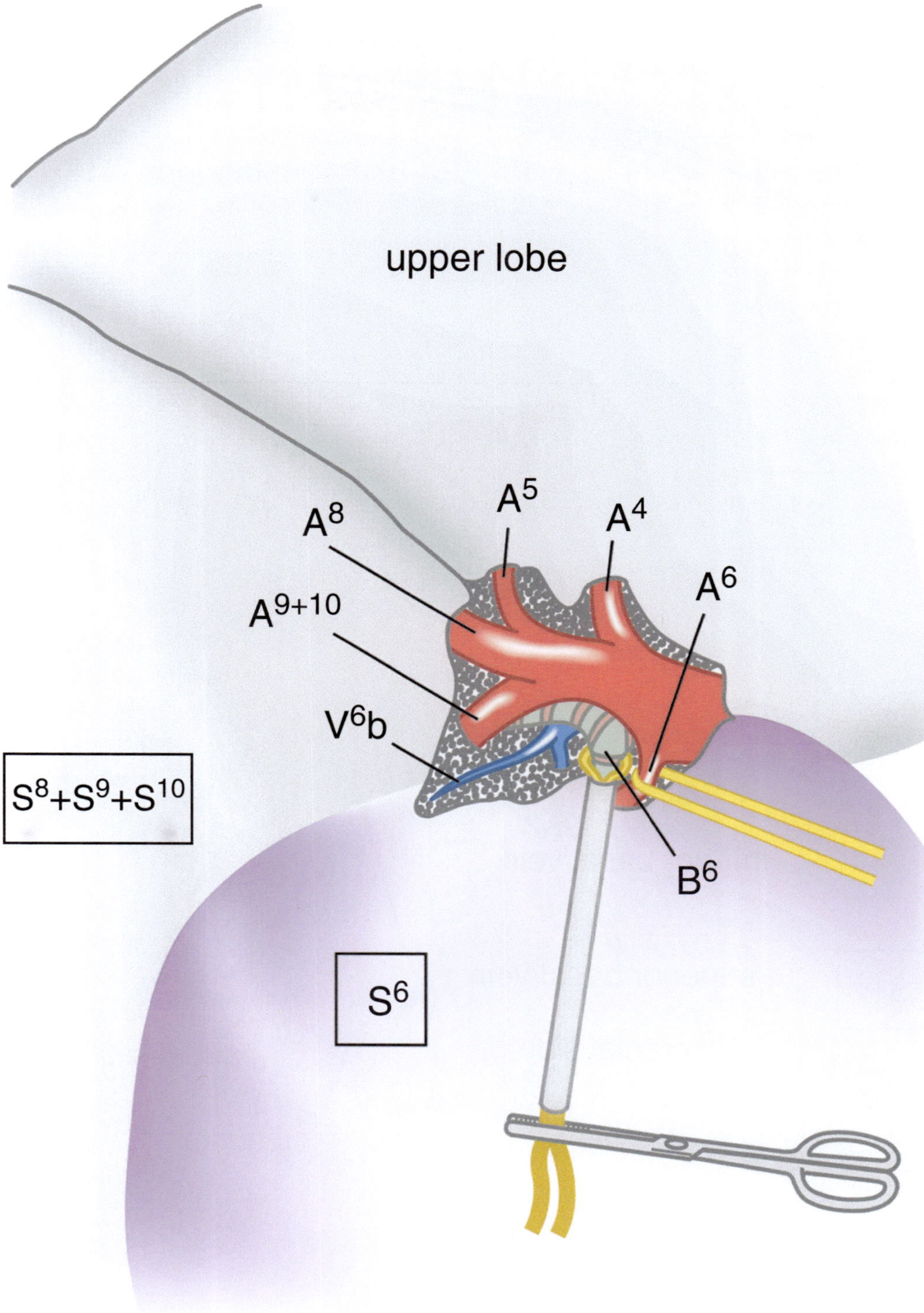

Fig. 6.4.10 Figures 6.4.10 and 6.4.11 show another approach to S^{10}-segmentectomy. The difficulties in the S^{10}-segmentectomy are exposing and identifying A^{10}. Because A^{10} runs dorsally and S^{10} does not face the interlobar fissure, the procedure described above with the approach only from the fissure can sometimes be rather complicated. The approach showing here is to divide S^{6} and S^{10} at first before exposing A^{10}. The concept is based on the followings: Because S^{6} and S^{10} are finally separated in S^{10}-segmentectomy, dividing them first is reasonable and also facilitates exposing A^{10}. To do that, A^{6} and B^{6} are exposed first, followed by taping B^{6} with using a tourniquet. B^{6} is clamped after jet ventilation of B^{6} to create an inflation–deflation line between the inflated S^{6} and deflated S^{8}+S^{9}+S^{10}.

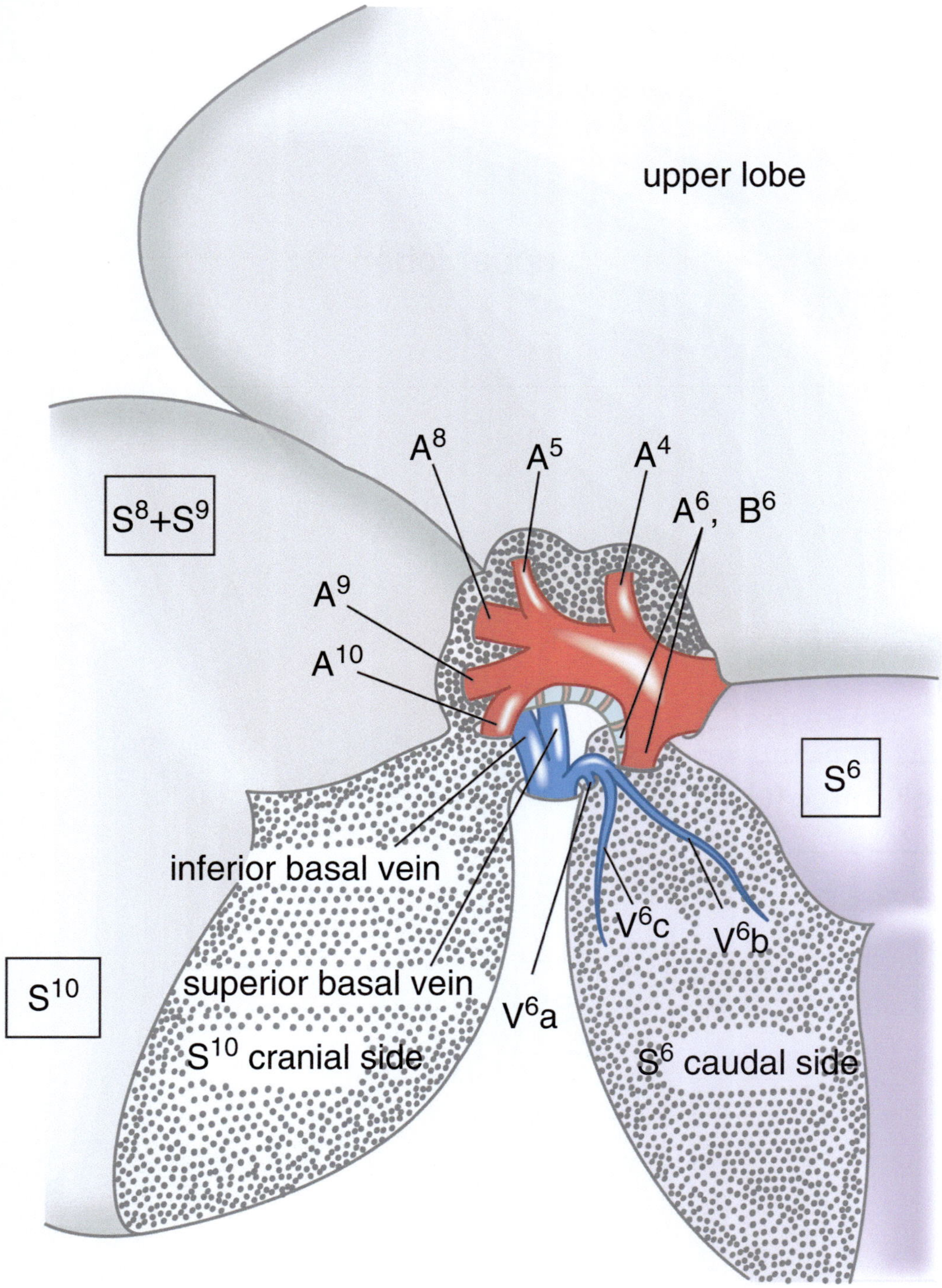

Fig. 6.4.11 The lung is cut along the inflation–deflation line between inflated S^6 and deflated $S^{8\text{-}10}$, which allows a clear view of A^9 and A^{10} from the dorsal direction and subsequent easy exposure and identification of these branches. The border between S^6 and S^8 can also be cut accurately along the inflation–deflation line between them using this technique.

6.5 Left S^9+S^{10} Segmentectomy

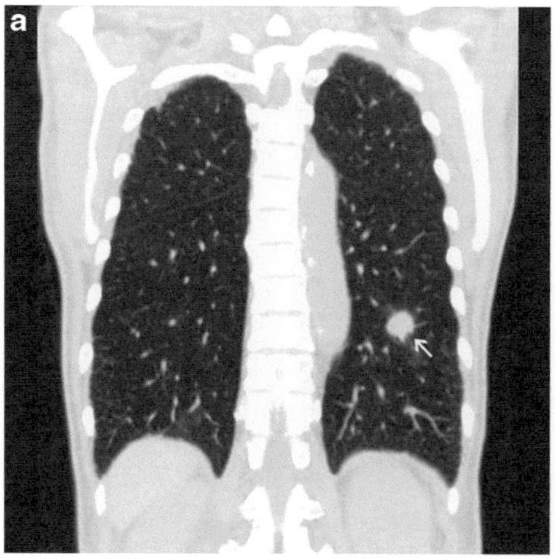

coronal view (CT scan)

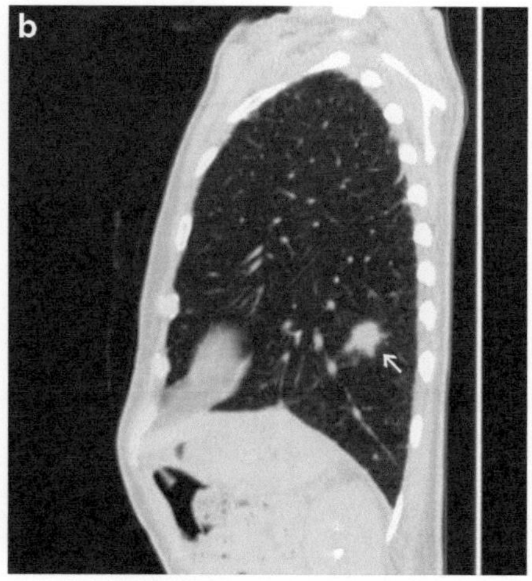

sagittal view (CT scan)

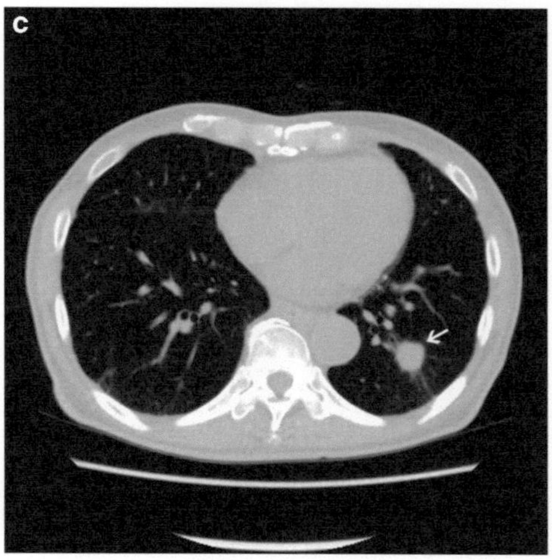

axial view (CT scan)

A CT scan of a 75-year-old male uncovered a solid 2.4-cm nodule located between S^9 and S^{10} that was diagnosed as adenocarcinoma from a bronchoscopic biopsy. Because of poor pulmonary function, S^{9+10}-segmentectomy was undertaken. The final pathological diagnosis was pT1bN0M0 papillary adenocarcinoma.

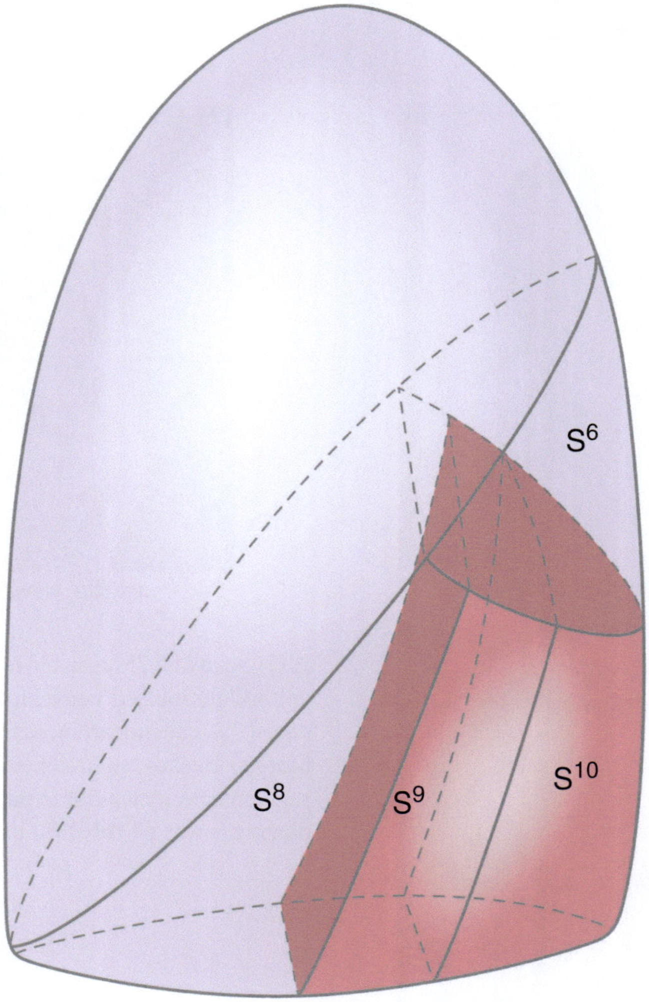

Fig. 6.5.1 The segmental arteries (A^{8-10}) and bronchi (B^{8-10}) are identified from axial, coronal, and sagittal views on HRCT. The branching and sizes of B^8, B^9, and B^{10} are further examined by bronchoscope after tracheal intubation. Figures in this session show the most frequent type of anatomical branching, i.e. two branches with B^8 and B^{9+10}. Lateral thoracotomy at the fifth intercostal space is generally appropriate for S^{9+10}-segmentectomy.

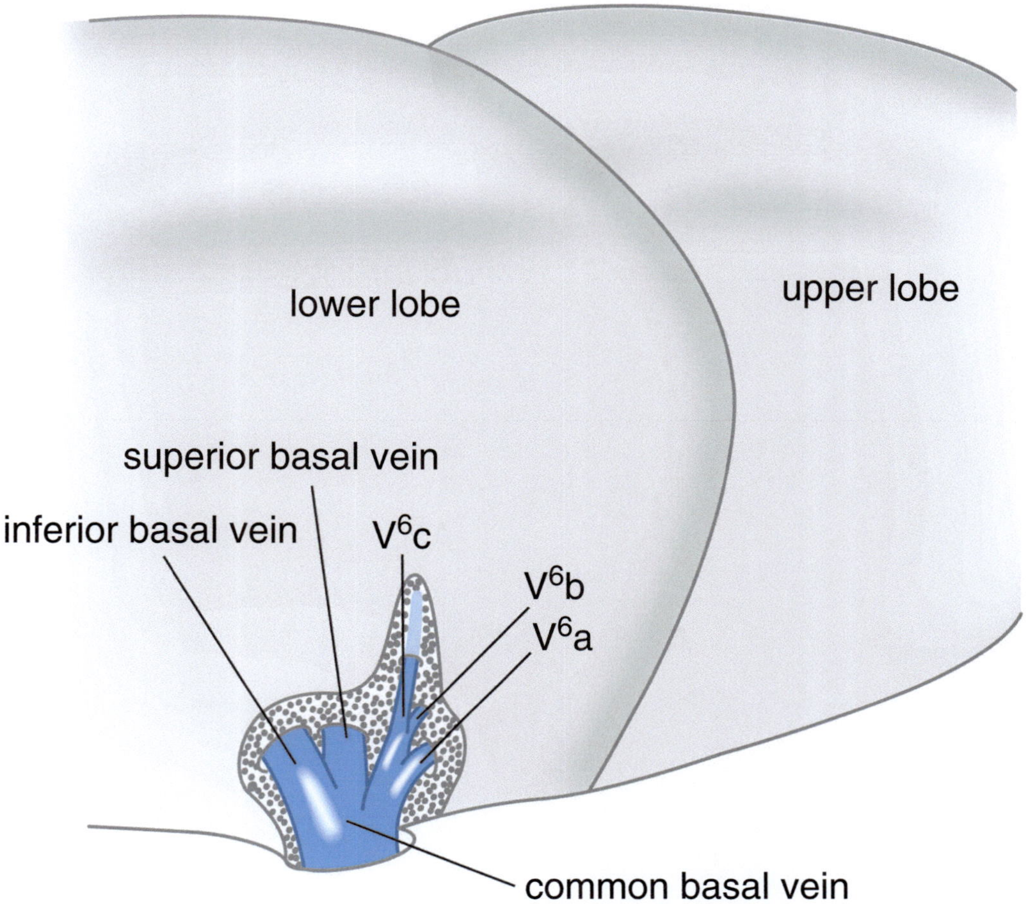

Fig. 6.5.2 The inferior pulmonary ligament is divided to expose V^6 and the common basal pulmonary vein. The inferior basal pulmonary vein should not be cut at this point, because V^{9+10} is usually not the inferior basal pulmonary vein. The frequency with which V^{9+10} is identical to the inferior basal pulmonary vein is only 24%.

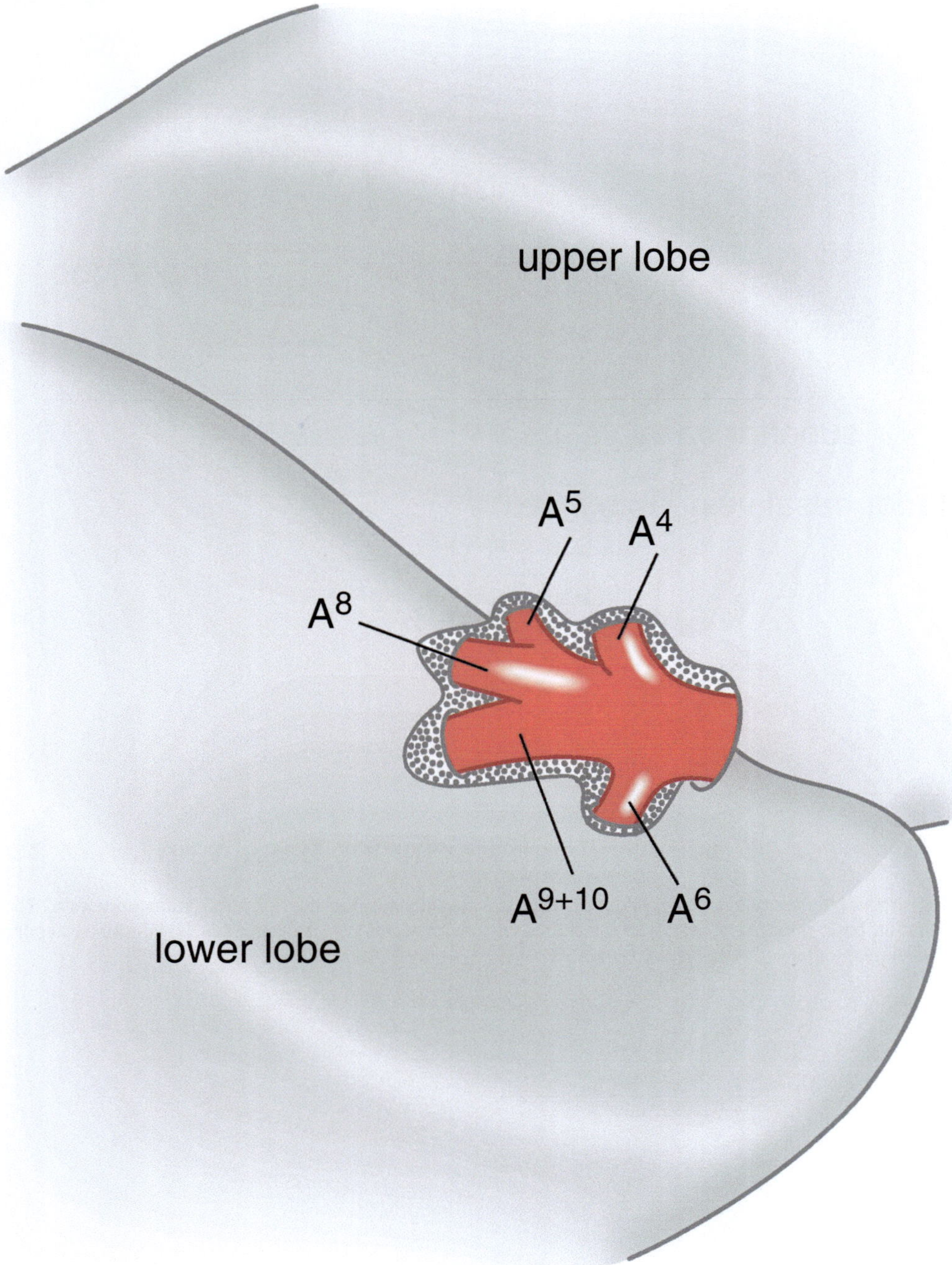

Fig. 6.5.3 The operator stands at the dorsal side of the patient. The branches of A^6, A^8 and A^{9+10} are exposed, which is important for S^8-, S^9, and S^{10}-segmentectomy to prevent misidentifying the pulmonary artery branches and also to facilitate hilar lymph node dissection later. The branching of A^8a and A^9a is sometimes complicated, such as A^8a branches from A^{9+10} and A^9a from A^8.

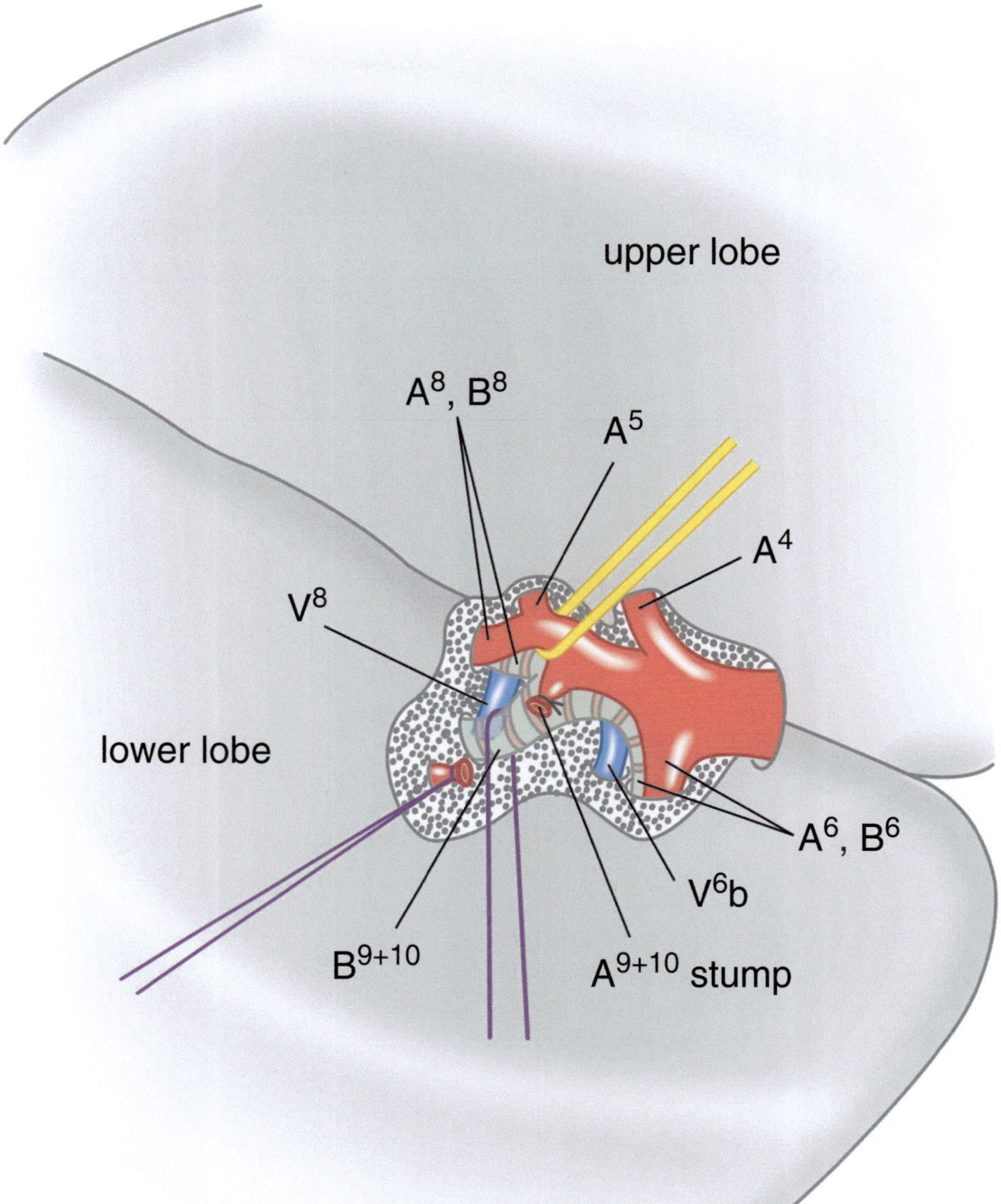

Fig. 6.5.4 Cutting A^{9+10} reveals B^{9+10} running at the back. B^{9+10} is carefully encircled with thread to avoid damage to V^{8-10} running behind it. The identification of B^{9+10} can be also confirmed by illumination from a bronchoscope inserted into B^8, B^9 and B^{10}.

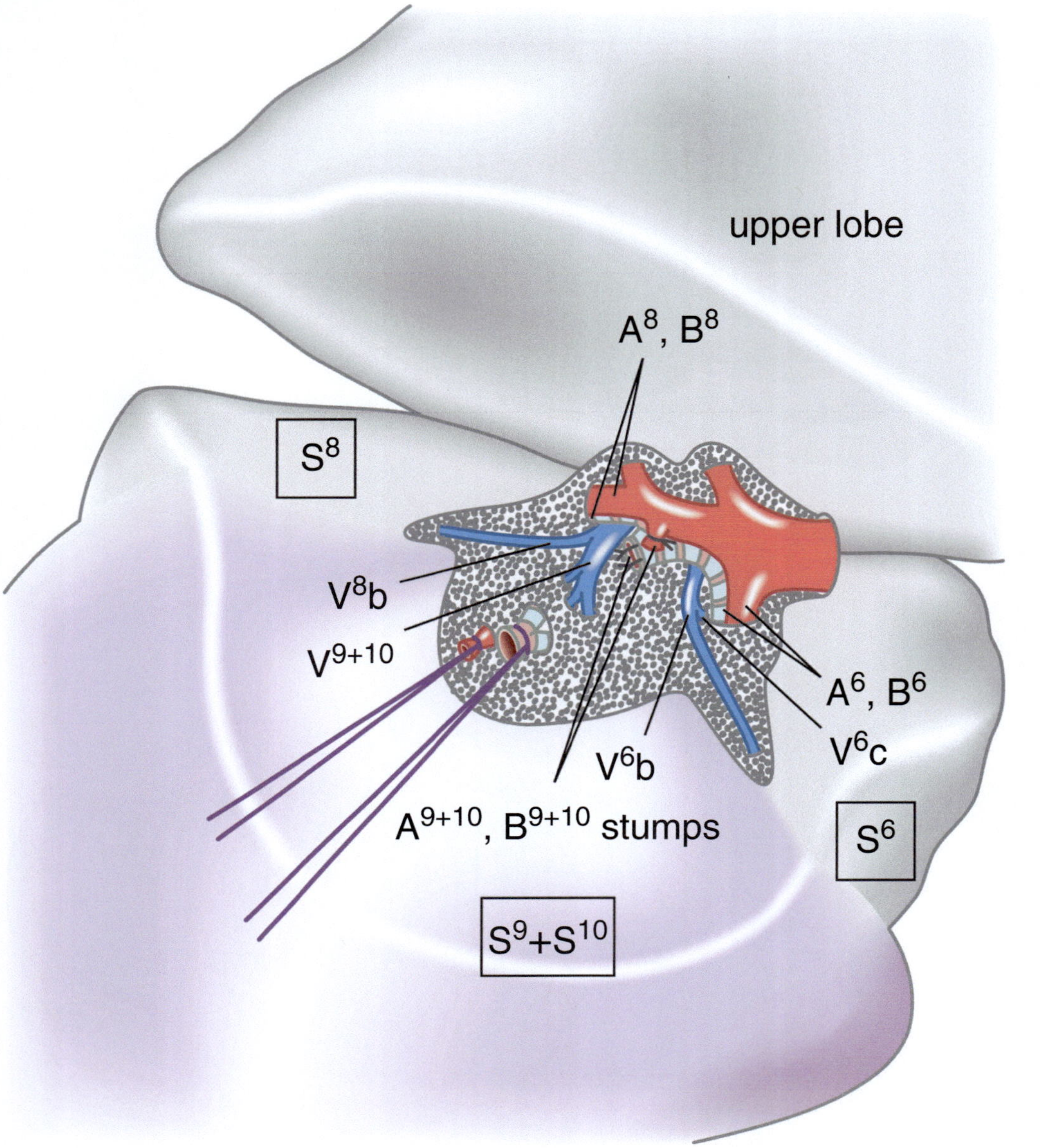

Fig. 6.5.5 S^9+S^{10} is selectively inflated by either inserting a bronchoscope into B^{9+10} followed by jet ventilation, or by cutting the B^{9+10} and inserting a catheter into the distal stump followed by air inflation. The distal stump is closed to trap air within S^9+S^{10}. The proximal stump of B^{9+10} is closed with suture or ligation. When S^9+S^{10} is inflated with jet ventilation via bronchoscope, B^{9+10} can be cut using a stapler. The distal stump of B^{9+10} is lifted and is denuded peripherally at its back to move it away from the hilum. Lifting the distal B^{9+10} stump exposes V^9 and V^{10} branches running into the S^9+S^{10}. Cutting these vein branches further elevates the distal stump of B^{9+10} together with lung tissues on the lateral side of the stump. The lung tissue of both sides of the stump is cut along the V^6c (between S^6 and S^{10}) and V^8b (between S^8 and S^9) and also towards the inflation–deflation line using electrocautery.

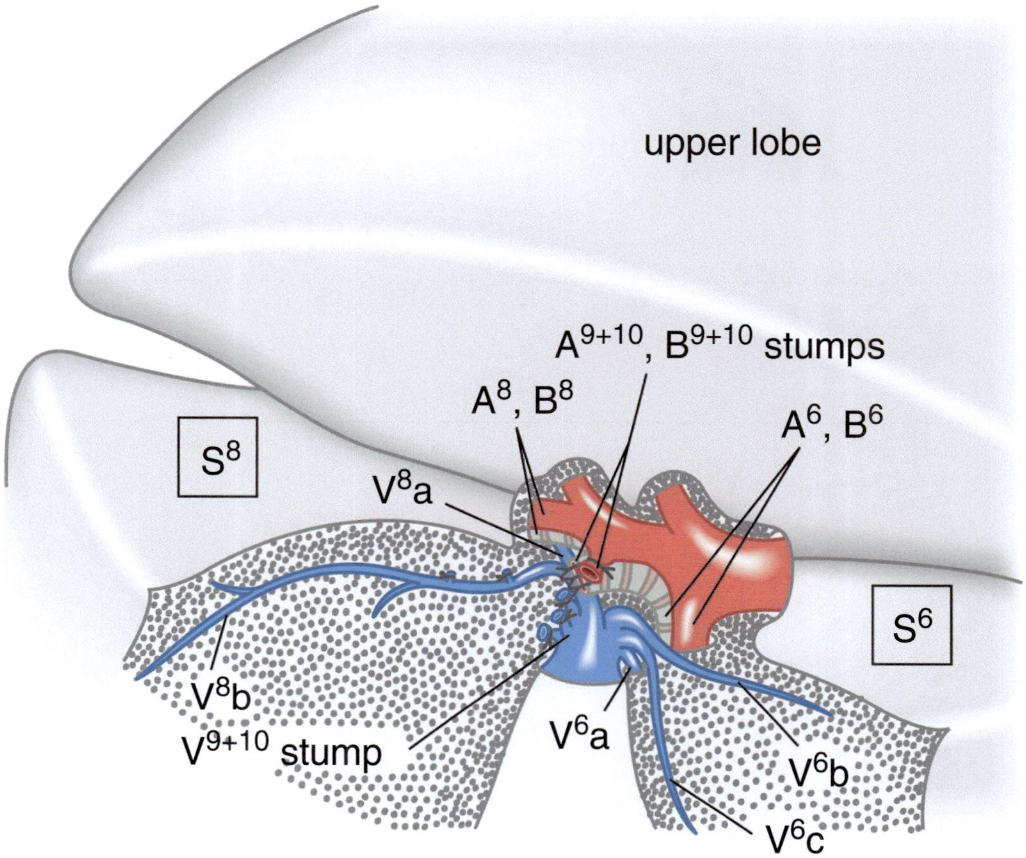

Fig. 6.5.6 After S^{9+10} resection, S^6 and S^8 are completely separated. V^6b and V^6c are preserved on S^6 and V^8b is preserved on S^8.

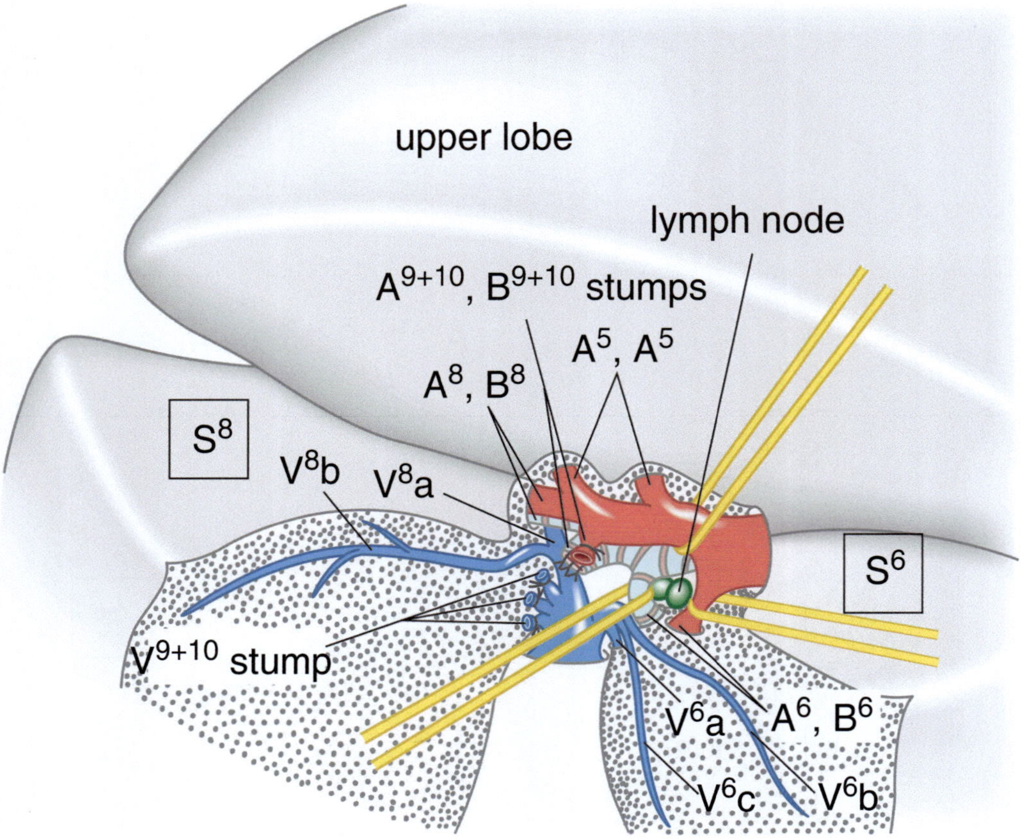

Fig. 6.5.7 B^6, A^6 and A^{8-10} are encircled with tape for hilar lymph node dissection and then the #12l and #13 (around B^6) nodes are dissected, which lie along the lymphatic chain from S^{9+10} towards the #7 node. A^4 and A^5 are encircled with tape and then the #11 lymph nodes are dissected.

7 Sleeve Segmentectomy

7.1 Left $S^{1+2}+S^3$ (Upper Division) Sleeve Segmentectomy

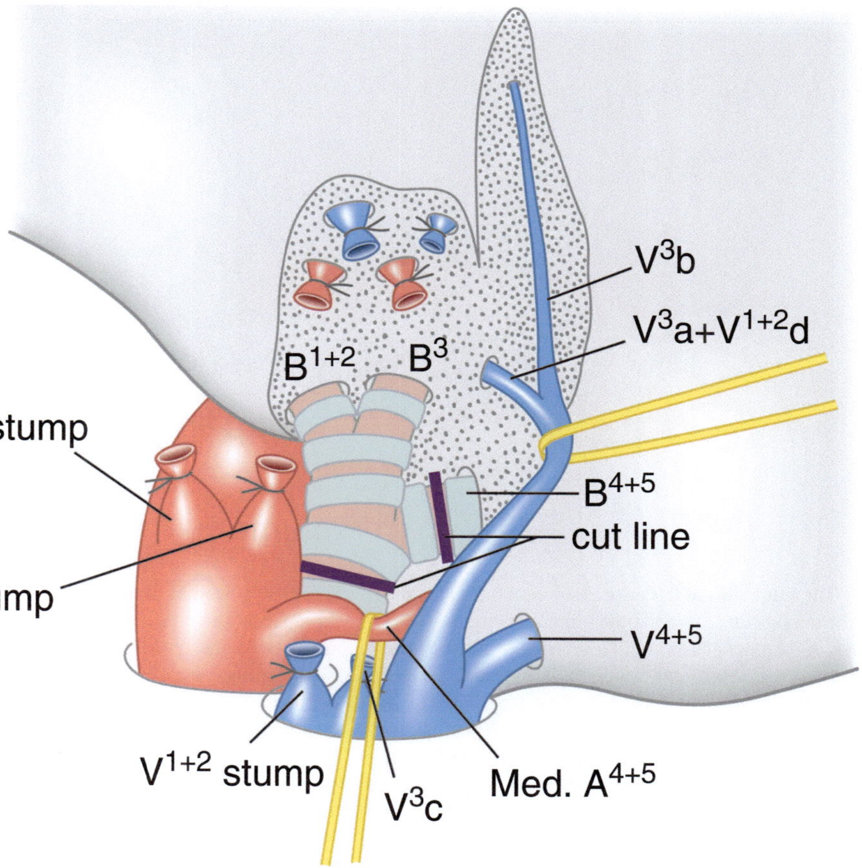

Fig. 7.1.1 The pulmonary arteries, pulmonary veins and bronchi are exposed as described for left upper division segmentectomy. The hilum of the left upper lobe is exposed from the ventral to the dorsal side, exposing the pulmonary vein, pulmonary artery, and bronchi. V^3b is identified, encircled with tape and exposed peripherally, which is the border of S^3b and S^4b. V^3a and V^{1+2}d, which usually form a common trunk branching from the back of V^3, is also identified and exposed. A mediastinal A^{4+5} (or A^5) should be preserved. All pulmonary veins from the upper division are exposed and then V^{1+2}, V^3c, V^{1+2}d and V^3a are cut, while the V^3b (between S^3b and S^4b) is preserved. The pulmonary artery branches to the upper division (A^3, A^{1+2}a+b, and A^{1+2}c) are cut. The upper lobar bronchus, B^{1-3} and B^{4+5} are identified and then a bronchoscope is inserted into B^{1-3}. S^{1-3} can be selectively inflated by jet-ventilation. When a tumor is located at the orifices of B^{1-3} and interrupts insertion of the bronchoscope into B^{1-3}, S^{4+5} can be inflated to detect the inflation–deflation line between S^{1-3} and S^{4+5} by inserting the bronchoscope into B^{4+5} followed by jet ventilation. B^{4+5} and the upper lobar bronchus are then cut to create sufficient surgical margins (sleeve resection). The rapid intraoperative pathologic examination of frozen sections can confirm that the cutting line is not involved with the tumor. The intersegmental plane between the $S^{1+2}+S^3$ and S^4+S^5 can usually be cut using electrocautery for complete removal of the upper division. The upper lobe bronchus and lingular bronchus is anastomosed using an absorbable suture.

H. Nomori and M. Okada, *Illustrated Anatomical Segmentectomy for Lung Cancer*,
DOI 10.1007/978-4-431-54144-8_7, © Springer Japan 2012

7.2 Left $S^4 + S^5$ (Lingular Division) Sleeve Segmentectomy

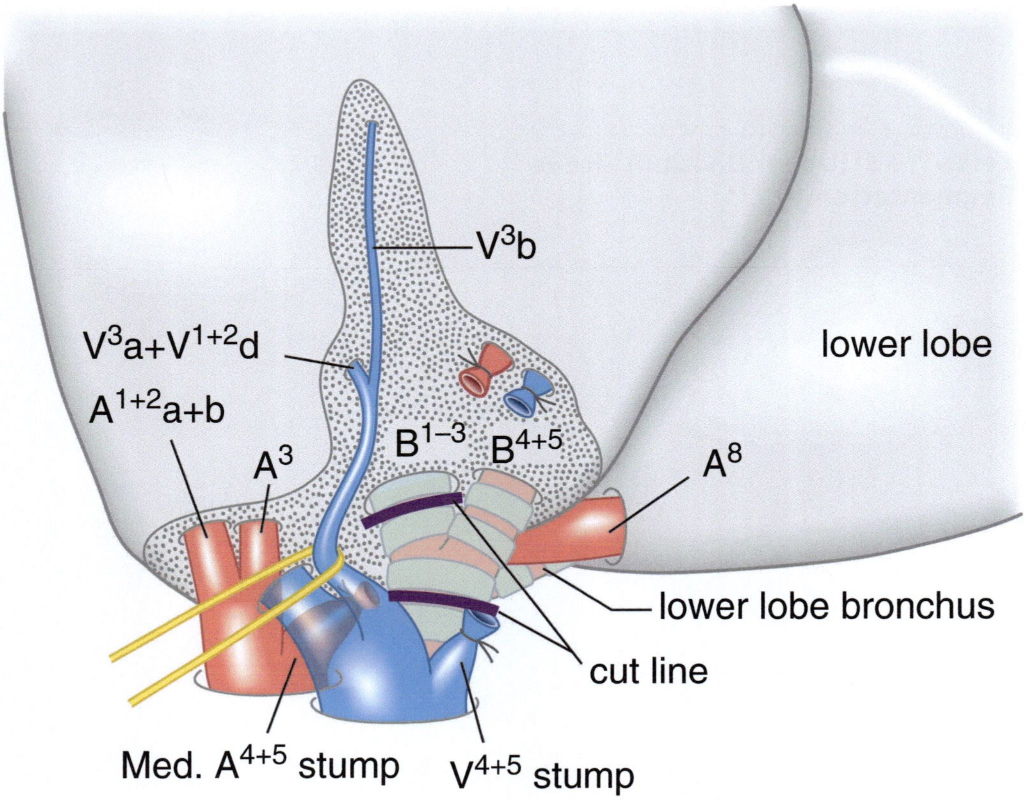

Fig. 7.2.1 The hilum of the left upper lobe is exposed from the ventral to the dorsal side, exposing the pulmonary veins, pulmonary arteries, and bronchi as in lingular division segmentectomy. V^3b is identified and taped and peripherally exposed, which is the border between S^3b and S^4b. A mediastinal A^{4+5} (or A^5) should be confirmed and cut if present. The branches of the pulmonary artery to the lingula (A^4 and A^5) are cut. All pulmonary veins from the lingula are exposed and V^4 and V^5 are cut, but V^3b (between S^3b and S^4b) is preserved. The upper lobar bronchus, B^{1-3} and B^{4+5} are identified and a bronchoscope is inserted into B^{4+5}. S^{4+5} can be selectively inflated by jet-ventilation. When a tumor located at the orifices of B^{4+5} interrupts insertion of the bronchoscope into B^{4+5}, S^{1-3} can be inflated to detect the inflation–deflation line between S^{1-3} and S^{4+5} by inserting the bronchoscope into B^{1-3}. B^{1-3} and upper lobar bronchus are cut with surgical margins (sleeve resection). The rapid intraoperative pathologic examination of frozen sections can confirm that the cutting line is not involved with tumor. The intersegmental plane between $S^{1+2}+S^3$ and S^4+S^5 can usually be cut using electrocautery for complete removal of the lingula. The upper division bronchus (B^{1-3}) and upper lobar bronchus are anastomosed using an absorbable suture.

7.3 Right S^6 Sleeve Segmentectomy

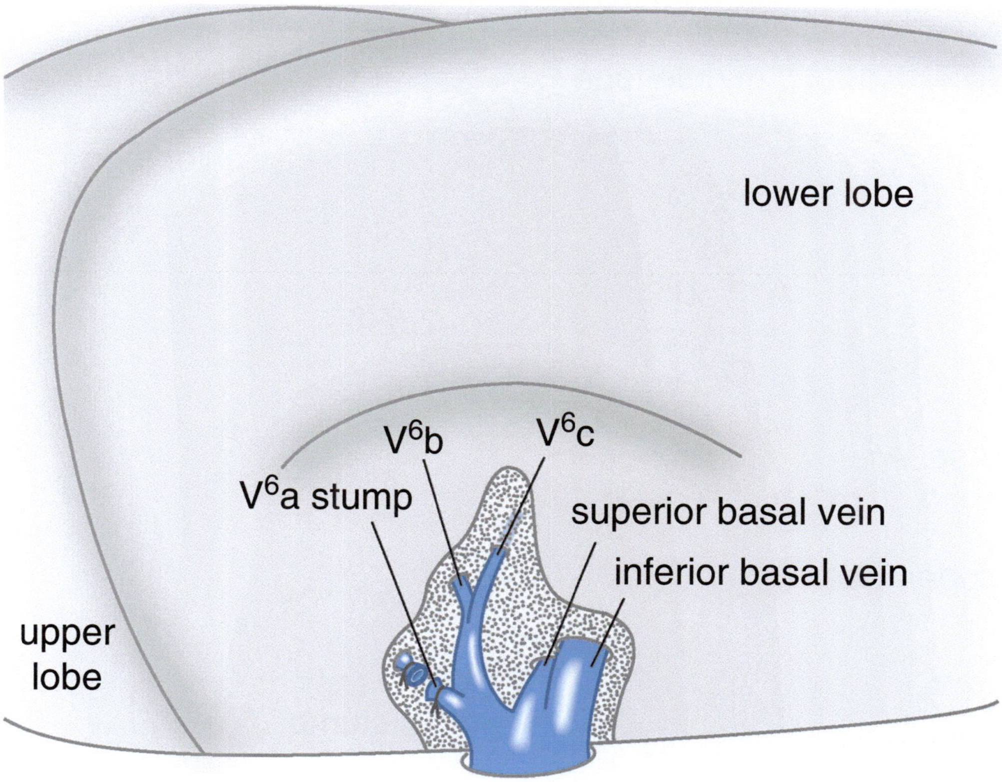

Fig. 7.3.1 The indications for sleeve segmentectomy are the most frequent in S^6. The procedures are similar to S^6-segmentectomy except for treatment of the bronchus. In principle, V^6a is cut, whereas V^6b and V^6c are exposed peripherally and finally preserved.

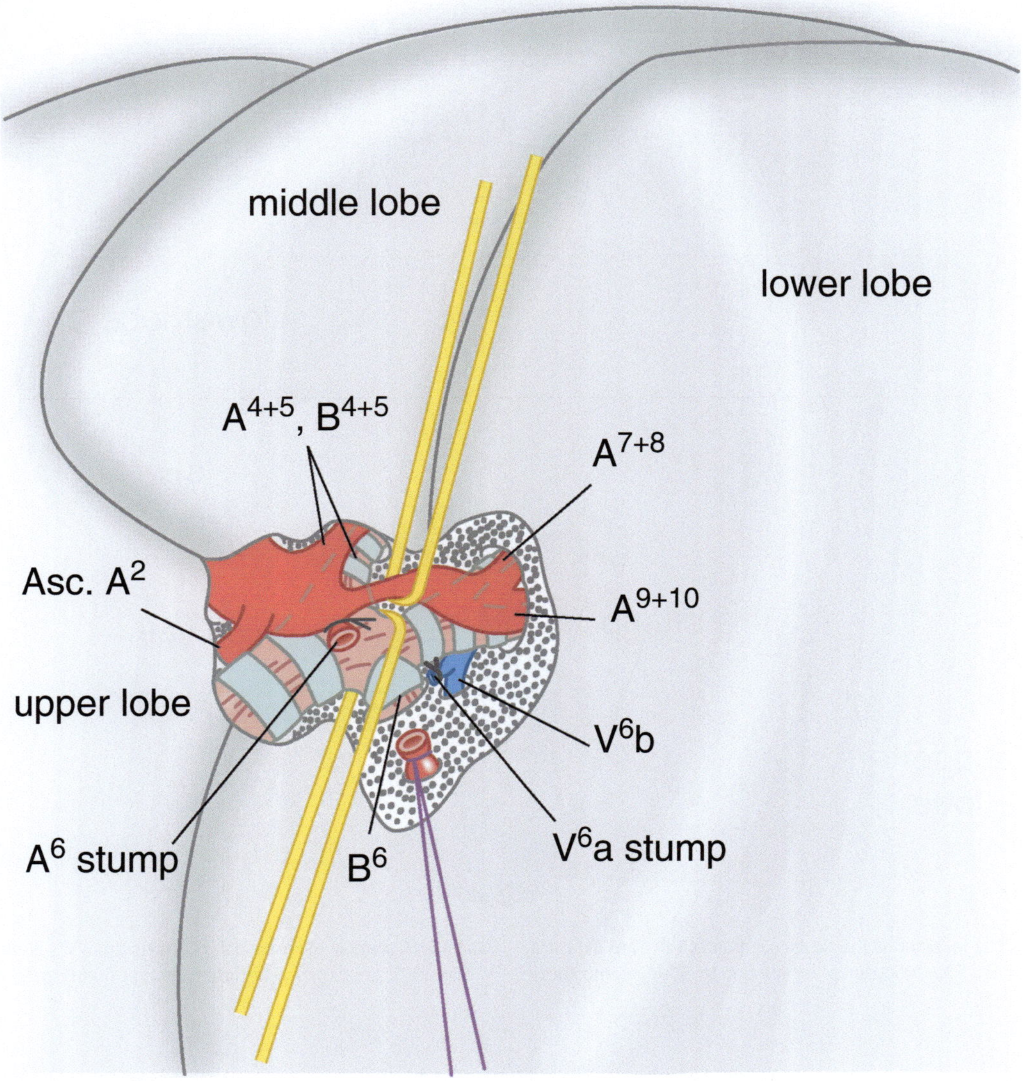

Fig. 7.3.2 The branches of ascending A^2, A^{4+5}, A^6, and A^{7-10} are exposed, A^6 is cut and A^{8-10} is encircled with tape. The tape is then pulled ventrally to expose the truncus intermediate bronchus. The truncus intermedius or the lower lobar bronchus is encircled with tape. V^6b can be visualized running behind B^6.

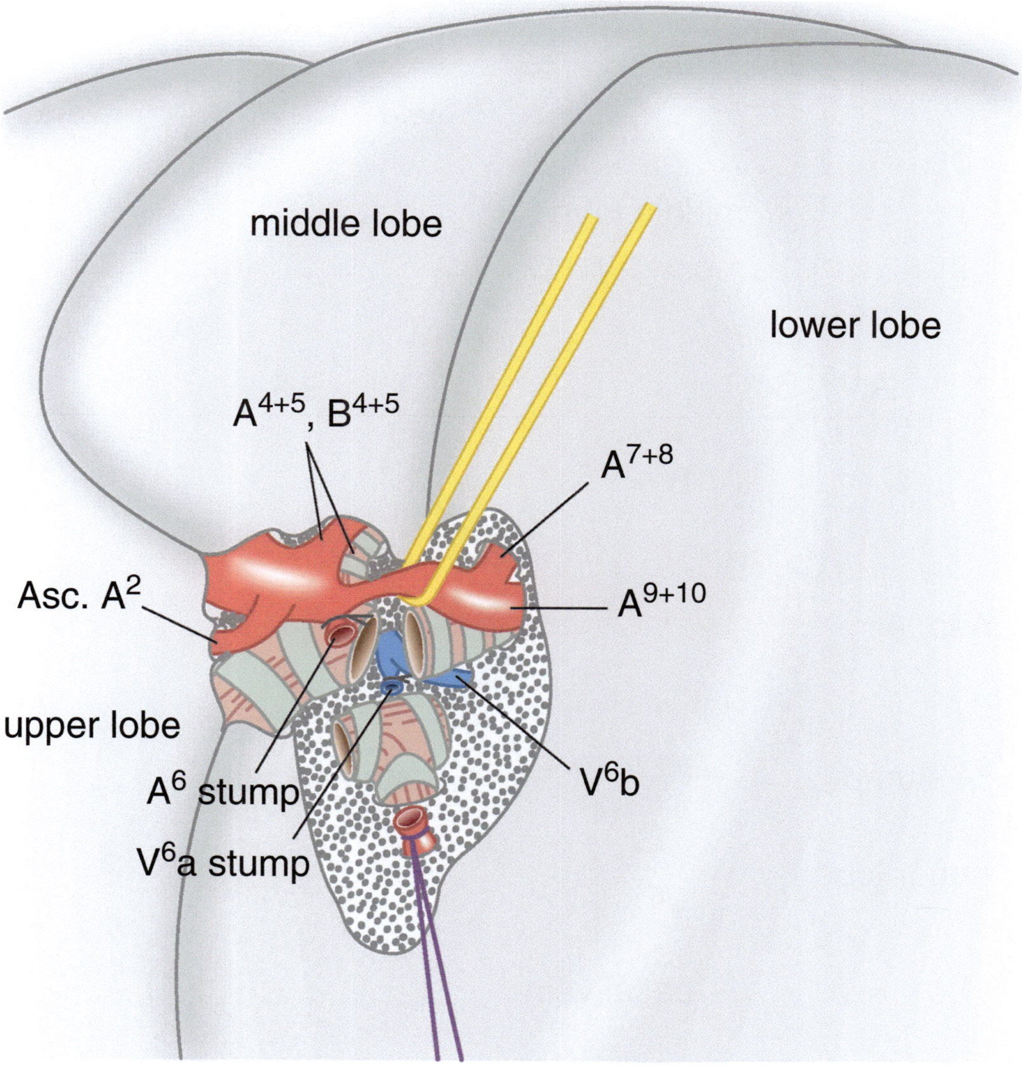

Fig. 7.3.3 Tumors obstructing B^6 are often indicated for this procedure, which makes difficulties with creating an inflation–deflation line with jet ventilation. Therefore, V^6b and V^6c are exposed peripherally to reveal the border of S^6. A^{8-10} is pulled in the ventral direction using tape. The truncus intermediate bronchus, the middle lobar bronchus, B^6 and the basal bronchus are exposed sufficiently, followed by sleeve resection.

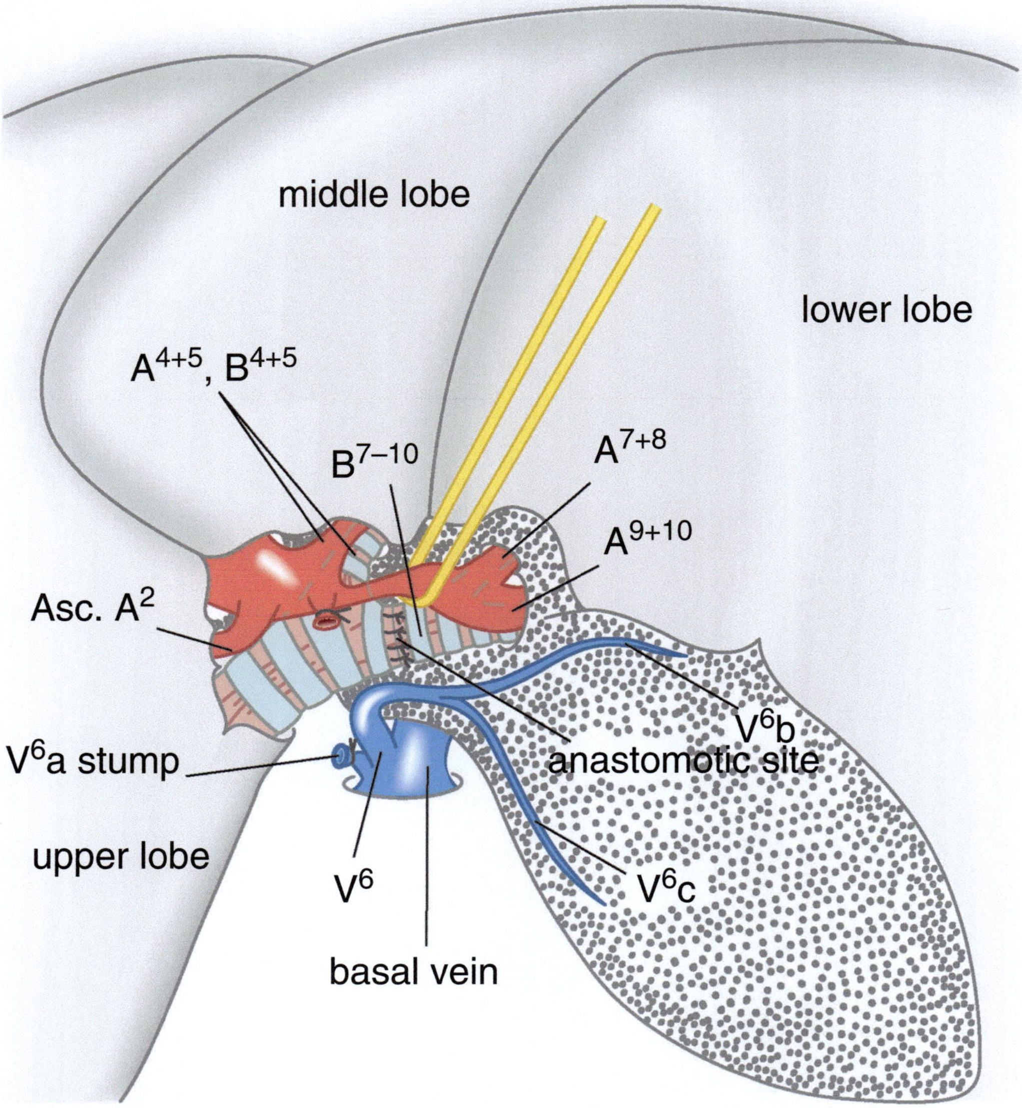

Fig. 7.3.4 Stumps of the bronchus are sutured using absorbable monofilament thread. The segmental bronchus is softer than the lobar bronchus, and thus stenosis at the anastomosis site should be carefully considered. Hilar lymph node dissection is similar to that of S^6-segmentectomy.

Bibliography

Pathophysiology

1. Nomori H, Shimosato Y, Kodama T, et al. Subtypes of small cell carcinoma of the lung. Hum Pathol. 1986;17:604–13.
2. Nomori H, Horinouchi H, Kaseda S, et al. Evaluation of the malignant grade of thymoma by morphometric analysis. Cancer. 1988;61:982–8.
3. Nomori H, Ishihara T, Torikata C. Malignant grading of cortical and medullary differentiated thymoma by morphometric analysis. Cancer. 1989;64:1694–9.
4. Nomori H, Nakajima T, Noguchi M, et al. Cytofluorometric analysis of metastases from lung adenocarcinoma with special reference to the difference between hematogenous and lymphatic metastases. Cancer. 1991;67:2941–7.
5. Nomori H, Hirohashi S, Noguchi M, et al. Tumor cell heterogeneity and subpopulations with metastatic ability in differentiated adenocarcinoma of the lung. Chest. 1991;99:934–40.
6. Nomori H, Horio H, Kobayashi R, et al. Protein 1 serum levels in lung cancer patients receiving chemotherapy. Eur Respir J. 1995;8:1654–7.
7. Nomori H, Horio H, Fuyuno G, et al. Protein 1(Clara cell protein) serum levels in healthy subjects and patients with bacterial pneumonia. Am J Respir Crit Care Med. 1995;152:746–50.
8. Nomori H, Horio H, Takagi M, et al. Clara cell protein correlation with hyperlipidemia. Chest. 1996;110:680–4.
9. Okada M, Nishio W, Sakamoto T, et al. Effect of histologic type and smoking status on the interpretation of serum carcinoembryonic antigen value in non-small cell lung carcinoma. Ann Thorac Surg. 2004;78:1004–9.
10. Mimura T, Ito A, Okada M, et al. Novel marker D2–40, combined with calretinin, CEA and TTF-1: an optimal set of immunodiagnostic markers for pleural mesothelioma. Cancer. 2007;109:933–8.
11. Yuki T, Sakuma T, Okada M, et al. Pleomorphic carcinoma of the lung. J Thorac Cardiovasc Surg. 2007;134:399–404.
12. Mori T, Nomori H, Ikeda K, et al. Microscopic-sized microthymoma in patients with myasthenia gravis. Chest. 2007;131:847–9.
13. Mori T, Nomori H, Ikeda K, et al. The distribution of parenchyma, follicles, and lymphocyte subsets in thymus of patients with myasthenia gravis with special reference to the remission after thymectomy. J Thorac Cardiovasc Surg. 2007;133:634–8.
14. Asakura K, Izumi Y, Nomori H, et al. Mediastinal germ cell tumor with somatic-type malignancy: report of 5 stage I/II cases. Ann Thorac Surg. 2010;90:1014–6.
15. Takahashi Y, Ishii G, Nomori H, et al. Fibrous stroma is associated with poorer prognosis in lung squamous cell carcinoma patients. J Thorac Oncol. 2011;6:1460–7.
16. Mimae T, Tsuta K, Okada M, et al. Steroid receptor expression in thymomas and thymic carcinomas. Cancer. 2011;117:4396–405.
17. Tanaka S, Hattori N, Okada M, et al. Krebs von den Lungen-6 (KL-6) is a prognostic biomarker in patients with surgically resected nonsmall cell lung cancer. Int J Cancer. 2012;130:377–87.
18. Mimae T, Okada M, Hagiyama M, et al. Upregulation of notch2 and six1 is associated with progression of early-stage lung adenocarcinoma and a more aggressive phenotype at advanced stages. Clin Cancer Res. 2012;18:945–55.
19. Tanaka S, Hattori N, Okada M, et al. Interferon (alpha, beta and omega) receptor 2 is a prognostic biomarker for lung cancer. Pathobiology. 2012;79:24–33.

H. Nomori and M. Okada, *Illustrated Anatomical Segmentectomy for Lung Cancer*,
DOI 10.1007/978-4-431-54144-8, © Springer Japan 2012

Pulmonary Function

1. Nomori H, Kobayashi R, Fuyuno G, et al. Preoperative respiratory muscle training. Chest. 1994; 105:1782–8.
2. Okada M, Ota T, Okada M, et al. Right ventricular dysfunction after major pulmonary resection. J Thorac Cardiovasc Surg. 1994;108:503–11.
3. Okada M, Okada M, Ishii N, et al. Right ventricular ejection fraction in the preoperative risk evaluation of candidates for pulmonary resection. J Thorac Cardiovasc Surg. 1996;112:364–70.
4. Nomori H, Horio H, Fuyuno G, et al. Respiratory muscle strength after lung resection with special reference to age and procedures of thoracotomy. Eur J Cardiothorac Surg. 1996;10:352–8.
5. Nomori H, Ishihara T. Pressure-controlled ventilation via a mini-tracheostomy tube for patients with neuromuscular disease. Neurology. 2000;55:698–702.
6. Nomori H, Horio H, Suemasu K. Assisted pressure control ventilation via a mini-tracheostomy tube for postoperative respiratory management of lung cancer patients. Respir Med. 2000;94:214–20.
7. Nomori H. Tracheostomy tube enabling speech during mechanical ventilation. Chest. 2004;125:1046–51.
8. Harada H, Okada M, Sakamoto T, et al. Functional advantage following radical segmentectomy over lobectomy for lung cancer. Ann Thorac Surg. 2005;80:2041–5.
9. Kashiwabara K, Nomori H, Mori T. Relationship between functional preservation after segmentectomy and volume-reduction effects after lobectomy in stage I non-small cell lung cancer patients with emphysema. J Thorac Oncol. 2009;4:1111–6.
10. Yoshimoto K, Nomori H, Mori T, et al. Prediction of pulmonary function after lung lobectomy by subsegments counting, computed tomography, single photon emission computed tomography and computed tomography: a comparative study. Eur J Cardiothorac Surg. 2009;35:408–13.
11. Yoshimoto K, Nomori H, Mori T, et al. Quantification the impact of segmentectomy on pulmonary function by perfusion SPECT/CT. J Thorac Cardiovasc Surg. 2009;137: 1200–5.
12. Yoshimoto K, Nomori H, Mori T, et al. Postoperative change in pulmonary function of the ipsilateral preserved lung after segmentectomy versus lobectomy. Eur J Cardiothorac Surg. 2010;37:36–9.

Diagnosis

1. Nomori H, Horio H, Fuyuno G, et al. Lung adenocarcinoma diagnosed by open lung or thoracoscopic vs. bronchoscopic biopsy. Chest. 1998;114:40–4.
2. Nomori H, Horio H, Naruke T, et al. Use of technetium-99 m tin colloid for sentinel lymph node identification in non-small cell lung cancer. J Thorac Cardiovasc Surg. 2002; 124:486–92.
3. Ohtsuka T, Nomori H, Horio H, et al. Radiological examination for peripheral lung cancers and benign nodules less than 10 mm. Lung Cancer. 2003;42:291–6.
4. Nomori H, Ohtsuka T, Naruke T, et al. Differentiating between atypical adenomatous hyperplasia and bronchiolo-alveolar carcinoma using the computed tomography number histogram. Ann Thorac Surg. 2003;76:867–71.
5. Nomori H, Ohtsuka T, Naruke T, et al. Histogram analysis of computed tomography numbers of clinical T1N0M0 lung adenocarcinoma, with special reference to lymph node metastasis and tumor invasiveness. J Thorac Cardiovasc Surg. 2003;126: 1584–9.
6. Okada M, Nishio W, Sakamoto T, et al. Discrepancy of computed tomographic image between lung and mediastinal windows as a prognostic implication in small lung adenocarcinoma. Ann Thorac Surg. 2003;76:1828–32.
7. Okada M, Nishio W, Sakamoto T, et al. Correlation between computed tomographic findings, bronchioloalveolar carcinoma component and the biologic behavior of small-sized lung adenocarcinomas. J Thorac Cardiovasc Surg. 2004;127:857–61.
8. Nomori H, Watanabe K, Ohtsuka T, et al. Evaluation of F-18 fluorodeoxyglucose(FDG) PET scanning for pulmonary nodules less than 3 cm in diameter, with special reference to the CT images. Lung Cancer. 2004;45:19–27.
9. Nomori H, Watanabe K, Ohtsuka T, et al. In vivo identification of sentinel lymph nodes for clinical stage I non-small cell lung cancer for abbreviation of mediastinal lymph node dissection. Lung Cancer. 2004;46:49–55.
10. Nomori H, Watanabe K, Ohtsuka T, et al. The size of metastatic foci and lymph nodes yielding false-negative and false-positive lymph node staging with positron emission tomography in patients with lung cancer. J Thorac Cardiovasc Surg. 2004; 127:1087–92.
11. Nomori H, Watanabe K, Ohtsuka T, et al. Fluorine 18-tagged fluorodeoxyglucose positron emission tomographic scanning to predict lymph node metastasis, invasiveness, or both, in clinical T1N0M0 lung adenocarcinoma. J Thorac Cardiovasc Surg. 2004;128: 396–401.
12. Watanabe K, Ohtsuka T, et al. Visual and semiquantitative analyses for F-18 fluorodeoxyglucose PET scanning in pulmonary nodules 1 cm to 3 cm in size. Ann Thorac Surg. 2005;79:984–8.

13. Nomori H, Kosaka N, Watanabe K, et al. ^{11}C-acetate positron emission tomography imaging for lung adenocarcinoma 1 to 3 cm in size with ground-glass opacity images on computed tomography. Ann Thorac Surg. 2005;80:2020–5.
14. Ohtsuka T, Nomori H, Watanabe K, et al. Positive imaging of thymoma by ^{11}C-acetate positron emission tomography. Ann Thorac Surg. 2006;81:1132–4.
15. Ohtsuka T, Nomori H, Watanabe K, et al. Prognostic significance of [^{18}F]fluorodeoxyglucose uptake on positron emission tomography in patients with pathological stage I lung adenocarcinoma. Cancer. 2006;107:2468–73.
16. Watanabe K, Nomori H, Ohtsuka T, et al. Usefulness and complications of computed tomography-guided lipiodol marking for fluoroscopy-assisted thoracoscopic resection of small pulmonary nodules: experience with 174 nodules. J Thorac Cardiovasc Surg. 2006;132:320–4.
17. Kaji M, Nomori H, Watanabe K, et al. ^{11}C-acetate and ^{18}F-fluorodeoxyglucose positron emission tomography of pulmonary adenocarcinoma. Ann Thorac Surg. 2007;83:312–4.
18. Ikeda K, Nomori H, Mori T, et al. Impalpable pulmonary nodules with ground-glass opacity: success for making pathological sections with preoperative marking by lipiodol. Chest. 2007;131:502–6.
19. Ikeda K, Awai K, Nomori H, et al. Differential diagnosis of ground-glass opacity nodules: CT number analysis by three-dimensional computerized quantification. Chest. 2007;132:984–90.
20. Nomori H, Ikeda K, Mori T, et al. Sentinel node identification in clinical stage Ia non-small cell lung cancer by a combined single photon emission computed tomography/computed tomography system. J Thorac Cardiovasc Surg. 2007;134:182–7.
21. Okada M, Tauchi S, Iwanaga K, et al. Associations among bronchioloalveolar carcinoma component, positron emission tomographic, computed tomographic findings and malignant behavior in small lung adenocarcinomas. J Thorac Cardiovasc Surg. 2007;133:1448–54.
22. Nomori H, Shibata H, Uno K, et al. ^{11}C-Acetate can be used in place of 18F-fluorodeoxyglucose for positron emission tomography imaging of non-small cell lung cancer with higher sensitivity for well-differentiated adenocarcinoma. J Thorac Oncol. 2008;3: 1427–32.
23. Mori T, Nomori H, Ikeda K, et al. Diffusion-weighted magnetic resonance imaging for diagnosing malignant pulmonary nodules/masses: comparison with positron emission tomography. J Thorac Oncol. 2008;3:358–64.
24. Ikeda K, Nomori H, Mori T, et al. Epidermal growth factor receptor mutations in multicentric lung adenocarcinomas and atypical adenomatous hyperplasias. J Thorac Oncol. 2008;3:467–71.
25. Ikeda K, Nomori H, et al. Novel germline mutation: EGFR V843I in patient with multiple lung adenocarcinomas and family members with lung cancer. Ann Thorac Surg. 2008;85:1430–2.
26. Nomori H, Mori T, Ikeda K, et al. Diffusion-weighted magnetic resonance imaging can be used in place of positron emission tomography for N staging of non-small cell lung cancer with fewer false-positive results. J Thorac Cardiovasc Surg. 2008; 135:816–22.
27. Shibata H, Nomori H, Uno K, et al. ^{11}C-acetate for positron emission tomography imaging of clinical stage IA lung adenocarcinoma: comparison with ^{18}F-fluorodeoxyglucose for imaging and evaluation of tumor aggressiveness. Ann Nucl Med. 2009; 23:609–16.
28. Ohba Y, Nomori H, et al. Evaluation of visual and semiquantitative assessments of fluorodeoxyglucose-uptake on PET scans for the diagnosis of pulmonary malignancies 1 to 3 cm in size. Ann Thorac Surg. 2009;87:886–91.
29. Nomori H, Ohba Y, Yoshimoto K, et al. Difference of sentinel lymph node identification between tin colloid and phytate in patients with non-small cell lung cancer. Ann Thorac Surg. 2009;87:906–10.
30. Shibata H, Nomori H, Uno K, et al. ^{18}F-fluorodeoxyglucose and ^{11}C-acetate positron emission tomography are useful modalities for diagnosing the histological type of thymoma. Cancer. 2009;115:2531–8.
31. Ohba Y, Nomori H, Mori T, et al. Is diffusion-weighted magnetic resonance imaging superior to fluorodeoxyglucose-positron emission tomography in non-small cell lung cancer? J Thorac Cardiovasc Surg. 2009;138:439–45.
32. Yamauchi Y, Izumi Y, Nomori H, et al. Diagnostic performance of percutaneous core-needle lung biopsy under CT scan fluoroscopic guidance for pulmonary lesions measuring ≤10 mm. Chest. 2011;140:1669–70.
33. Yamauchi Y, Izumi Y, Nomori H, et al. Percutaneous cryoablation for pulmonary nodules in the residual lung after pneumonectomy: report of two cases. Chest. 2011; 140:1633–7.
34. Nakayama H, Okumura S, Okada M, et al. Value of integrated positron emission tomography revised using a phantom to evaluate malignancy grade of lung adenocarcinoma: a multicenter study. Cancer. 2010;111:3170–7.
35. Okada M, Nakayama H, Okumura S, et al. Multicenter analysis of HR-CT and PET/CT findings to choose therapeutic strategies for clinical stage IA lung adenocarcinoma. J Thorac Cardiovasc Surg. 2011;141:1384–91.
36. Tsutani Y, MiyataY, Okada M, et al. Difference in prognostic significance of maximum standardized uptake value on [18F]-fluoro-2-deoxyglucose positron emission tomography between adenocarcinoma and squamous cell carcinoma of the lung. Jpn J Clin Oncol. 2011;41:890–6.
37. Tsutani Y, Miyata Y, Okada M, et al. Prognostic significance of using solid versus whole tumor size on high-resolution computed tomography for predicting pathologic malignant grade of tumors in clinical stage IA lung adenocarcinoma: a multicenter study. J Thorac Cardiovasc Surg. 2012 ;143:607–12.

Surgery

1. Nomori H, Kaseda S, Kobayashi K, et al. Adenoid cystic carcinoma of the trachea and main-stem bronchus. J Thorac Cardiovasc Surg. 1988;96:271–7.
2. Nomori H, Kobayashi R, Kodera K, et al. Indications for an expandable metallic stent for tracheobronchial stenosis. Ann Thorac Surg. 1993;56:1324–8.
3. Okada K, Okada M, Yamamoto S, et al. Successful resection of a recurrent leiomyosarcoma of the pulmonary trunk. Ann Thorac Surg. 1993;55:1009–12.
4. Nomori H, Morinaga S, Kobayashi R, et al. Cervical thymic cancer infiltrating the trachea and thyroid. Eur J Cardiothorac Surg. 1994;8:222–4.
5. Nomori H, Hasegawa T, Kobayashi R, et al. The "reversed" latissimus dorsi muscle flap with conditioning delay for closure of a lower thoracic tuberculous empyema. Thorac Cardiovasc Surg. 1994;42:182–4.
6. Okada M, Tsubota N, Yoshimura M, et al. Simultaneous occurrence of three primary lung cancers. Chest. 1994;105:631–2.
7. Nomori H, Kobayashi R, Hasegawa T. Intrathoracic transposition of the musculocutaneous flap in treating empyema. Thorac Cardiovasc Surg. 1995;43:171–5.
8. Nomori H, Horio H, Nara S. Synchronous reconstruction of the trachea and innominate artery in thyroid carcinoma. Ann Thorac Surg. 1995;60:1421–2.
9. Nomori H, Nara S, Horio H. Modified trap-door thoracotomy for malignancies invading the subclavian and innominate vessels. Thorac Cardiovasc Surg. 1995;43:204–7.
10. Okada M, Nishio W, Sakamoto T, et al. Sleeve lobectomy for lung carcinoma in a patient with muscular dystrophy. Thorac Cardiovasc Surg. 1996;44:264–5.
11. Nomori H, Horio H. Endofinger for tactile localization of pulmonary nodules during thoracoscopic resection. Thorac Cardiovasc Surg. 1996;44:50–3.
12. Nomori H, Horio H. Colored collagen is a long-lasting point marker for small pulmonary nodules in thoracoscopic operations. Ann Thorac Surg. 1996;61: 1070–3.
13. Okada M, Kawaraya N, Kujime K, et al. Omentopexy for anastomotic dehiscence after tracheal sleeve pneumonectomy. Thorac Cardiovasc Surg. 1997;45:144–5.
14. Nomori H, Horio H. Gelatin-resorcinol-formaldehyde-glutaraldehyde glue-spread stapler prevents air leakage from the lung. Ann Thorac Surg. 1997;63:352–5.
15. Nomori H, Horio H, Fuyuno G, Kobayashi R. Non-serratus-sparing antero-axillary thoracotomy with disconnection of anterior rib cartilage. Chest. 1997;111:572–6.
16. Nomori H, Horio H, Hasegawa T. Chest wall reconstruction using a titanium hollow screw reconstruction plate. Thorac Cardiovasc Surg. 1997;45:35–7.
17. Nomori H, Horio H, Fuyuno G, et al. Opening of infectious bulla with use of video-assisted thoracoscopic surgery. Chest. 1997;112:1670–3.
18. Nomori H, Horio H, Fuyuno G, Morinaga S. Contacting metastasis of a fibrous tumor of the pleura. Eur J Cardiothorac Surg. 1997;12:928–30.
19. Nomori H, Horio H, Suemasu K. Daily and long-term balloon dilatation via minitracheostomy in cicatric bronchial stenosis. Ann Thorac Surg. 1998;66:2100–2.
20. Nomori H, Horio H, Imazu Y, et al. De-epithelialization for esophageal cyst by video-assisted thoracoscopic surgery monitored by esophagoscopy. Thorac Cardiovasc Surg. 1998;46:107–8.
21. Nomori H, Nara S, Morinaga S, et al. Primary malignant lymphoma of superior vena cava. Ann Thorac Surg. 1998;66:1423–4.
22. Okada M, Tsubota N, Yoshimura M, et al. Operative approach for multiple primary lung carcinomas. J Thorac Cardiovasc Surg. 1998;115:836–40.
23. Okada M, Tsubota N, Yoshimura M, et al. Proposal for reasonable mediastinal lymphadenectomy in bronchogenic carcinomas. J Thorac Cardiovasc Surg. 1998;116:949–53.
24. Okada M, Tsubota N, Yoshimura M, et al. How should interlobar pleural invasion be classified? Prognosis of resected T3 non-small cell lung cancer? Ann Thorac Surg. 1999;68:2049–52.
25. Okada M, Tsubota N, Yoshimura M, et al. Evaluation of TNM classification for lung carcinoma with ipsilateral intrapulmonary metastasis. Ann Thorac Surg. 1999;68:326–30.
26. Okada M, Tsubota N, Yoshimura M, et al. Prognosis of completely resected pN2 non–small cell lung carcinomas. J Thorac Cardiovasc Surg. 1999;118:270–5.
27. Okada M, Tsubota N, Yoshimura M, et al. Extended sleeve lobectomy for lung cancer: the avoidance of pneumonectomy. J Thorac Cardiovasc Surg. 1999;118:710–3.
28. Okada M, Tsubota N, Yoshimura M, et al. Role of pleural lavage cytology before resection for primary lung carcinoma. Ann Surg. 1999;229:579–84.
29. Nomori H, Horio S, Morinaga S, Suemasu K. Gelatin-resorcinol formaldehyde-glutaraldehyde(GRFG) glue for sealing pulmonary air leakage during thoracoscopic surgery. Ann Thorac Surg. 1999;67:212–6.
30. Nomori H, Horio H, Suemasu K. Dumon stent placement via tracheal tube. Chest. 1999;115: 582–3.

31. Nomori H, Horio S, Suemasu K. Anterior limited thoracotomy with intrathoracic illumination for lung cancer: its advantages over antero-axillary and posterolateral thoracotomy. Chest. 1999;115:874–80.
32. Nomori H, Horio H, Suemasu K. Mixing collagen with fibrin glue to strengthen the sealing effect for pulmonary air leakage. Ann Thorac Surg. 2000;70:1666–70.
33. Nomori H, Horio H, Imazu Y, Suemasu K. Double stenting for esophageal and tracheobronchial stenosis. Ann Thorac Surg. 2000;70:1803–7.
34. Nomori H, Horio H, Suemasu K. The efficacy and side effects of gelatin-resorcinol formaldehyde glutaraldehyde (GRFG) glue for preventing and sealing pulmonary air leakage. Surg Today. 2000;30:244–8.
35. Okada M, Tsubota N, Yoshimura M, et al. Induction therapy for non-small cell lung cancer with involved mediastinal nodes in multiple stations. Chest. 2000;118:123–8.
36. Okada M, Tsubota N, Yoshimura M, et al. Survival related to lymph node involvement in lung cancer after sleeve lobectomy compared with pneumonectomy. J Thorac Cardiovasc Surg. 2000;119:814–9.
37. Okada M, Yoshikawa K, Hatta T, et al. Is segmentectomy with lymph node assessment an alternative to lobectomy for non-small cell lung cancer of 2 cm or smaller? Ann Thorac Surg. 2001;71:956–60.
38. Nomori H, Horio H, Suemasu K. Early removal of chest drainage tubes and oxygen support after a lobectomy for lung cancer facilities earlier recovery of the 6-minute walking distance. Surg Today. 2001;31:395–9.
39. Nomori H, Horio H, Naruke T, Suemasu K. Posterolateral thoracotomy is behind limited thoracotomy and thoracoscopic surgery in terms of postoperative pulmonary function and walking capacity. Eur J Cardiothorac Surg. 2001;21:155–6.
40. Nomori H, Horio H, Suemasu K. Comparison of short-term versus long-term epidural analgesia after limited thoracotomy with special reference to pain score, pulmonary function, and respiratory muscle strength. Surg Today. 2001;31:191–5.
41. Nomori H, Horio H, Suemasu K. Differentiating early malignant lung tumors from inflammatory nodules to minimize the use of video-assisted thoracoscopic surgery or open biopsy to establish a diagnosis. Surg Today. 2001;31:102–7.
42. Nomori H, Horio H, Naruke T, Suemasu K. What is the advantage of a thoracoscopic lobectomy over a limited thoracotomy procedure for lung cancer surgery? Ann Thorac Surg. 2001; 72:879–84.
43. Nomori H, Horio H, Naruke T, Suemasu K. Fluoroscopy-assisted thoracoscopic resection of lung nodules marked with lipiodol. Ann Thorac Surg. 2001;74:170–3.
44. Nomori H, Horio H, Suemasu K. Intrathoracic transposition of a pectoralis major and pectoralis minor muscle flap for empyema in patients previously subjected to posterolateral thoracotomy. Surg Today. 2001;31:295–9.
45. Nomori H, Ohtsuka T, Horio H, Naruke T, Suemasu K. Thoracoscopic lobectomy for lung cancer with a largely fused fissure. Chest. 2003;123:619–22.
46. Okada M, Sakamoto T, Nishio W, et al. Characteristics and prognosis of patients after resection of non-small cell lung carcinoma measuring 2 cm or less in greatest dimension. Cancer. 2003;98:535–41.
47. Okada M, Sakamoto T, Nishio W, et al. Pleural lavage cytology in non-small cell lung cancer. J Thorac Cardiovasc Surg. 2003; 126:1911–5.
48. Okada M, Nishio W, Sakamoto T, et al. Long-term survival and prognostic factors of 5-year survivors with complete resection of non-small cell lung carcinoma. J Thorac Cardiovasc Surg. 2003;126:558–62.
49. Matsuoka H, Nishio W, Okada M, et al. Resection of chest wall invasion in patients with non-small cell lung cancer. Eur J Cardiothorac Surg. 2004;26:1200–4.
50. Ohtsuka T, Nomori H, Horio H, Naruke T, Suemasu K. Is major pulmonary resection by video-assisted thoracic surgery an adequate procedure in clinical stage I lung cancer? Chest. 2004;125:1742–6.
51. Okada M, Nishio W, Sakamoto T, et al. Evolution of surgical outcomes for non-small cell lung cancer. Ann Thorac Surg. 2004;77:1926–30.
52. Okada M, Nishio W, Sakamoto T, et al. Prognostic significance of perioperative serum carcinoembryonic antigen in non-small cell lung cancer. Ann Thorac Surg. 2004;78: 216–21.
53. Okada M, Nishio W, Sakamoto T, et al. Sleeve segmentectomy for non-small cell lung carcinoma. J Thorac Cardiovasc Surg. 2004;128:420–4.
54. Matsuoka H, Okada M, Sakamoto T, et al. Complications and outcomes after pulmonary resection for cancer in patients 80 to 89 years of age. Eur J Cardiothorac Surg. 2005;28:380–3.
55. Okada M, Sakamoto T, Yuki T, et al. Hybrid surgical approach of video-assisted minithoracotomy for lung cancer. Chest. 2005;128:2696–701.
56. Okada M, Sakamoto T, Yuki T, et al. Border between N1 and N2 stations in lung carcinoma. J Thorac Cardiovasc Surg. 2005;129:825–30.
57. Okada M, Nishio W, Sakamoto T, et al. Effect of tumor size on prognosis in non-small cell lung cancer. J Thorac Cardiovasc Surg. 2005;129:87–93.
58. Nomori H, Imazu Y, Watanabe K, et al. Radiofrequency ablation of pulmonary tumors and normal lung tissue in Swine and rabbits. Chest. 2005;127:973–7.
59. Ikeda K, Nomori H, Mori T, et al. Size of metastatic and non-metastatic mediastinal lymph nodes in non-small cell lung cancer. J Thorac Oncol. 2006;1:949–52.
60. Okada M, Sakamoto T, Yuki T, et al. Selective mediastinal lymphadenectomy for clinico-surgical stage I non-small cell lung cancer. Ann Thorac Surg. 2006;81:1028–32.

61. Okada M, Koike T, Higashiyama M, et al. Radical sublobar resection for small-sized non-small cell lung cancer. J Thorac Cardiovasc Surg. 2006;132:769–75.
62. Okada M, Mimura T, Ikegaki J, et al. A novel video-assisted anatomical segmentectomy technique-selective segmental inflation via bronchofiberoptic jet followed by cautery cutting. J Thorac Cardiovasc Surg. 2007;133:753–8.
63. Nomori H, Ikeda K, Mori T, et al. Sentinel node navigation segmentectomy for c-T1N0M0 non-small cell lung cancer. J Thorac Cardiovasc Surg. 2007;133:780–5.
64. Okada M, Mimura T, Ohbayashi C, et al. Radical surgery for malignant pleural mesothelioma. Interact Cardiovasc Thorac Surg. 2008;7:102–6.
65. Okada M. Radical sublobar resection for lung cancer. Gen Thorac Cardiovasc Surg. 2008;56:151–7.
66. Nomori H. Sentinel node mapping in lung cancer. The Japanese experience. Semin Thorac Cardiovasc Surg. 2009;21:316–22.
67. Kobayashi H, Nomori H, Mori T, et al. Extrapleural pneumonectomy with reconstruction of diaphragm and pericardium using autologous materials. Ann Thorac Surg. 2009;87:1630–2.
68. Nomori H, Ohba Y, Shibata H, et al. Required area of lymph node sampling during segmentectomy for clinical stage IA non-small cell lung cancer. J Thorac Cardiovasc Surg. 2010;139:38–42.
69. Mimae T, Hirayasu T, Okada M, et al. Advantage of absorbable suture material for pulmonary artery ligation. Gen Thorac Cardiovasc Surg. 2010;58:511–5.
70. Lim E, Clough R, Okada M, et al. Impact of positive pleural lavage cytology on survival in patients having lung resection for non-small-cell lung cancer: an international individual patient data meta-analysis. J Thorac Cardiovasc Surg. 2010;139: 1441–6.
71. Nakamura K, Saji H, Okada M, et al. A phase III randomized trial of lobectomy versus limited resection for small-sized peripheral non-small cell lung cancer. Jpn J Clin Oncol. 2010;40:271–4.
72. Miyoshi K, Mimura T, Okada M, et al. Surgical treatment of clinical N1 non-small cell lung cancer: ongoing controversy over diagnosis and prognosis. Surg Today. 2010;40: 428–32.
73. Miyata Y, Okada M. Hybrid video-assisted thoracic surgery basilar (S9–10) segmentectomy. Semin Thorac Cardiovasc Surg. 2011;23:73–7.
74. Asakura K, Nomori H, Izumi Y, et al. Effect of cutting technique at the intersegmental plane during segmentectomy on expansion of the preserved segment: comparison between staplers and scissors in ex vivo pig lung. Eur J Cardiothorac Surg. 2011; 40:e34–8.
75. Fukutomi T, Kohno M, Nomori H, et al. Sentinel node microscopic metastasis detected after segmentectomy for lung cancer followed by completion lobectomy: two case reports. Thorac Cardiovasc Surg. 2011 May 12 [Epub ahead of print].
76. Horinouchi H, Nomori H, Izumi Y, et al. How many pathological T1N0M0 non-small cell lung cancers can be completely resected in one segment? Special reference to high-resolution computed tomography findings. Surg Today. 2011;41:1062–6.
77. Nomori H, Kohno M, Izumi Y, et al. Sentinel nodes in lung cancer: our 10 years-experience. Surg Today. 2011;41:889–95.
78. Nomori H, Mori T, Iyama K, et al. Risk of bronchioloalveolar carcinoma in patients with human T-cell lymphotropic virus type 1 (HTLV-I): case–control study results. Ann Thorac Cardiovasc Surg. 2011;17:19–23.
79. Nomori H, Mori T, Izumi Y, et al. Is completion lobectomy merited for unanticipated nodal metastases after radical segmentectomy for cT1N0M0/pN1–2 non-small cell lung cancer? J Thorac Cardiovasc Surg. 2011 Nov 19 [Epub ahead of print].
80. Okui M, Kohno M, Nomori H, et al. Combined subsegmentectomy for S(2)(b) (horizontal subsegment of the posterior segment) and S(3)(a) (lateral subsegment of the anterior segment) in the right upper pulmonary lobe. Gen Thorac Cardiovasc Surg. 2011; 59:632–5.
81. Nakayama T, Kohno M, Nomori H, et al. Innovative segmentectomy to remove the posterior segment of the lower lobe (S^{10}) of the lung. Surg Today. 2012;42:104–6.
82. Okada M, Tsutani Y, Ikeda T, et al. Radical hybrid video-assisted thoracic segmentectomy: long-term results of minimally invasive anatomical sublobar resection for treating lung cancer. Interact Cardiovasc Thorac Surg. 2012;14:5–11.
83. Nomori H, Mori T, Ikeda K, et al. Segmentectomy for cT1N0M0 non-small cell lung cancer: a prospective study at a single institute. J Thorac Cardiovasc Surg. 2012;144:87–93.
84. Ikeda T, Miyata Y, Okada M, et al. Fibrinogen/thrombin-based collagen fleece [TachoComb(R)] promotes regeneration in pulmonary arterial injury. Eur J Cardiothorac Surg. 2012;41:926–32.

MIX
Papier aus verantwortungsvollen Quellen
Paper from responsible sources
FSC® C105338

If you have any concerns about our products,
you can contact us on
ProductSafety@springernature.com

In case Publisher is established outside the EU,
the EU authorized representative is:
Springer Nature Customer Service Center GmbH
Europaplatz 3, 69115 Heidelberg, Germany

Printed by Libri Plureos GmbH
in Hamburg, Germany